Patellofemoral Pain and Instability

Beth E. Shubin Stein • Sabrina M. Strickland
Editors

Patellofemoral Pain and Instability

Etiology, Diagnosis and Management

Springer

Editors
Beth E. Shubin Stein, MD
Department of Orthopedic Surgery
Hospital for Special Surgery
New York, NY, USA

Sabrina M. Strickland, MD
Hospital for Special Surgery
New York, NY, USA

ISBN 978-3-319-97639-6 ISBN 978-3-319-97640-2 (eBook)
https://doi.org/10.1007/978-3-319-97640-2

Library of Congress Control Number: 2018964721

This Springer imprint is published by the registered company Springer Nature Switzerland AG
The registered company address is: Gewerbestrasse 11, 6330 Cham, Switzerland

Preface

Patellofemoral Pain and Instability: Etiology, Diagnosis and Management is a clear and concise text intended to be useful for all health care professionals caring for patients with patellofemoral dysfunction.

Interest in patellofemoral disorders has increased in recent years as new studies and new technologies have emerged, helping guide us in terms of diagnosis and best practices in treatment. Although many patellofemoral disorders have historically been considered complex and difficult to treat, use of the most up-to-date research and practical guidelines has helped simplify the diagnosis and the treatment options available. Understanding the etiology and evolving high-level literature on patellofemoral instability, as well as the modern treatment options for patients with patellofemoral pain and arthritis, is essential to diagnosing and treating the broad spectrum of patellofemoral disease.

The patellofemoral joint is unique in every patient. However, the basic principles of this joint and its form and function can help us understand the underlying etiology of the pathology as well as the appropriate treatment options to decrease pain and restore function.

This book presents best practices in diagnosis and treatment of patients with what have previously been considered to be complex patellofemoral disorders. We know this book will be an invaluable and practical guide to all physicians and medical professionals caring for patients with patellofemoral disorders.

New York, NY, USA

Beth E. Shubin Stein, MD
Sabrina M. Strickland, MD

Contents

Contributors

Christopher S. Ahmad, MD Columbia University Medical Center, Department of Orthopedic Surgery, New York, NY, USA

Jacqueline Munch Brady, MD Department of Orthopaedics and Rehabilitation, Oregon Health and Science University, Portland, OR, USA

Daniel M. Dean, MD Department of Orthopedic Surgery, Georgetown University Hospital, Washington, DC, USA

David R. Diduch, MD Department of Orthopedic Surgery, Universtiy of Virginia, Charlottesville, VA, USA

Brandon J. Erickson, MD Hospital for Special Surgery, Division of Sports and Shoulder, New York, NY, USA

Andreas H. Gomoll, MD Hospital for Special Surgery, Division of Sports and Shoulder, New York, NY, USA

Daniel W. Green, MD, MS, FAAP, FACS Hospital for Special Surgery, New York, NY, USA

Alex A. Johnson, MD Department of Orthopedic Surgery, The Johns Hopkins University, Baltimore, MD, USA

Vivek Kalia, MD, MPH, MS Hospital for Special Surgery, New York, NY, USA

Michael S. Laidlaw, MD Department of Orthopedic Surgery, Universtiy of Virginia, Charlottesville, VA, USA

Douglas N. Mintz, MD Hospital for Special Surgery, New York, NY, USA

Joseph Moloney, PT, MS, SCS, CSCS Hospital for Special Surgery, New York, NY, USA

Ryan S. Murray, MD Department of Orthopedic Surgery, Georgetown University Hospital, Washington, DC, USA

Meghan J. Price, BS Duke University School of Medicine, Durham, NC, USA

Lauren H. Redler, MD Columbia University Medical Center, Department of Orthopedic Surgery, New York, NY, USA

Beth E. Shubin Stein, MD Sports Medicine and Shoulder Service, Hospital for Special Surgery, New York, NY, USA

Sabrina M. Strickland, MD Sports Medicine and Shoulder Service, Hospital for Special Surgery, New York, NY, USA

Miho J. Tanaka, MD Department of Orthopedic Surgery, The Johns Hopkins University, Baltimore, MD, USA

Dean Wang, MD Sports Medicine and Shoulder Service, Hospital for Special Surgery, New York, NY, USA

Brian C. Werner, MD Department of Orthopedic Surgery, Universtiy of Virginia, Charlottesville, VA, USA

Robin West, MD Inova Sports Medicine, Georgetown University Medical Center, Washington, DC, USA

Virginia Commonwealth University School of Medicine, Richmond, VA, USA

Part I
Patellofemoral Pain

Chapter 1
PF Pain in the Skeletally Immature Patient: Diagnosis and Management

Meghan J. Price, Joseph Moloney, and Daniel W. Green

Introduction

The focus of this chapter is on the differential diagnoses of anterior patellofemoral knee pain in children and adolescents. The discrete causes of anterior knee pain that we discuss are listed in Table 1.1; however, many patients will present with anterior knee pain without a discrete diagnosis. These are the patients who fall into the broader diagnostic categories of anterior knee pain in adolescents and patellofemoral pain syndrome. Historically, these conditions have been referred to in the literature by the overarching diagnosis of chondromalacia. At a certain point, chondromalacia was so commonly associated with anterior knee pain that it was the accepted clinical diagnosis for anterior patellofemoral pain [1, 2]. However, now diagnosis of chondromalacia of the patella requires radiographic or arthroscopic proof of soft or damaged articular cartilage. This distinction has led to more effective and specific treatment and physical therapy plans for the causes of patellofemoral knee pain that are unrelated to cartilage damage.

This chapter will review common diagnoses of anterior knee pain in children and adolescents. Patellofemoral pain secondary to instability and malalignment will be discussed elsewhere in this textbook.

M. J. Price
Duke University School of Medicine, Durham, NC, USA

J. Moloney · D. W. Green (✉)
Hospital for Special Surgery, New York, NY, USA
e-mail: greend@hss.edu

B. E. Shubin Stein, S. M. Strickland (eds.), *Patellofemoral Pain and Instability*,
https://doi.org/10.1007/978-3-319-97640-2_1

Table 1.1 List of differential diagnoses for pediatric anterior patellofemoral knee pain

Anterior knee pain in adolescents
Patellofemoral pain syndrome (PFPS)
Osgood-Schlatter's disease
Tibial tubercle fracture
Sinding-Larsen-Johansson syndrome
Patellar sleeve fracture
Bipartite patella
Trochlear JOCD
Patellar JOCD
Hoffa's fat pad impingement
Plica syndrome
Chondromalacia of the patella
Prepatellar bursitis
Patellar tendonitis
Patellar stress fracture
Patellofemoral maltracking/malalignment
Patellofemoral instability
Pain syndromes
Avascular necrosis
Bone bruise/bone contusion
Inflammatory arthritis
Tumor

Anterior Knee Pain of the Adolescent

When young adolescents present with anterior patellofemoral knee pain that cannot be given a discrete diagnosis, we often use the term adolescent anterior knee pain. This condition typically occurs in adolescents who are active and participate in sports. It is considered an overuse injury that often results from a training routine that does not include sufficient strengthening and stabilizing routines for the knee and the surrounding hip and core muscles.

Patients with anterior knee pain of the adolescent typically experience a dull, achy pain that presents over time and worsens with activities, particularly those that involve flexion and extension such as jumping, squatting, sprinting, etc. other typical symptoms are pain with repetitive bending of the knee, when climbing stairs or after prolonged periods of sitting. Physical examination should include an evaluation of lower leg alignment, kneecap position, tightness of the heel cord, flexibility of the feet, knee stability, hip rotation, range of motion (ROM) of knees and hips, kneecap palpation, and strength, flexibility, firmness, and tone of the quadriceps and hamstrings. Plain radiographs and MRIs can help exclude a more concrete diagnosis; however, radiography will typically appear normal in patients with anterior knee pain of the adolescent.

In most cases, temporary activity modification, short-term use of nonsteroidal anti-inflammatory drugs (NSAIDs) and ice to address pain, and a strengthening and flexibility routine will be successful in providing relief. Patients can work with their physicians to establish an activity regimen that limits the duration and intensity of athletic activities and rather focuses on low-impact sports such as biking and swimming. In addition, a physical therapy regimen that includes exercises to help increase hamstring flexibility and strength of the core and hip muscles supporting the knee is important. Trainers and physical therapists can also help address any issues in exercise technique that could be causing this persistent knee pain. It is important that patients develop good exercise habits including wearing proper athletic shoes, warming up thoroughly before practice, stretching before and after physical activity, and establishing a routine which supports hip and core strength.

Patellofemoral Pain Syndrome (PFPS)

We acknowledge that there is significant overlap between anterior knee pain of the adolescent and patellofemoral pain syndrome (PFPS) – so much that some physicians do not distinguish between the two. However, PFPS often comes with the implication of mild patellofemoral instability (without dislocation) and/or patellofemoral overloading (without obvious articular cartilage damage).

Patients with PFPS typically present with pain and stiffness in the front of the knee around the patella. This pain can worsen when climbing stairs, kneeling, squatting, or performing everyday tasks. Patients often report cracking or popping sounds when changing position or climbing stairs and also experience pain during repeated knee bending. PFPS is a non-specific diagnosis that is given when all other differential diagnoses can be ruled out by the appropriate clinical and radiographic exams.

Symptoms are most often relieved with conservative treatment including activity modification, rest, ice, temporary compression, and short-term use of NSAIDs. Patients are advised to decrease the intensity and duration of physical activities and to initiate physical therapy exercises that improve range of motion, strength, and endurance. Core, hip, and quadriceps strength and hamstring flexibility are particularly important as they help optimize patellofemoral tracking.

Osgood-Schlatter's Disease

Osgood-Schlatter's is characterized as a traction apophysitis of the proximal tibial tubercle at the insertion of the patellar tendon. Osgood-Schlatter's was first described in 1903 by Robert Osgood, and its etiology is widely accepted as repetitive strain and chronic avulsion of the secondary ossification center of the tibial tuberosity [3]. The specifics of this etiology have not been widely accepted, but several hypotheses have been presented in the literature. Ogden and Southwick suggested that as the tuberosity matures, if the growing ossification center cannot withstand the forces from the patellar tendon, Osgood-Schlatter's disease avulsion can result in extra bone migration between the fragments [4]. Lancourt and Cristini proposed that a shorter patellar ligament in children with patella infera could cause increased stress on the secondary ossification center [5]. Pronated feet, genu valgum, internal rotation [6], and increased external tibial rotation [7] have also been associated with Osgood-Schlatter's.

Osgood-Schlatter's typically develops during peak growth (ages 8–12 for girls, 12–15 for boys) with a higher prevalence in athletes (21% of adolescents) than non-athletes (4.5% of adolescents) [8]. Common sports that exacerbate Osgood-Schlatter's include soccer, football, basketball, volleyball, gymnastics, and figure skating as they involve sprinting, cutting, and jumping. These activities result in repetitive patellar tendon strain from the strong pull of the quadriceps muscle. Patients usually present with a gradual onset of pain, tenderness, and swelling at the tibial tubercle. There is often an area of prominence at the tibial tuberosity, and pain intensifies with extension of knee against resistance or squatting with the knee in full flexion. straight leg raise is typically painless [9].

Diagnosis of Osgood-Schlatter's is made by clinical examination; however, radiographs are recommended in unilateral cases to rule out other differential diagnoses. Plain radiographs (lateral view of the knee with leg internally rotated 10–20°) are the most useful radiograph for diagnosis of OSS. Typical findings are irregularity of the apophysis with separation from the tibial tuberosity nearly stages and fragmentation in later stages [10] (Fig. 1.1). While radiographic findings may be difficult to distinguish from normal variation in ossification of the tubercle, the tibial tubercle in OSS may also appear elevated from the shaft and irregular, fragmented, or particularly dense. A superficial ossicle, calcification, or thickening may be seen in the patellar tendon [9]. While magnetic resonance imaging (MRI) is typically more useful for identifying atypical presentations of OSS, Hirano et al.

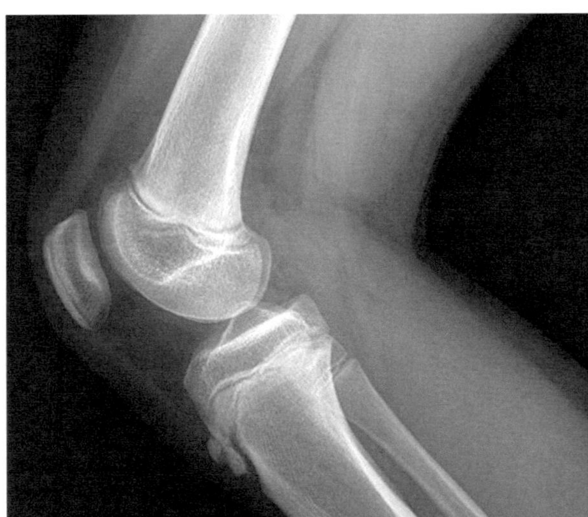

Fig. 1.1 Lateral radiograph

proposed five stages of classification for typical OSS on MRI: normal, early, progressive, terminal, and healing. [11]. The patient presents with symptoms in the normal and early stage but no inflammation or avulsion on MRI. The progressive stage reveals partial cartilaginous avulsion from the secondary ossification center, and the terminal stage includes the separated ossicles. Osseous healing is evident in the fifth, healing, stage without separated ossicles [11].

It is important to be aware of nondisplaced tibial tubercle fracture as a differential diagnosis. These fractures appear similar to Osgood-Schlatter's on radiograph; however, clinically patients present with severe pain and an inability to do a straight leg raise.

Osgood-Schlatter's is a self-limiting condition with expected recovery in well over 90% of patients [12]. A non-operative treatment plan that includes ice, limitation of activities, NSAIDs, knee protection, and a physical therapy plan for strength and flexibility is recommended. For patients who present with severe pain, stopping physical activity until acute pain subsides is recommended. For patients who present with mild to moderate pain (majority of patients), continued athletic participation in moderation is appropriate. Typically the pre-pain activity level of the patient is reviewed and the overall hours spent doing rigorous sprinting and jumping is decreased. Rest days and flexibility exercises are recommended between episodes of strenuous activity.

The vast majority of symptoms resolve when the proximal tibial growth plate closes. However, in less than 1–2% of patients, pain and tenderness over the tibial tubercle persist. Indications for surgery in these patients include skeletal maturity and a persistence of symptoms with a free fragment/ossicle seen on radiograph [13]. The literature has identified surgical procedures to treat rare cases of Osgood-Schlatter's that remain symptomatic in skeletally mature patients. These procedures typically include excision of the prominent portion of the tibial tubercle via a longitudinal incision in the patellar tendon and excision of the ununited ossicles and cartilaginous pieces [14–18].

Sinding-Larsen-Johansson (SLJ) Syndrome

Sinding-Larsen-Johansson (SLJ) syndrome or overuse of distal patellar apophyseal traction is a painful condition that occurs at the junction of the patellar tendon and the lower margin of the patella. First described independently by both Sinding-Larsen and Johansson, this condition shares many similarities with Osgood-Schlatter's [19, 20]. SLJ is an uncommon cause of anterior PF pain with a reported incidence of about 4.8% [21]. SLJ typically occurs when young rapidly growing adolescents overstrain themselves in activities involving repetitive traction exerted by the patellar tendon on the patella such as sprinting or jumping. The repetitive stress and microtrauma from this traction are thought to be the source of pain [22].

Clinically, patients present between ages 10 and 12 with tenderness and/or swelling at the inferior pole of the patella. Pain is accentuated by resistance to quadriceps

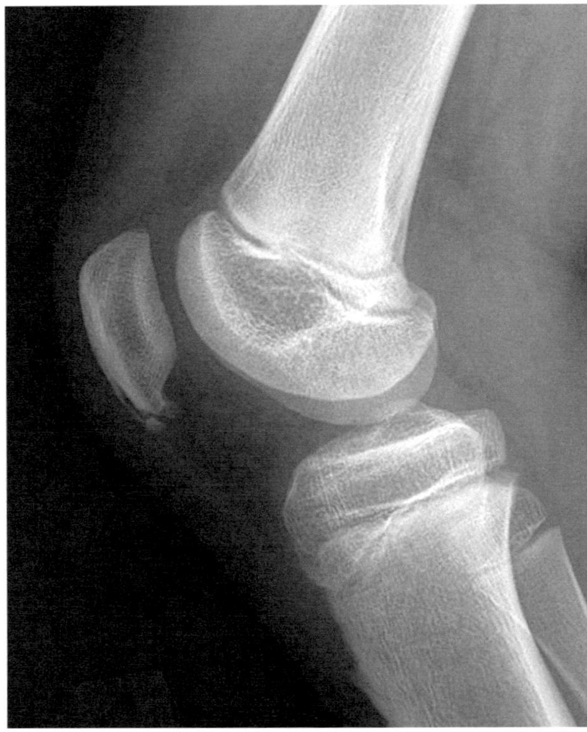

Fig. 1.2 A 12-year-old male who plays squash and runs cross-country competitively presents with ongoing complaints of aching right knee pain for the last 6 months with no history of acute injury. Pain occurs in the distal aspect of his patella. Lateral radiographs demonstrate mild bony changes on the distal pole of the patella consistent with SLJ

contraction and patellar loading during flexion [23, 24]. Patellar tendon thickening and infrapatellar bursitis may also be observed [23]. Typically imaging is not necessary to diagnose SLJ, but plain radiographs of the knee are recommended in unilateral cases to rule out tibial apophyseal fracture, tumor, or infection (Fig. 1.2). Plain radiographs of SLJ can show slight separation and elongation, fragmentation, and/or irregular calcification of the distal patella ossification centers [22, 25]. Medlar et al described staging of the SLJ on radiograph with the following findings: Stage 1 normal findings, Stage 2 irregular calcifications at the inferior pole of the patella, Stage 3 coalescence of calcification, Stage 4A incorporation of the calcification into the patella, and Stage 4B a calcification mass separate from the patella [25].

An important differential diagnosis to be aware of are patellar sleeve fractures (discussed later in this chapter) as they look very similar to SLJ on radiographs. The distinction is the clinical presentation. Patellar sleeve fractures typically present after acute trauma, and the patient has severe pain with knee motion. They are also unable to extend the knee. If there is any doubt as to which condition the patient has, an MRI should be obtained. The distinction between these two conditions is important as treatment for sleeve fractures involves immobilization while treatment for SLJ does not.

SLJ is a self-limiting syndrome that typically resolves on its own within 12–18 months of presentation with the typical duration coinciding with heightened growth. Following presentation, patients are recommended to follow conservative treatment plans with activity modification, application of ice, and use of nonsteroidal anti-inflammatory drugs NSAIDS for acute pain and swelling [26]. Once initial pain has subsided, a rehabilitation program focused on increasing strength and flexibility of quadriceps, iliotibial band, gastrocnemius, and hamstring muscles is recommended. We believe an important risk factor for SLJ is tight hamstrings, so increasing the flexibility of these muscles is particularly important. If pain does not abate, patients may benefit from rest and physical therapy followed by a slow return to sports with a supportive patellar sleeve [10].

Surgical treatments are very uncommon with SLJ, but they may be necessary in patients whose pain does not subside and continues into adulthood. Only one case report documenting successful surgical treatment of SLJ was found in the literature [27].

Bipartite Patella

Bipartite or tripartite patella is a congenital anomaly that is typically asymptomatic but can present with painful symptoms in the superolateral or lateral portion of the patella after overuse during activities or after trauma [28–30]. Of particular interest, bipartite patella is one of the only sources of superolateral knee pain and tenderness at presentation. The patella is the largest sesamoid bone in the body and typically develops with one center of ossification; bipartite patella occurs when one ossification center does not fuse with the main patella. Incidence is reported to be as low as 0.2–6% and as high as 60% [31–33]. Bipartite patella is more common in males than females with male to female ratios reported anywhere from 4:1 to 9:1 [33–35]. Symptomatic knees present more frequently in athletic, active adolescents than in inactive ones. Iossifidis et al. proposed that the etiology of painful bipartite patella was the disruption of the fibrocartilaginous zone between the patella and the accessory bipartite fragment due to direct or indirect injury [30].

History, clinical examination, and squatting skyline radiographs are used to diagnose bipartite patella. Ishikawa et al. described the squatting skyline view as most effective for viewing the bipartite patella and ruling out other causes of patellofemoral pain including hypoplasia, patellar instability, or abnormal patellar tracking [36]. On radiographs, bipartite patella appears in two parts with smooth, well-corticated borders (Fig. 1.3). Saupe developed a classification system for the location of the secondary ossification center. Type III is the most common at 75% incidence and appears in the superolateral region. Type II occurs in 20% of cases in the lateral or vertical region, and Type I in the inferior pole is least common at 5% [37]. MRI is also recommended for surgical patients. In addition, Kavanagh et al. indicated that MRI is particularly useful in young males with gradual onset of pain due to overuse and secondary abnormal patellofemoral tracking [38]. In these cases, MRI is not required to make the diagnosis of bipartite patella but may be useful to show the degree of edema at the synchondrosis of the bipartite patella and to evaluate the quality of the articular cartilage. All radiographs should be correlated with clinical

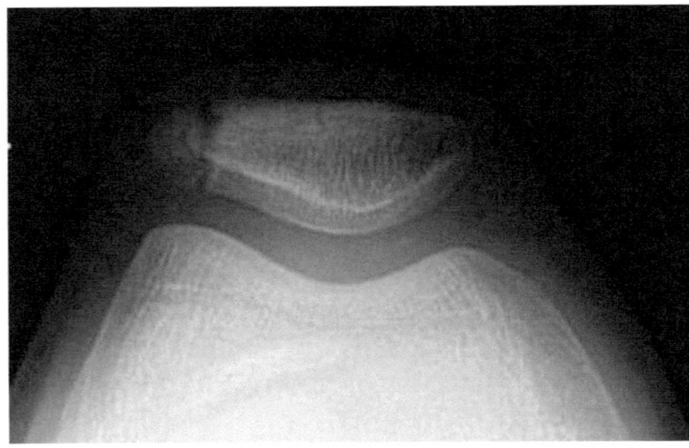

Fig. 1.3 Classic case of bipartite patella in a 13-year-old female

findings of tenderness and/or bony prominence over the lateral or superolateral portion of the patella. Symptoms typically worsen during knee extension when walking, jumping, and climbing stairs and during knee flexion.

This condition is typically self-limiting and most do not require surgery. Initial conservative treatments including NSAIDs, activity modification, local corticosteroid injections, and rehabilitation to increase quadriceps flexibility are recommended [33, 35]. In a meta-analysis of surgical treatment of bipartite patella, Matic et al. reported treatment of 130 knees in 125 patients with 90 out of 96 knees failing initial conservative treatment [34]. Surgical techniques including excision of the accessory fragment, lateral retinacular release [39], or vastus lateralis release [40] are indicated after conservative treatment fails at 6 months. For larger lesions in which excision would destabilize the patellofemoral joint, open reduction and internal fixation are recommended [28, 35]. Vaishya et al. report positive results in a case study of five patients undergoing excision or open reduction and internal fixation. All patients were pain- and symptom-free at average follow-up of 13 months [41]. Matic's meta-analysis also reports positive results with 105 of the 125 patients who underwent either surgical or conservative treatments being symptom-free and able to return to sports after intervention.

Trochlear and Patellar Juvenile Osteochondritis Dissecans (JOCD) of the Knee

Juvenile osteochondritis dissecans (JOCD) is an idiopathic condition characterized by the development of lesions in the subchondral bone of skeletally immature patients. This condition may or may not involve the overlying articular cartilage. JOCD is a fairly common cause of knee pain in athletic children and young adolescents with a reported rate of 15 to 29 cases per 100,000 [42, 43]. There is not yet a consensus on the etiology of OCD; however, several authors have proposed that OCD of the knee is an overuse injury from repetitive microtrauma to an area of vulnerable subchondral bone [44]. Once injured, loading and stress on this area can result in avascular necrosis and potential non-union [44, 45]. This makes athletic children are more vulnerable to OCD; however, many cases of OCD occur in non-active children and recent genetic studies showing potential links between several DNA loci and OCD suggest a familial etiology [46]. The most common area in which OCD develops is the lateral aspect of the medial femoral condyle (50–80%) with trochlear and patellar lesions occurring at much lower incidence rates of 1% and 5–10%, respectively [44, 45, 47].

Patients typically present with knee pain and tenderness in the anterior medial part of the knee and swelling related to activity. They may walk with an antalgic gait or with the leg externally rotated. In terms of radiography, merchant and AP and lateral radiographs are the most helpful in diagnosing trochlear OCD [48, 49]. Once OCD is suspected, an MRI of the knee should be taken to confirm the diagnosis and track post-treatment progress (Fig. 1.4a–d).

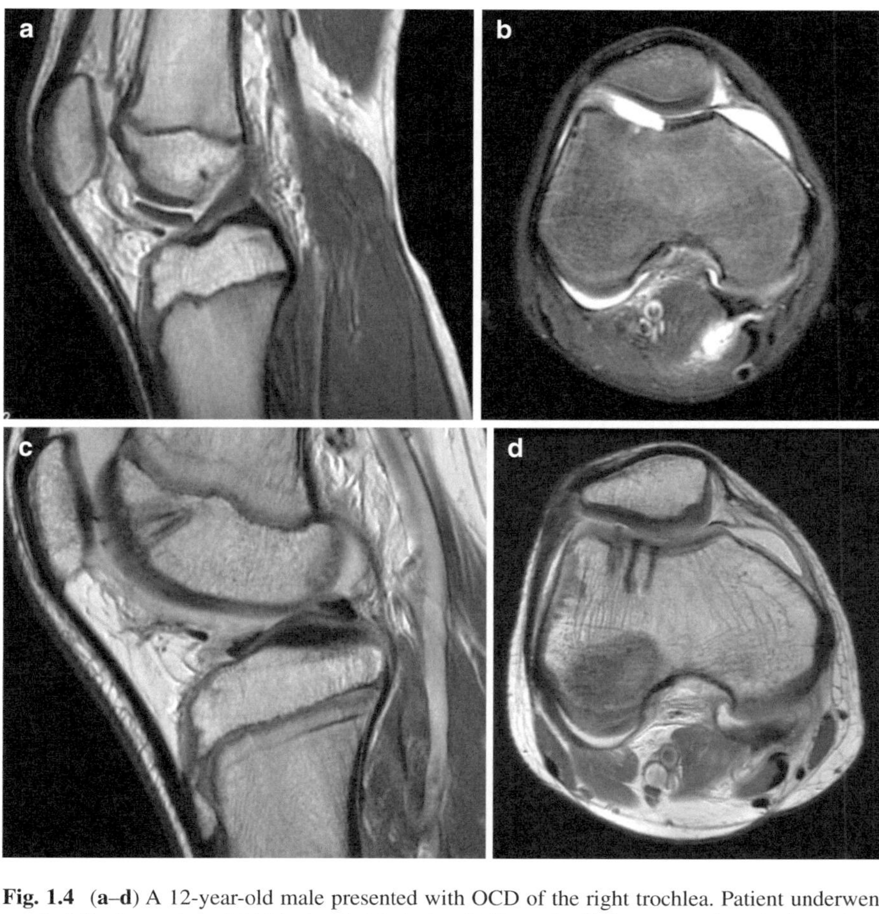

Fig. 1.4 **(a–d)** A 12-year-old male presented with OCD of the right trochlea. Patient underwent surgical fixation using eight bioabsorbable tacks. At 8 months follow-up, patient denies pain or symptoms and shows radiographic healing and incorporation. (Fig. 1.6a, b pre-op; Fig. 1.6c, d post-op)

Most studies on treatment for OCD have reported on femoral condyle lesions, and the American Academy of Orthopedic Surgeons (AAOS) clinical practice guidelines for treatment of OCD do not address trochlear lesions [50]. Due to the paucity of studies on its etiology and treatment, standardized treatments for trochlear OCD have not yet been established [51–54]. Due to the unique forces exerted on the patellofemoral joint, the diagnosis and treatment of trochlear OCD may differ from that of the femoral condyle. However, in the absence of conclusive studies, similar treatment guidelines as those for OCD of the femoral condyle are typically followed. Stable OCD lesions in skeletally immature patients respond well to non-operative treatment such as immobilization, non-weightbearing, or activity modification [55]. Operative intervention is indicated for patients with mechanical symptoms and evidence of loose body or unstable articular surface or those with closed growth plates. The goals of surgery are to reestablish the subchondral interface and preserve the overlying articular cartilage, ensure early motion, ideally preserve the bone without use of allograft, and achieve rigid fixation. Procedures include arthroscopy, chondroplasty, drilling, removal of loose bodies, lateral retinacular release, fixation, and allograft implantation. Postoperative management includes lateral retinacular stretching, patellar taping, and vastus medialis obliquus muscle exercises [56].

There is a paucity of literature reporting on the outcomes of surgical treatment for trochlear JOCD. Aside from several case reports, Wall et al. conducted a multicenter study of 24 cases of trochlear OCD treated either operatively (50%) or nonoperatively ([51–53]). Of the operative patients, eight had surgical signs of healing and were able to return to sports. To better understand this rare condition, we conducted a retrospective cohort study of 30 patients with 34 trochlear JOCD lesions and report good short-term surgical outcomes. We also have found that there is an association with patients' participation in sports, specifically basketball and soccer that involve loading of the patellofemoral joint [57].

Similar to trochlear JOCD, the etiology and treatment for patellar JOCD are not well understood as it is also an uncommon location for lesions [44, 47, 58]. Patients typically present with anterior patellar pain similar to those with trochlear lesions. On imaging the lesion is typically seen on the posterior surface of the patella involving the overlying cartilage (Fig. 1.5a, b). Kramer et al. conducted one of the only studies evaluating treatment of both trochlear and patellar JOCD lesions. This surgical case series included 17 trochlear JOCD cases and 12 patellar JOCD and reported good clinical outcomes with 48% pain-free and 48% left with mild residual pain. At last follow-up, 85% of patients were able to return to sports, and the satisfaction scores and pedi-IKDC scores were positive [56]. In contrast to this study, some literature has reported less successful surgical outcomes for patellar OCD.

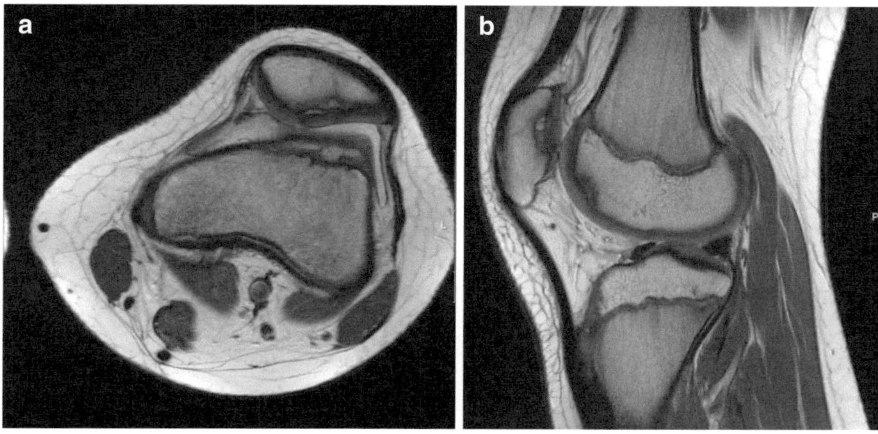

Fig. 1.5 (**a**, **b**) Preoperative images from a 12-year-old male presenting with unstable patellar OCD lesion of the left knee and a stable OCD lesion of the trochlea. Patient complains of anterior knee pain

Hoffa's Fat Pad Impingement

The knee joint is composed of three main fat pads: the anterior or infrapatellar fat pad (IFP), the intracapsular or quadriceps fat pad, and the extrasynovial or prefemoral fat pad. The infrapatellar fat pad (IFP) or Hoffa's fat pad is an intracapsular but extrasynovial wedge-shaped mass in the anterior region of the knee. The IFP extends from the inferior pole of the patella to the upper tibia and infrapatellar bursa and is delimited anteriorly by the patellar tendon and joint capsule and posteriorly by synovial membrane [59]. This structure acts as a shock absorber and guide for the patellar tendon. Hoffa's disease was first described by Albert Hoffa in 1904 as a cause of anterior knee pain resulting from impingement and inflammation of the IFP [60]. This impingement can be caused by multiple factors including patellar tendinitis, direct trauma such as sleeve fractures, or IFP tumors [61]. While tumors (typically benign) have been shown to be a source of pain in adult populations, they are far less common in children; however, it is important to be aware of tumors as a differential diagnosis [61]. In the absence of these underlying factors, fat pad impingement can often result after a hyperextension injury in which the fat pad is pinched. This injury can be caused by an acute closed degloving called the Morel-Lavallee lesion or by chronic exposure to repetitive shear forces and overuse [62]. Both of these types of injuries are most commonly seen in athletes such as dancers, gymnasts, or swimmers, whose activities require full knee extension. In response to impingement, the IFP becomes inflamed and swollen. If Hoffa's fat pad impingement is not addressed, it can result in fibrotic changes in cartilaginous or bony tissue including ossification of the fat pad [62].

Upon physical exam and patellar tendon palpation, patients present with tenderness along either side of the patellar tendon. This pain typically intensifies during flexion and extension [26]. In terms of radiography, plain radiographs are typically normal unless the condition has progressed into a chronic stage in which ossification is present. MRI is more helpful in diagnosing painfully impinged IFP as these cases often exhibit edema on MRI. Increased signal intensity on T2-weighted MRI of Hoffa's fat pad between the patellar ligament and lateral femoral condyle has been described as diagnostic of an impinged Hoffa's fat pad [63–65]. However several studies have shown that while edema in the superolateral region of Hoffa's fat pad is associated with clinical fat pad impingement, edema can also appear in patients without clinical pain [66, 67].

Several studies have also looked at the association of patellofemoral malalignment with Hoffa's fat pad impingement. Campagnes et al. report two types of patellofemoral malalignment that may be associated with impingement: a high-riding patella and an increased TT-TG distance, which may be associated with impingement [68, 69]. Campagna hypothesized that a high-riding patella could allow the patellar ligament to lie in front of the lateral trochlear facet and result in pressure between the patellar ligament and bone during motion [70]. Chung et al. also proposed that abnormal narrowing between the patellar ligament and bone could be associated with Hoffa's fat pad impingement [71]. Campagna et al. supported this study by observing an increase in patellar tendinopathy and decrease in the distance from the patellar tendon to bone in patients with edema due to impingement [70].

Initial treatment of impingement of Hoffa's fat pad typically involves physical therapy paired with NSAIDs to combat inflammation. If the impingement resulted from hyperextension, exercises targeting hamstring strength typically reduce the risk of repeated impingement. Injections of corticosteroids have been used in some clinics in an attempt to relieve pain in more extreme cases [72]. For patients who do not experience relief of symptoms with conservative treatment, surgical excision of the fat pad can provide relief [60, 72–74]. In addition, if a secondary morbidity such as an ossifying chondroma presents, a surgical arthroscopic resection is recommended [75].

Plica Syndrome

Plica syndrome or inflammation and thickening of the synovial folds around the patella typically occur in the medial superior portion of the medial retinaculum radiating toward the medial quadriceps tendon. "Synovial plicae" refer to four defined intracapsular folds in the synovial lining of the knee. These folds are remnants of septum-like divisions in the knee present during embryonic development [76, 77]. If these embryonic remnants fail to be reabsorbed as part of normal development, they become plica folds in adulthood [78]. These plicae are typically asymptomatic; however, blunt trauma, twisting injuries, or repetitive mechanical irritation from flexion extension activities can result in inflammation. Inflammation of the synovial plica of the medial patella in particular results in the anteromedial knee pain associated with plica syndrome [79–83]. If not treated after initial presentation of symptoms, the symptomatic plica can become fibrotic and subsequently lose elasticity. This often results in the painful impingement against nearby intraarticular structures that is characteristic of plica syndrome. The incidence of symptomatic plicae remains unclear, and different investigators report vastly different numbers depending on age and various criteria [84–86].

Patients with plica syndrome may present with intermittent, dull medial pain or combined medial and anterior pain that worsens with running, squatting, kneeling, and walking up and down the stairs. The injured knee often pops when flexed and patients can feel instability, stiffness, catching, and locking upon moving. Clinically, palpation may reveal thickened, tender regions in the medial superior part of the knee and tenderness over the medial femoral condyle or patellar facet. Patients may also experience swelling and a firm, tender ridge parallel to the medial edges of the patella. Additionally, some studies that measure a difference in thigh circumference report mild to moderate quadriceps atrophy of about 0.5–1 inch in 50% or more of patients [87, 88]. MRI can show enlarged plicae and associated bone edema at the distal medial trochlea in most patients. It can also help rule out meniscal tears and articular cartilage injuries; however, MRI does not help distinguish normal thickening of the synovial tissue and plica syndrome. Arthroscopy provides a definitive diagnosis of plica syndrome as it reveals thickened, white, fibrotic plicae, but arthroscopy is only recommended when conservative treatment fails [80, 83] (Fig. 1.6).

For initial treatment of plica syndrome, we recommend two phases of conservative treatment. Conservative techniques are particularly successful in younger patients with a short duration of symptoms associated with acute trauma [87, 89].

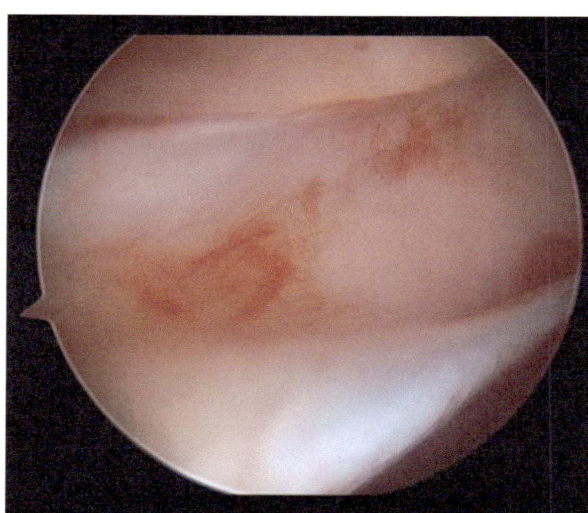

Fig. 1.6 Arthroscopy photo of a 14-year-old female with symptomatic plica. The image demonstrates two large plicas in the superior medial aspect of the knee

To combat acute painful symptoms, patients should apply ice and use NSAIDs for short-term relief. They should also reduce activities that exacerbate the plica. Patients who present with severe pain or limping should avoid all running and jumping activities. Those who have more mild pain can work with their physician to establish a plan to modify activity by decreasing duration and intensity of activity. Several physicians have reported success by applying an upward and lateralized pull on the patella via taping [90]. In terms of physical therapy, programs focused on quadriceps strengthening and increasing the flexibility of the hamstrings have been shown to be successful [89, 91, 92]. While not the first line of treatment, corticosteroids injected intraarticularly or into the symptomatic plica have been shown to be effective [90]. These injections are typically most successful if implemented early in the disease process. Surgical arthroscopic excision of the symptomatic plica is recommended if pain persists or if the plica has undergone permanent changes in morphology [90]. Postoperative reports have generally had positive results following excision of pathological plicae [88, 91, 93].

Tibial Tubercle Fracture

Occurring at the anterior tibial ossification center, tibial tubercle fracture is an important differential diagnosis for Osgood-Schlatter's. The incidence of these injuries is quite low, representing 3% of all epiphyseal and 1% of all physeal injuries in adolescents [94–96]. When they do occur, these fractures are most common in adolescent males from ages 12 to 17 after acute injuries in which the quadriceps is forcefully contracted during a jump or sprint or when the knee is violently flexed during quadriceps contraction as in landing from a jump [97, 98]. These incidences tend to cause injury in male adolescents of this age range because they are mechanically vulnerable at this stage of development. During this time, male adolescents are experiencing rapid growth of the proximal tibia, which extends distally toward the tibial tubercle [99]. Developing from a secondary ossification center in the proximal aspect of the tibia, the tibial tubercle develops in traction, which leaves it more sensitive to tensile forces [4]. By the time males go through this vulnerable stage of developmental growth, they are larger and heavier and have stronger quadriceps than females. These factors combine to make the tibial tubercle more vulnerable to these potentially damaging forces.

Clinically, patients present with acute pain, swelling, knee effusion, and decreased extension of the knee. Plain lateral radiographs of the knee show the fracture. A classification system of three types of tibial tubercle fractures was established by Sir Reginald Watson-Jones in 1955 and has since been expanded upon by several authors [97]. Watson-Jones defined a Type I fracture as an avulsion of a small part of the tibial tubercle, distal to the proximal tibial physis. Type II was classified as a fracture that crosses the physis but does not enter the knee joint. Type III was defined as an avulsion proximal to the physis that extended into the knee [97]. Ogden et al. supplemented this classification system by defining displacement and comminution to help delineate different treatment strategies and more specific fracture patterns [100]. Subsequently Types III, IV, V, and IIIB have been added to the classification system. Ryu and Debenham defined a Type IV fracture as an avulsion of the entire proximal epiphysis that extends posteriorly along the proximal tibial physis [101]. Type III refers to fractures that are also associated with patella ligament avulsions [102], and Type V fractures are described as those that combine Type III and Type IV to make a "Y" appearance [99, 103]. Plain radiographs are typically sufficient to establish these classifications; however, complicated fractures may require additional imaging such as computerized tomography (CT) or MRI. This type of imaging is particularly useful for irreducible fractures that may have entrapped periosteum [104].

Proper classification of tibial tubercle fractures is important for establishing appropriate treatment recommendations. Nondisplaced fractures can be treated with immobilization for about 4 weeks. This immobilization should be followed by rehabilitation to achieve full ROM by 8 weeks. Displaced fractures should be treated with surgical open reduction and internal fixation. Use of cannulated screws for this procedure is the most common, and the literature reports positive results and rehabilitation. In addition more severe nondisplaced fractures can be treated using percutaneous screws [105]. With a careful physical therapy regiment to help regain ROM and muscle strength, patients should be able to return to normal activity at about 3–4 months following surgery. It is important to be aware of some of the complications that rarely accompany tibial tubercle fractures including compartment syndrome upon initial presentation, meniscal tears, and knee stiffness and genu recurvatum following treatment [106]. A recent meta-analysis of the literature on outcomes and complications of 336 tibial tubercle fractures in pediatrics reported compartment syndrome in 3.57% [107]. Meniscal tears with tibial tubercle avulsions, while rare, have been reported in a small number of patients with Type III fractures [108].

Patellar Sleeve Fracture

A potential differential diagnosis for SLJ syndrome (SLJ), patellar sleeve fractures are characterized by an avulsion of a small bony fragment attached to the cartilage, periosteum, and retinaculum from the distal pole of the patella. These fractures are specific to children and have a very low incidence rate of 1–6.5% [109, 110]. Direct trauma and patellar subluxation or dislocation are common causes of these fractures [111].

Clinically, patients present with very tender and swollen knees. A palpable gap may be apparent upon physical examination if the fracture is significantly displaced [110, 112]. A lateral plain radiograph can show the avulsed bone fragment and patella alta (Fig. 1.7); however, if the fragment is composed mainly of the cartilage, it can be missed in the diagnosis [110, 113, 114]. AP or lateral radiographs can also rule out bipartite patella, accessory ossification centers, and SLJ, which appear very

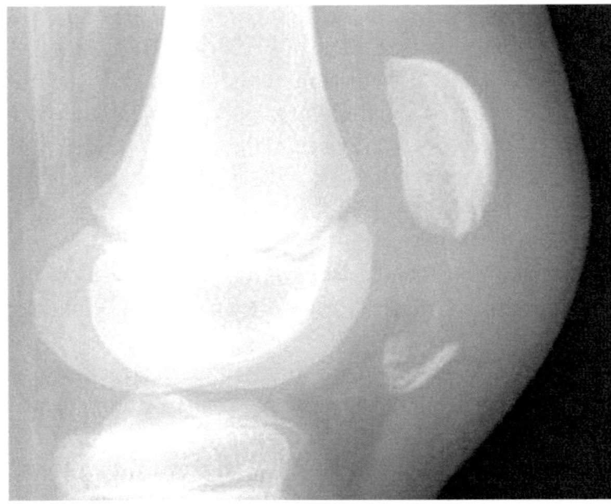

Fig. 1.7 Patellar sleeve fracture with displacement

similar to patella sleeve fractures. If the injury is clear on plain radiographs, there is no need to obtain MRIs; however, sagittal plane T2-weighted images of sleeve fractures in the line of the patellar tendon can provide useful information about the extent of the cartilaginous injury and the location of the fracture fragments [113, 115]. The fracture line typically appears with high signal intensity which contrasts well against the low signal cartilage.

Unlike SLJ, patellar sleeve fractures should not be treated conservatively. If a patient is misdiagnosed and managed non-operatively with conservative treatment, he/she tends to develop extensor lag, deformity of the patella, prominence, and potential reduced knee flexion if immobilization was used as the initial conservative measure [116–118]. Surgical options ranging from irrigation and debridement to open reduction and internal fixation are recommended for displaced patellar sleeve fractures. If the extensor retinaculum is torn, it should also be repaired. A surgical complication to be aware of is an excessive exposure or unintentional injury to the anterior surface of the distal pole of the patella. As this is a major source of blood for the growing patella, injury to this structure could lead to avascular necrosis of the proximal pole [119].

Rehabilitation of Patellofemoral Pain

A guiding principle to effective treatment of patellofemoral pain in the pediatric and adolescent population is to perform all exercises without pain. In addition, day-to-day activities should be modified so that the patient is as symptom-free as possible [120]. While painful activities should be avoided, they should also be replaced, so as not to create unnecessary deconditioning. Generally, nonimpact activities can be pursued, such as swimming, biking, and use of an elliptical machine. Regarding treatment, open chain isometric exercises tend to create the least amount of irritation. Straight leg raises can be performed in different directions to facilitate knee and hip strength. These can be performed lying down or standing using elastic bands. Tight muscle groups, typically hamstrings and quadriceps, iliotibial band, and hip flexors, should be stretched. Care should be taken though to identify hyperlaxity/hypermobility, and if present, not to advance it. When beginning closed chain exercises, start static with only as much knee flexion as able without pain during or after the activity. As symptoms resolve the amount of knee flexion can be advanced. During closed chain exercises, it is important to utilize a hip strategy to engage gluteal and hamstring musculature, thereby decreasing patellofemoral loading. When static exercises in knee flexion can be performed without pain, movement can be introduced in short pain-free ranges. Progress should go from double to single leg activities, from low load short duration activities to low load increased duration activities to high load short duration activities to high load long duration activities, and then to progressive impact activities emphasizing soft landings.

During closed chain exercises, proper lower extremity alignment should be addressed [121]. In order for neutral alignment to be achieved, the foot must be positioned properly, which can be accomplished through active as well as external positioning. Active positioning can be taught. In cases where pes planus is present, the patient is instructed to actively maintain an appropriate arch, keeping the first metatarsal head on the floor rather than simply rolling the foot into inversion. Foot intrinsic muscle strengthening can assist in forming a strong base upon which the extremity can function. Towel crunches, as well as marble pickups via toe splaying rather than curling, are useful techniques. The use of proper footwear and an arch support or formal orthotics can assist in optimizing alignment. The hip and core also play an important role [122–125]. Exercises of those body parts can be initiated immediately without symptom provocation. Simple exercises such as hip abduction and clamshells for the hip as well as prone and side planks for the core can be utilized.

Other components of effective treatment include examination of running technique. Patients who tend to make initial contact via heel strike can be trained in low-impact running which utilizes a forefoot/midfoot initial contact. This reduces impact forces on the knee. Footwear is also important. Suboptimal footwear such as old shoes, or incorrect design for the individual (such as a minimalist running shoe for a patient who pronates significantly), can also be a contributing factor to symptom provocation. Guidance on matching the footwear with conditions is also helpful (wearing turf shoes on hard dry grass fields rather than cleats). In order to maximize the speed of recovery and to prevent future recurrence, establishing a long-term home program is vital [126]. Compliance can be maximized through prescribing a limited number of essential exercises which are to be performed daily, working with the patient to link the performance of exercises to a daily activity or time as well as establishing monitoring mechanisms such as informing parents that exercises have been performed (this places the locus of control on the patient, rather than having the parent ask) and addressing compliance at each visit. The provider should have an open and honest dialogue with the patient and approach the discussion in a supportive, non-threatening way, which aims to assist in the development of effective strategies. Other methods include an exercise log/diary and utilization of reminders such as a post-it note on a bedroom mirror or alarm on an electronic device such as a phone or touch pad. Regarding the use of modalities, ultrasound and electrical stimulation are discouraged due to concerns about their potential impact on growth centers. Ice can be useful, and heat is generally discouraged.

References

1. Bentley G, Dowd G. Current concepts of etiology and treatment of chondromalacia patellae. Clin Orthop Relat Res. 1984;189:209–28.
2. Insall J, Falvo KA, Wise DW. Chondromalacia patellae. A prospective study. J Bone Joint Surg Am. 1976;58(1):1–8.
3. Osgood RB. Lesions of the tibial tubercle occurring during adolescence. Bost Med Surg J. 1903;148:114.
4. Ogden JA, Southwick WO. Osgood-Schlatter's disease and tibial tuberosity development. Clin Orthop Relat Res. 1976;116:180–9.
5. Lancourt JE, Cristini JA. Patella Alta and patella infera. Their etiological role in patellar dislocation, chondromalacia, and apophysitis of the tibial tubercle. J Bone Joint Surg Am. 1975;57(8):1112–5.
6. Willner P. Osgood-Schlatter's disease: etiology and treatment. Clin Orthop Relat Res. 1969;62:178–9.
7. Gigante A, Bevilacqua C, Bonetti MG, Greco F. Increased external tibial torsion in Osgood-Schlatter disease. Acta Orthop Scand. 2003;74(4):431–6. https://doi.org/10.1080/00016470310017749.
8. Kujala UM, Kvist M, Heinonen O. Osgood-Schlatter's disease in adolescent athletes. Retrospective study of incidence and duration. Am J Sports Med. 1985;13(4):236–41.
9. Dunn JF. Osgood-Schlatter disease. Am Fam Physician. 1990;41(1):173–6.
10. Gholve PA, Scher DM, Khakharia S, Widmann RF, Green DW. Osgood Schlatter syndrome. Curr Opin Pediatr. 2007;19(1):44–50. https://doi.org/10.1097/MOP.0b013e328013dbea.
11. Hirano A, Fukubayashi T, Ishii T, Ochiai N. Magnetic resonance imaging of Osgood-Schlatter disease: the course of the disease. Skelet Radiol. 2002;31(6):334–42. https://doi.org/10.1007/s00256-002-0486-z.
12. Krause BL, Williams JP, Catterall A. Natural history of Osgood-Schlatter disease. J Pediatr Orthop. 1990;10(1):65–8.
13. Mital MA, Matza RA, Cohen J. The so-called unresolved Osgood-Schlatter lesion: a concept based on fifteen surgically treated lesions. J Bone Joint Surg Am. 1980;62(5):732–9.
14. Orava S, Malinen L, Karpakka J, et al. Results of surgical treatment of unresolved Osgood-Schlatter lesion. Ann Chir Gynaecol. 2000;89(4):298–302.
15. Flowers MJ, Bhadreshwar DR. Tibial tuberosity excision for symptomatic Osgood-Schlatter disease. J Pediatr Orthop. 1995;15(3):292–7.
16. FERCIOT CF. Surgical management of anterior tibial epiphysis. Clin Orthop. 1955;5:204–6.
17. Glynn MK, Regan BF. Surgical treatment of Osgood-Schlatter's disease. J Pediatr Orthop. 1983;3(2):216–9.
18. Bosworth DM. Lesions of the tibial tubercle and their treatment. Am J Surg. 1939;43(2):526–31. https://doi.org/10.1016/S0002-9610(39)90874-3.
19. Sinding-Larsen M. A hitherto unknown affection of the patella in children. Acta Radiol. 1921;1:171.
20. Johansson S. En forut icke beskriven sjukdom patella. Hygie. 1922;84:161.

21. Foss KDB, Myer GD, Magnussen RA, Hewett TE. Diagnostic differences for anterior knee pain between sexes in adolescent basketball players. J Athl Enhanc. 2014;3(1):1814. https://doi.org/10.4172/2324-9080.1000139.
22. Bernhardt D. Overuse injuries of the knee. In: Harris SS, Anderson SJ, editors. Care of the young athlete. 2nd ed. Elk Grove Village: American Academy of Pediatrics; 2010. p. 421.
23. Valentino M, Quiligotti C, Ruggirello M. Sinding-Larsen-Johansson syndrome: a case report. J Ultrasound. 2012;15(2):127–9. https://doi.org/10.1016/j.jus.2012.03.001.
24. Cook C, Hegedus E, Hawkins R, Scovell F, Wyland D. Diagnostic accuracy and association to disability of clinical test findings associated with patellofemoral pain syndrome. Physiother Can Physiothér Can. 2010;62(1):17–24. https://doi.org/10.3138/physio.62.1.17.
25. Medlar RC, Lyne ED. Sinding-Larsen-Johansson disease. Its etiology and natural history. J Bone Jt Surg. 1978;60(8):1113–6.
26. Duri ZA, Patel DV, Aichroth PM. The immature athlete. Clin Sports Med. 2002;21(3):461–82. https://doi.org/10.1016/S0278-5919(01)00008-4.
27. Kajetanek C, Thaunat M, Guimaraes T, Carnesecchi O, Daggett M, Sonnery-Cottet B. Arthroscopic treatment of painful Sinding-Larsen-Johansson syndrome in a professional handball player. Orthop Traumatol Surg Res. 2016;102(5):677–80. https://doi.org/10.1016/j.otsr.2016.05.011.
28. Atesok K, Doral MN, Lowe J, Finsterbush A. Symptomatic bipartite patella: treatment alternatives. J Am Acad Orthop Surg. 2008;16(8):455–61.
29. Weaver JK. Bipartite patellae as a cause of disability in the athlete. Am J Sports Med. 1977;5(4):137–43.
30. Iossifidis A, Brueton RN. Painful bipartite patella following injury. Injury. 1995;26(3):175–6.
31. Sponseller P, Stanitski C. Fractures and dislocation. In: Beaty B, Kasser J, editors. Rockwood and Wilkin's fractures in children. Phladelphia: Lippincott Williams & Wilkins; 2001. p. 981.
32. Melvin JS, Mehta S. Patellar fractures in adults. J Am Acad Orthop Surg. 2011;19(4):198–207.
33. Oohashi Y, Koshino T, Oohashi Y. Clinical features and classification of bipartite or tripartite patella. Knee Surg Sports Traumatol Arthrosc. 2010;18(11):1465–9. https://doi.org/10.1007/s00167-010-1047-y.
34. Matic GT, Flanigan DC. Return to activity among athletes with a symptomatic bipartite patella: a systematic review. Knee. 2015;22(4):280–5. https://doi.org/10.1016/j.knee.2015.01.005.
35. Gaheer RS, Kapoor S, Rysavy M. Contemporary management of symptomatic bipartite patella. Orthopedics. 2009;32(11):850–1. https://doi.org/10.3928/01477447-20091101-04.
36. Ishikawa H, Sakurai A, Hirata S, et al. Painful bipartite patella in young athletes. The diagnostic value of skyline views taken in squatting position and the results of surgical excision. Clin Orthop Relat Res. 1994;305:223–8.
37. Saupe H. Primäre Krochenmark serelung der kniescheibe. Dtsch Z Chir. 1943;258:386–92.
38. Kavanagh EC, Zoga A, Omar I, Ford S, Schweitzer M, Eustace S. MRI findings in bipartite patella. Skelet Radiol. 2007;36(3):209–14. https://doi.org/10.1007/s00256-006-0232-z.
39. Mori Y, Okumo H, Iketani H, Kuroki Y. Efficacy of lateral retinacular release for painful bipartite patella. Am J Sports Med. 1995;23(1):13–8.
40. Adachi N, Ochi M, Yamaguchi H, Uchio Y, Kuriwaka M. Vastus lateralis release for painful bipartite patella. Arthroscopy. 2002;18(4):404–11.
41. Vaishya R, Chopra S, Vijay V, Vaish A. Bipartite patella causing knee pain in young adults: a report of 5 cases. J Orthop Surg (Hong Kong). 2015;23(1):127–30.
42. Hughston JC, Hergenroeder PT, Courtenay BG. Osteochondritis dissecans of the femoral condyles. J Bone Joint Surg Am. 1984;66(9):1340–8.
43. Linden B. The incidence of osteochondritis dissecans in the condyles of the femur. Acta Orthop Scand. 1976;47(6):664–7.
44. Flynn JM, Kocher MS, Ganley TJ. Osteochondritis dissecans of the knee. J Pediatr Orthop. 2004;24(4):434–43.
45. Kocher MS, Tucker R, Ganley TJ, Flynn JM. Management of osteochondritis dissecans of the knee: current concepts review. Am J Sports Med. 2006;34(7):1181–91. https://doi.org/10.1177/0363546506290127.

46. Yellin JL, Gans I, Carey JL, Shea KG, Ganley TJ. The surgical management of osteochondritis dissecans of the knee in the skeletally immature: a survey of the pediatric orthopedic society of North America (POSNA) membership. J Pediatr Orthop. 2015;37:491. https://doi.org/10.1097/BPO.0000000000000696.
47. Hixon AL, Gibbs LM. Osteochondritis dissecans: a diagnosis not to miss. Am Fam Physician. 2000;61(1):151–6. 158
48. Bohndorf K. Osteochondritis (osteochondrosis) dissecans: a review and new MRI classification. Eur Radiol. 1998;8(1):103–12. https://doi.org/10.1007/s003300050348.
49. Schenck RC, Goodnight JM. Osteochondritis dissecans. J Bone Joint Surg Am. 1996;78(3):439–56.
50. Chambers HG, Shea KG, Carey JL. AAOS clinical practice guideline: diagnosis and treatment of osteochondritis dissecans. J Am Acad Orthop Surg. 2011;19(5):307–9.
51. Kurzweil PR, Zambetti GJ, Hamilton WG. Osteochondritis dissecans in the lateral patellofemoral groove. Am J Sports Med. 1988;16(3):308–10.
52. Luessenhop S, Behrens P, Bruns J, Rehder U. Bilateral osteochondritis dissecans of the medial trochlea femoris: an unusual case of patellofemoral pain. Knee Surg Sports Traumatol Arthrosc. 1993;1(3–4):187–8.
53. Mori Y, Kubo M, Shimokoube J, Kuroki Y. Osteochondritis dissecans of the patellofemoral groove in athletes: unusual cases of patellofemoral pain. Knee Surg Sports Traumatol Arthrosc. 1994;2(4):242–4.
54. Ronga M, Zappalà G, Cherubino M, Genovese EA, Bulgheroni P. Osteochondritis dissecans of the entire femoral trochlea. Am J Sports Med. 2006;34(9):1508–11. https://doi.org/10.1177/0363546506286342.
55. Twyman RS, Desai K, Aichroth PM. Osteochondritis dissecans of the knee. A long-term study. J Bone Joint Surg Br. 1991;73(3):461–4.
56. Kramer DE, Yen Y-M, Simoni MK, et al. Surgical management of osteochondritis dissecans lesions of the patella and trochlea in the pediatric and adolescent population. Am J Sports Med. 2015;43(3):654–62. https://doi.org/10.1177/0363546514562174.
57. Price MJ, Tuca M, Nguyen J, et al. Juvenile osteochondritis dissecans of the trochlea. J Pediatr Orthop. 2018;38:176–80. https://doi.org/10.1097/BPO.0000000000001174.
58. Kocher MS, Micheli LJ, Yaniv M, Zurakowski D, Ames A, Adrignolo AA. Functional and radiographic outcome of juvenile osteochondritis dissecans of the knee treated with transarticular arthroscopic drilling. Am J Sports Med. 2001;29(5):562–6.
59. Maurel B, Le Corroller T, Cohen M, et al. Infrapatellar fat pad: anterior crossroads of the knee. J Radiol. 2010;91(9 Pt 1):841–55.
60. Hoffa A. Influence of adipose tissue with regard to the pathology of the knee joint. JAMA. 1904;43:795–6.
61. Albergo JI, Gaston CLL, Davies M, et al. Hoffa's fat pad tumours: what do we know about them? Int Orthop. 2013;37(11):2225–9. https://doi.org/10.1007/s00264-013-2041-z.
62. Lapègue F, Sans N, Brun C, et al. Imaging of traumatic injury and impingement of anterior knee fat. Diagn Interv Imaging. 2016;97(7–8):789–807. https://doi.org/10.1016/j.diii.2016.02.012.
63. Subhawong TK, Eng J, Carrino JA, Chhabra A. Superolateral Hoffa's fat pad edema: association with patellofemoral maltracking and impingement. AJR Am J Roentgenol. 2010;195(6):1367–73. https://doi.org/10.2214/AJR.10.4668.
64. Chhabra A, Subhawong TK, Carrino JA. A systematised MRI approach to evaluating the patellofemoral joint. Skelet Radiol. 2011;40(4):375–87. https://doi.org/10.1007/s00256-010-0909-1.
65. Saddik D, McNally EG, Richardson M. MRI of Hoffa's fat pad. Skelet Radiol. 2004;33(8):433–44. https://doi.org/10.1007/s00256-003-0724-z.
66. De Smet AA, Davis KW, Dahab KS, Blankenbaker DG, del Rio AM, Bernhardt DT. Is there an association between superolateral Hoffa fat pad edema on MRI and clinical evidence of fat

pad impingement? AJR Am J Roentgenol. 2012;199(5):1099–104. https://doi.org/10.2214/AJR.12.8798.
67. Tsavalas N, Karantanas AH. Suprapatellar fat-pad mass effect: MRI findings and correlation with anterior knee pain. Am J Roentgenol. 2013;200(3):W291–6. https://doi.org/10.2214/AJR.12.8821.
68. Dejour H, Walch G, Nove-Josserand L, Guier C. Factors of patellar instability: an anatomic radiographic study. Knee Surg Sports Traumatol Arthrosc. 1994;2(1):19–26.
69. Kannus PA. Long patellar tendon: radiographic sign of patellofemoral pain syndrome--a prospective study. Radiology. 1992;185(3):859–63. https://doi.org/10.1148/radiology.185.3.1438776.
70. Campagna R, Pessis E, Biau DJ, et al. Is superolateral Hoffa fat pad edema a consequence of impingement between lateral femoral condyle and patellar ligament? Radiology. 2012;263(2):469–74. https://doi.org/10.1148/radiol.12111066.
71. Chung CB, Skaf A, Roger B, Campos J, Stump X, Resnick D. Patellar tendon-lateral femoral condyle friction syndrome: MR imaging in 42 patients. Skelet Radiol. 2001;30(12):694–7. https://doi.org/10.1007/s002560100409.
72. Larbi A, Cyteval C, Hamoui M, et al. Hoffa's disease: a report on 5 cases. Diagn Interv Imaging. 2014;95:1079–84. https://doi.org/10.1016/j.diii.2014.06.009.
73. Smilie IS. Lesions of the infrapatellar fat pad and synovial fringes: Hoff's disease. Acta Orthop Scand. 1963;33:371–7.
74. Metheny JA, Mayor MB. Hoffa disease: chronic impingement of the infra-patellar fat pad. Am J Knee Surg. 1988;1:134–9.
75. Krebs VE, Parker RD. Arthroscopic resection of an extrasynovial ossifying chondroma of the infrapatellar fat pad: end-stage Hoffa's disease? Arthroscopy. 1994;10(3):301–4.
76. Gray DJ, Gardner E. Prenatal development of the human knee and superior tibiofibular joints. Am J Anat. 1950;86(2):235–87. https://doi.org/10.1002/aja.1000860204.
77. Ogata S, Uhthoff HK. The development of synovial plicae in human knee joints: an embryologic study. Arthroscopy. 1990;6(4):315–21.
78. Pipkin G. Knee injuries: the role of the suprapatellar plica and suprapatellar bursa in simulating internal derangements. Clin Orthop Relat Res. 1971;74:161–76.
79. Mital MA, Hayden J. Pain in the knee in children: the medial plica shelf syndrome. Orthop Clin North Am. 1979;10(3):713–22.
80. Møller H. Incarcerating mediopatellar synovial plica syndrome. Acta Orthop Scand. 1981;52(3):357–61.
81. Munzinger U, Ruckstuhl J, Scherrer H, Gschwend N. Internal derangement of the knee joint due to pathologic synovial folds: the mediopatellar plica syndrome. Clin Orthop Relat Res. 1981;155:59–64.
82. Nottage WM, Sprague NF, Auerbach BJ, Shahriaree H. The medial patellar plica syndrome. Am J Sports Med. 1983;11(4):211–4.
83. Patel D. Plica as a cause of anterior knee pain. Orthop Clin North Am. 1986;17(2):273–7.
84. Barber FA. Fenestrated medial patella plica. Arthroscopy. 1987;3(4):253–7.
85. Nakayama A, Sugita T, Aizawa T, Takahashi A, Honma T. Incidence of medial plica in 3,889 knee joints in the Japanese population. Arthroscopy. 2011;27(11):1523–7. https://doi.org/10.1016/j.arthro.2011.06.022.
86. Jackson RW, Marshall DJ, Fujisawa Y. The pathologic medical shelf. Orthop Clin North Am. 1982;13(2):307–12.
87. Hardaker WT, Whipple TL, Bassett FH. Diagnosis and treatment of the plica syndrome of the knee. J Bone Joint Surg Am. 1980;62(2):221–5.
88. Richmond JC, McGinty JB. Segmental arthroscopic resection of the hypertrophic mediopatellar plica. Clin Orthop Relat Res. 1983;178:185–9.
89. Griffith CJ, LaPrade RF. Medial plica irritation: diagnosis and treatment. Curr Rev Musculoskelet Med. 2008;1(1):53–60. https://doi.org/10.1007/s12178-007-9006-z.

90. Schindler OS. "The sneaky plica" revisited: morphology, pathophysiology and treatment of synovial plicae of the knee. Knee Surg Sports Traumatol Arthrosc. 2014;22(2):247–62. https://doi.org/10.1007/s00167-013-2368-4.
91. Dorchak JD, Barrack RL, Kneisl JS, Alexander AH. Arthroscopic treatment of symptomatic synovial plica of the knee. Long-term followup. Am J Sports Med. 1991;19(5):503–7.
92. Amatuzzi MM, Fazzi A, Varella MH. Pathologic synovial plica of the knee. Results of conservative treatment. Am J Sports Med. 1990;18(5):466–9.
93. Klein W. The medial shelf of the knee. A follow-up study. Arch Orthop Trauma surgery Arch für orthopädische und Unfall-Chirurgie. 1983;102(2):67–72.
94. Osgood RB. Lesions of the tibial tubercle occurring during adolescence. 1903. Clin Orthop Relat Res. 1993;286:4–9.
95. Frey S, Hosalkar H, Cameron DB, Heath A, David Horn B, Ganley TJ. Tibial tuberosity fractures in adolescents. J Child Orthop. 2008;2(6):469–74. https://doi.org/10.1007/s11832-008-0131-z.
96. Abalo A, Akakpo-numado KG, Dossim A, Walla A, Gnassingbe K, Tekou AH. Avulsion fractures of the tibial tubercle. J Orthop Surg (Hong Kong). 2008;16(3):308–11.
97. Watson-Jones R. The classic: "fractures and joint injuries" by sir Reginald Watson-Jones, taken from "fractures and joint injuries," by R. Watson-Jones, vol. II, 4th ed., Baltimore, Williams and Wilkins Company. Clin Orthop Relat Res. 1955;105:4–10.
98. Levi JH, Coleman CR. Fracture of the tibial tubercle. Am J Sports Med. 1976;4(6):254–63.
99. McKoy BE, Stanitski CL. Acute tibial tubercle avulsion fractures. Orthop Clin North Am. 2003;34(3):397–403.
100. Ogden JA, Tross RB, Murphy MJ. Fractures of the tibial tuberosity in adolescents. J Bone Joint Surg Am. 1980;62(2):205–15.
101. Ryu RK, Debenham JO. An unusual avulsion fracture of the proximal tibial epiphysis. Case report and proposed addition to the Watson-Jones classification. Clin Orthop Relat Res. 1985;194:181–4.
102. Frankl U, Wasilewski SA, Healy WL. Avulsion fracture of the tibial tubercle with avulsion of the patellar ligament. Report of two cases. J Bone Joint Surg Am. 1990;72(9):1411–3.
103. Curtis JF. Type IV tibial tubercle fracture revisited: a case report. Clin Orthop Relat Res. 2001;389:191–5.
104. Whan A, Breidahl W, Janes G. MRI of trapped periosteum in a proximal tibial physeal injury of a pediatric patient. AJR Am J Roentgenol. 2003;181(5):1397–9. https://doi.org/10.2214/ajr.181.5.1811397.
105. Ozkayin N, Aktuglu K. Avulsion fractures of tibial tuberosity in adolescents. Treatment with closed reduction and percutaneous screwing, using MRI to identify combined intraarticular lesions. Saudi Med J. 2005;26(10):1636–9.
106. Pape JM, Goulet JA, Hensinger RN. Compartment syndrome complicating tibial tubercle avulsion. Clin Orthop Relat Res. 1993;295:201–4.
107. Pretell-Mazzini J, Kelly DM, Sawyer JR, et al. Outcomes and complications of tibial tubercle fractures in pediatric patients: a systematic review of the literature. J Pediatr Orthop. 2016;36(5):440–6. https://doi.org/10.1097/BPO.0000000000000488.
108. Choi NH, Kim NM. Tibial tuberosity avulsion fracture combined with meniscal tear. Arthroscopy. 1999;15(7):766–9.
109. Kimball MJ, Kumar NS, Jakoi AM, Tom JA. Subacute superior patellar pole sleeve fracture. Am J Orthop (Belle Mead NJ). 2014;43(1):29–32.
110. Ray JM, Hendrix J. Incidence, mechanism of injury, and treatment of fractures of the patella in children. J Trauma. 1992;32(4):464–7.
111. Heckman JD, Alkire CC. Distal patellar pole fractures. A proposed common mechanism of injury. Am J Sports Med. 1984;12(6):424–8.
112. Sponsellar PD, Beaty JH. Fractures and dislocations of the knee. Fract Patella Chlild. 1996;3:1284–90.

113. Bates DG, Hresko MT, Jaramillo D. Patellar sleeve fracture: demonstration with MR imaging. Radiology. 1994;193(3):825–7. https://doi.org/10.1148/radiology.193.3.7972832.
114. Gao GX, Mahadev A, Lee EH. Sleeve fracture of the patella in children. J Orthop Surg (Hong Kong). 2008;16(1):43–6.
115. Yu JS, Petersilge C, Sartoris DJ, Pathria MN, Resnick D. MR imaging of injuries of the extensor mechanism of the knee. Radiographics. 1994;14(3):541–51.
116. Bruijn JD, Sanders RJ, Jansen BR. Ossification in the patellar tendon and patella Alta following sports injuries in children. Complications of sleeve fractures after conservative treatment. Arch Orthop Trauma Surg. 1993;112(3):157–8.
117. Houghton G, Ackroyd C. Sleeve fractures of the patella in children: a report of three cases. Bone Joint J. 1979;61-B(2):165–8.
118. Dai LY, Zhang WM. Fractures of the patella in children. Knee Surg Sports Traumatol Arthrosc. 1999;7(4):243–5. https://doi.org/10.1007/s001670050156.
119. Shands PA, McQueen DA. Demonstration of avulsion fracture of the inferior pole of the patella by magnetic resonance imaging. A case report. J Bone Joint Surg Am. 1995;77(11):1721–3.
120. Gorman McNerney ML, Arendt EA. Anterior knee pain in the active and athletic adolescent. Curr Sports Med Rep. 2013;12(6):404–10. https://doi.org/10.1249/JSR.0000000000000013.
121. Noehren B, Pohl MB, Sanchez Z, Cunningham T, Lattermann C. Proximal and distal kinematics in female runners with patellofemoral pain. Clin Biomech. 2012;27(4):366–71. https://doi.org/10.1016/j.clinbiomech.2011.10.005.
122. Crossley KM, van Middelkoop M, Callaghan MJ, Collins NJ, Rathleff MS, Barton CJ. 2016 patellofemoral pain consensus statement from the 4th international patellofemoral pain research retreat, Manchester. Part 2: recommended physical interventions (exercise, taping, bracing, foot orthoses and combined interventions). Br J Sports Med. 2016;50(14):844–52. https://doi.org/10.1136/bjsports-2016-096268.
123. Ferber R, Bolgla L, Earl-Boehm JE, Emery C, Hamstra-Wright K. Strengthening of the hip and Core versus knee muscles for the treatment of patellofemoral pain: a multicenter randomized controlled trial. J Athl Train. 2015;50(4):366–77. https://doi.org/10.4085/1062-6050-49.3.70.
124. Bloomer BA, Durall CJ. Does the addition of hip strengthening to a knee-focused exercise program improve outcomes in patients with patellofemoral pain syndrome? J Sport Rehabil. 2015;24(4):428–33. https://doi.org/10.1123/jsr.2014-0184.
125. Khayambashi K, Ghoddosi N, Straub RK, Powers CM. Hip muscle strength predicts noncontact anterior cruciate ligament injury in male and female athletes: a prospective study. Am J Sports Med. 2016;44(2):355–61. https://doi.org/10.1177/0363546515616237.
126. Rathleff MS, Bandholm T, McGirr KA, Harring SI, Sørensen AS, Thorborg K. New exercise-integrated technology can monitor the dosage and quality of exercise performed against an elastic resistance band by adolescents with patellofemoral pain: an observational study. J Physiother. 2016;62(3):159–63. https://doi.org/10.1016/j.jphys.2016.05.016.

Chapter 2
Anterior Knee Pain

Alex A. Johnson and Miho J. Tanaka

Abbreviations

ACI	Autologous chondrocyte implantation
CT	Computed tomography
ESWT	Extracorporeal shock-wave therapy
GAGPS	Glycosaminoglycan polysulfate
HA	Hyaluronic acid
ITBS	Iliotibial band syndrome
LPFC	Lateral patellofemoral compression
MPP	Medial patellar plica
MRI	Magnetic resonance imaging
PRP	Platelet-rich plasma
TTO	Tibial tuberosity osteotomy
VMO	Vastus medialis obliquus

Epidemiology

Anterior knee pain is one of the most common orthopedic conditions [1, 2]. It is estimated to affect 25% of athletes, occurring primarily in young patients [3]. For those presenting to a sports medicine clinic, 70% of diagnosed cases of patellofemoral pain are in patients aged 16–25 years [4]. The prevalence in the general young population has been reported as 13.5%, with the condition disproportionately

A. A. Johnson · M. J. Tanaka (✉)
Department of Orthopedic Surgery,
The Johns Hopkins University, Baltimore, MD, USA
e-mail: Mtanaka4@jhmi.edu

B. E. Shubin Stein, S. M. Strickland (eds.), *Patellofemoral Pain and Instability*,
https://doi.org/10.1007/978-3-319-97640-2_2

affecting women more than men by approximately 25% [5]. Anterior knee pain is a condition every orthopedic surgeon will encounter; therefore, clinicians should have a firm understanding of the various causes of pain, the ability to delineate and diagnose these causes, and the competency to treat them.

Etiology

Anterior knee pain encompasses a wide range of clinical entities but is most commonly synonymous with patellofemoral pain syndrome. This is characterized by pain in the patellofemoral joint that occurs in the absence of substantial structural or mechanical pathology, including patellofemoral instability. This condition can be frustrating and puzzling to treat because we do not have a complete understanding of its causes. Several theories on the causes of anterior knee pain have provided a framework of understanding for patellofemoral pain and dysfunction in most patients and are discussed in this chapter.

Afferent nerves can be affected in three ways to produce a signal that can be perceived as pain. The first is inherent damage or alteration to the afferent nerves, such as in a demyelinating, fibrotic, or inflammatory process. The abnormal nerves can send altered signals that are felt as pain. Inherent changes within the afferent nerves of the patellofemoral complex have been identified as a source of anterior knee pain. In histological studies of patients with anterior knee pain, degenerative nerve changes have been identified throughout the lateral retinaculum. Some have likened these changes to those seen in Morton neuroma of the foot. Interestingly, these neuromas may be more prevalent in patients with anterior knee pain than in those without [6]. Damage to proprioceptive nerve fibers has also been reported in patients with anterior knee pain [7]. Patellar dislocation leads to a decrease in proprioception at the knee and is thought to be caused by damage to the proprioceptive nerves [8]. However, unlike inherent changes in the afferent nerves, loss of proprioception acts indirectly on the pain pathway. A lack of effective proprioception results in suboptimal stabilization of the patellofemoral complex, creating pain-generating conditions such as subluxation and asymmetric loading.

The second phenomenon leading to peripheral pain is when an increased quantity of sensory nerves is available to transmit a painful signal. A bigger "cable" results in a more powerful signal transmission. This hyper-innervation has been shown to play a substantial role in pain generation in the patellofemoral complex. Patients with severe anterior knee pain have been shown to have increased sensory innervation in the lateral retinaculum compared with patients experiencing less pain [9]. Furthermore, compared with nerves of the medial retinaculum, nerves of the lateral retinaculum, which are thought to play a major role in development of anterior knee pain syndrome, have more of the nociceptive substance P [6]. It has been postulated that this hyper-innervation, which is primarily perivascular, is caused by tissue ischemia and release of vascular endothelial growth factor [9]. It has also been suggested that this ischemia could have mechanical causes, including retraction or tightening of the lateral retinaculum [9]. This hyper-innervation theory, in conjunction with the histological changes seen in the nerves of the lateral retinaculum, represents the "neural model" of anterior knee pain.

The third method of peripheral pain generation is when afferent nerves are stimulated by a noxious source, such as overloading of the subchondral bone or alterations of innervated soft tissue. Many "mechanical" theories have been proposed to explain this method of peripheral pain generation in the patellofemoral complex. Early theories investigated changes in the articular cartilage of the patella as the source of pain. It was felt that although cartilage itself does not generate pain, the subsequent overloading of nerve-rich subchondral bone generates pain in the anterior knee. However, this theory has been disputed because the presence of patellar chondral lesions does not correlate well with anterior knee pain [10–12].The patellofemoral malalignment theory proposed a mechanical basis for anterior knee pain related to a tight lateral retinaculum. This tight lateral retinaculum was believed to create an imbalance in the facets of the patella, resulting in increased pressure on the lateral side and decreased pressure on the medial side, both being detrimental to the cartilage [13]. However, Fulkerson [14] was careful not to view cartilage damage as the main source of pain in the patellofemoral malalignment theory. In a prospective study of 78 knees with patellofemoral pain, only 29% of patients had visible chondromalacia on arthroscopy. Fulkerson proposed that the lateral retinaculum itself is a pain generator as it undergoes chronic irritation from constant stress on the tight retinaculum with knee flexion and centering of the patella in the trochlea. This emphasis on the lateral retinaculum overlapped with the abovementioned neural theory as Fulkerson [14] discussed both the rich innervation of the lateral retinaculum and the painful nerve changes seen in histological studies. Despite the topics addressed by this theory, it failed to account for patients with malalignment who have no pain and patients with relatively good alignment but with substantial pain. This led to a broadening of the patellofemoral malalignment theory of anterior knee pain and the development of the tissue homeostasis theory [15].

This theory, proposed by Dye [16], introduced the idea of an "envelope of function," in which the patellofemoral joint can operate without pain. Anatomic, kinematic, physiologic, and treatment factors determine the envelope of function, according to Dye [16]. Anatomic factors include the biomechanical arrangement of the knee and patellofemoral joint. Kinematic factors pertain to these morphological characteristics in action under loading conditions and active control by the nervous system in terms of proprioception and coordination. Physiologic factors relate to the ability of the body to adapt to and heal injury to the patellofemoral complex. Treatment factors include any operative or nonoperative remedy aimed at altering the previous three factors and the overall envelope of function. This envelope of function determines the amount of load the patellofemoral complex can "absorb" before becoming symptomatic. Relatively "normal" knees can become symptomatic if subjected to consistent "supraphysiologic" loading as is commonly seen in young healthy patients with pain from overuse. Furthermore, "abnormal" or unbalanced knees can be asymptomatic if subjected to minimal loading. The envelope of function can shift with changes in any of the four previously mentioned factors.

This theory incorporates what we know to be true concerning patellofemoral malalignment as a pain generator and also explains anterior knee pain in patients without identifiable anatomic, kinematic, or physiologic abnormality.

Recent research has demonstrated which of these factors defining the envelope of function are most important for young, athletic patients. In a prospective study of 282 young men and women participating in a standard physical education program, Witvrouw et al. [17] diagnosed patellofemoral pain syndrome in 35 participants (12%) over a 2-year period. After investigating factors including physical fitness, joint laxity, static and dynamic patellofemoral alignment characteristics, and psychological parameters, they found the only significant factors to be decreased muscular flexibility in the quadriceps, abnormal vastus medialis obliquus (VMO) muscle reflex response, reduction in vertical jump performance, and increased medial patellar mobility. This study highlights the importance of dynamic factors, primarily in the quadriceps and VMO, in determining the envelope of function in young, athletic patients.

Despite these theories of how pain can be generated peripherally in the patellofemoral joint, some believe there is psychological aspect to anterior knee pain. Domenech et al. [18] investigated the role of psychological factors in disability and pain in patients with anterior knee pain. In an evaluation of psychological variables, including anxiety, depression, pain coping strategies, catastrophizing, and fear of movement in 97 patients with anterior knee pain, they found that catastrophizing played a significant role in pain and disability. Catastrophizing, which is the belief that pain will never get better, has also been shown to be associated with increased activity in the pain centers of the brain, including emotional processing and anticipation on functional magnetic resonance imaging (MRI) studies [19]. Even in patients with underlying neuroanatomic reasons for anterior knee pain, these psychological aspects should not be ignored because addressing them may be the difference between a transient event and a chronic pain condition.

Evaluation of Anterior Knee Pain

History

Most causes of anterior knee pain are atraumatic, although patellofemoral pain or chondral pathology may develop as a result of traumatic injury, particularly in which the patient falls and lands directly on the knee. Factors that increase repetitive stress within the patellofemoral joint should be identified, including activities that involve running, jumping, or squatting. Biomechanical studies have shown that the first contact between the patella and femur occurs between 10° and 20° of flexion, and contact continues to increase past 90°. Maximum patellar contact pressure occurs when the knee reaches 90° of flexion. Increased contact surface area helps offset some of the load at higher levels of flexion but cannot compensate fully for the increased stress; thus, greater contact pressure is seen at higher flexion angles [20]. This explains the aggravation of pain with activities involving bending of the knee. Patients often report that sudden increases in activity or running mileage preceded their symptoms. Changes in weight at the onset of symptoms should be identified, because some studies have reported an association between body mass index and patellofemoral pain syndrome [21, 22]. However, one recent study [23] found no relationship between body composition or body mass index and patellofemoral pain. Alterations in gait and/or shoes can change the distribution of loads across the patellofemoral joint and should be explored as part of history taking [24–26].

The nature of the patient's pain should be described in terms of quality, location, and associated symptoms, while ruling out other conditions such as radicular pain or chronic exertional compartment syndrome, which often present with additional symptoms such as numbness and tingling. Patients often describe pain with squatting, running, and walking down stairs. The "theater sign" is often described as pain over the anterior knee that becomes more pronounced when sitting with the knee in a flexed position for prolonged periods of time [27].

The presence of effusions should be identified in terms of onset, size, and frequency and should be distinguished from generalized swelling. Patients may report mechanical symptoms such as popping or clicking. It is critical to rule out a history of patellar dislocation because the treatment for this is different. Functional "giving way" of the knee should be carefully differentiated from knee instability or patellar dislocation.

Clinical Examination

The evaluation of patellofemoral pain begins with an assessment of alignment. Standing alignment is often reflective of bony malalignment that can contribute to anterior knee pain. Femoral anteversion, which has been associated with patellofemoral disorders, can be detected on standing assessment, in which the feet are in neutral position but the patellae are facing each other [24, 28, 29]. This is also referred to as "squinting patellae." Femoral anteversion can also be assessed in the prone position by comparing hip rotation. The Q-angle is a measurement of malalignment that reflects the lateral pull of the extensor mechanism relative to the axis of the knee [30]. This is measured by the angle formed between a line from the anterior superior iliac spine to the center of the patella and a line from the center of the patella to the tibial tuberosity (Fig. 2.1). This has been described in both sitting and supine positions [31], with normal values reported as 12°–18° [32, 33]. Q-angle has long been considered a risk factor for patellofemoral pain; however, recent studies have questioned this. Studies [17, 34] have demonstrated greater Q-angle to be associated with less abduction moment and impulse during running, leading authors to suggest that it may not be implicated in patellofemoral pain syndrome. Even in light of these studies, Q-angle should be evaluated in patients with patellofemoral pain as an indicator of malalignment that may contribute to abnormal patellofemoral kinematics. The presence of pes planus and pronation of the foot should also be assessed because these can contribute to the valgus moment of the knee [25, 26].

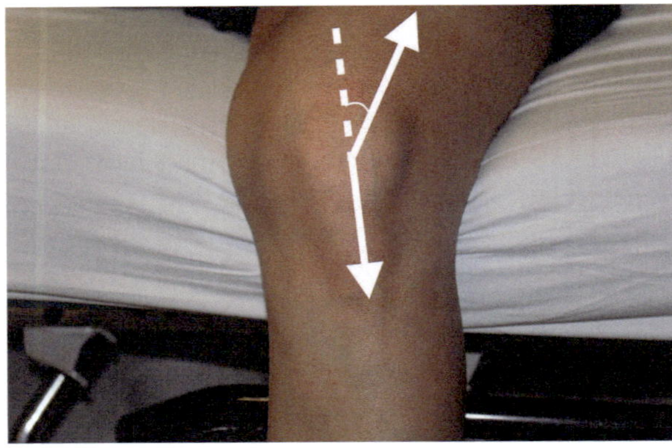

Fig. 2.1 The Q-angle is a measurement of malalignment that reflects the lateral pull of the extensor mechanism relative to the axis of the knee. This is measured by the angle formed between a line from the anterior superior iliac spine to the center of the patella and a line from the center of the patella to the tibial tuberosity

Functional assessment is critical in identifying slight deficiencies in strength, coordination, or flexibility that may be contributing to the patient's pain. The patient's gait is assessed for any abnormality. The functional assessment of the hip and leg can be accomplished by asking the patient to perform a single-leg squat. The evaluator should assess for symmetry to the contralateral side, including trunk lean, hip drop, knee valgus, or pronation of the foot during this motion, any of which can indicate weakness of the dynamic stabilizers of the knee. Strength testing of the hip external rotators and quadriceps against resistance can be helpful because eccentric hip abduction and adduction peak torque have been demonstrated in female patients with patellofemoral pain syndrome versus controls [35]. The presence of VMO atrophy may serve as another indicator of weakness.

Flexibility, or lack or flexibility, can indicate pathology or contribute to knee dysfunction. Hamstring tightness has been associated with patellofemoral pain [36]. In a case-control study, patients with patellofemoral pain syndrome were found to have less flexibility of the gastrocnemius, soleus, quadriceps, and hamstrings compared with sex-matched controls. Hamstring flexibility can be assessed with the patient in a supine position and with passive hip flexion with the knee extended. This should be compared with the contralateral side. The Ober test is performed to identify iliotibial band tightness, which can also be the cause or be associated with existing pathology [37].

Ligamentous laxity has also been associated with patellofemoral pain [38]. A series of criteria known as the Beighton score can be calculated to help diagnose hypermobility. The score includes 1 point for each of the following: (1) the ability to place the palms on the ground when bending forward with the legs straight in a standing position, (2) each elbow that hyperextends, (3) each knee that hyperextends, (4) each thumb that can be bent backward to touch the forearm, and (5) each little finger that can be bent backward past 90° [39].

The knee examination begins with a standard assessment of the skin, range of motion, and ligamentous stability. The presence of an effusion can indicate chondral pathology in a young patient. Pain or crepitus with patellar loading can be elicited by placing direct pressure on the patella while asking the patient to actively contract the quadriceps. This may be performed with the leg resting in extension, with active contraction of the quadriceps mechanism, or in a sitting position while bending the knee actively from flexion to extension. Pain with this maneuver is considered pathognomonic for patellofemoral pain. Medial and lateral patellar stability should be assessed. The tightness of the lateral retinaculum should be assessed carefully. This is performed while assessing for medial excursion of the patella, which may be limited by a tight lateral retinaculum. There may also be visibly increased tilt in the patella and inability to evert the patella to neutral. Examination should always be compared with the contralateral, asymptomatic knee when possible. In a systematic review of 22 patellofemoral tests in nine studies, Cook et al. [40] found positive likelihood ratios to be the strongest for the active instability test, pain during climbing, Clarke's test (pain with activation of the quadriceps with manual pressure from the examiner on the superior pole of the patella), pain during prolonged sitting, and patellar inferior pole tilt.

The location of pain and/or tenderness should be elicited carefully during physical examination (Fig. 2.2). This includes palpation of the medial and lateral facets of the patella, the inferior pole of patella, and the patellar tendon. Tenderness over the patellar tendon should be differentiated between proximal, middle, or distal over the tuberosity. Joint line tenderness should be assessed using standard examination techniques. Patients with symptomatic plica may have tenderness slightly proximal to the medial joint line, and this should be differentiated carefully from medial joint line pain. Patients with plica syndrome may report catching and pain over the medial joint line, which may be mistaken for meniscal symptoms. Careful examination should also be performed for tenderness over Gerdy's tubercle, the iliotibial band, and pes anserine tendons. The location of the patient's symptoms can serve as an important guide for diagnosis.

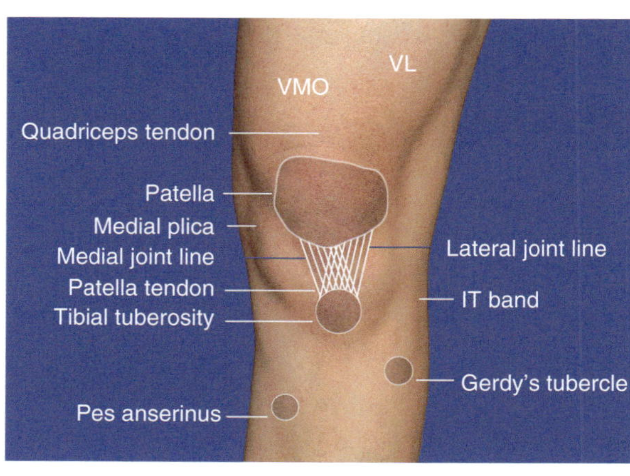

Fig. 2.2 Characteristic locations for patellofemoral tenderness. IT iliotibial, VL vastus lateralis, VMO vastus medialis obliquus

Imaging

Radiographs of the knee are typically taken during assessment of anterior knee pain to look for signs of bony pathology and to assess alignment. Anteroposterior views should be taken during weightbearing, with posteroanterior flexion views if needed to assess for tibiofemoral arthritis. A standard lateral view should be assessed carefully for patellofemoral morphology and alignment, including patella alta and trochlear dysplasia. Soft-tissue disorders, such as Osgood-Schlatter disease, as well as Sinding-Larsen-Johansson syndrome (discussed in the previous chapter), can be seen on lateral radiographs. Axial views can be obtained at 20°, 30°, or 45° of flexion [41–43]. This can show patellar lateralization, tilt, and degenerative joint disease. An example of increased patellar tilt is shown in Fig. 2.3.

MRI is typically reserved for recalcitrant cases or cases of unexplained effusions. MRI can be useful in evaluating the chondral surfaces of the patellofemoral joint. However, it should be noted that the presence of chondral thinning is not necessarily symptomatic. Full-thickness, focal chondral defects may be an indication for further intervention. Anterior or Hoffa's fat pad edema is a frequent finding in patients with patellar malalignment and has been significantly associated with larger patellar tendon–patellar length ratios and loosely associated with increased lateral patellar tilt and a shallow trochlear sulcus [44]. Although plica may not always be seen on MRI, trochlear morphology is usually well visualized. Tendinosis may appear as increased uptake within the midsubstance or insertion of the tendon, and partial tendon tears may be identified. These abnormalities of tendons can also be evaluated at the iliotibial band insertion and the pes anserine insertions. Computed tomography (CT) is typically reserved for cases in which the bone healing or quality needs to be assessed. Most providers prefer MRI to CT because of MRI's enhanced soft-tissue visualization and lower radiation exposure.

Dynamic imaging has been reported for its utility in evaluating anterior knee pain [45, 46]. In a comparison of motion-triggered cine MRI and traditional radiography, dynamic MRI was superior as a prognostication tool for determining success with patellar realignment surgery. Similarly, dynamic CT has been described for its utility in characterizing maltracking patterns [46, 47].

Fig. 2.3 Radiographic sunrise views of the knees show bilaterally increased patellar tilt in a patient with lateral patellofemoral compression syndrome

Rehabilitation Concepts in Anterior Knee Pain

Most rehabilitation regimens for anterior knee pain are based on the tissue homeostasis theory ("envelope of function") described above. Whereas many surgical remedies for patellofemoral pain seek to address anatomic factors, the primary focus of rehabilitation is on the kinematic factors affecting the envelope of function. The elements of a rehabilitation regimen seek to address a specific derangement affecting dynamic patellofemoral function, such as quadriceps or hip weakness. Addressing these deficiencies brings the patella into improved functional alignment under dynamic conditions, thus favorably shifting the envelope of function and decreasing symptoms. Many studies have shown these kinematic factors, including quadriceps weakness, hip weakness, decreased lower-extremity flexibility, and abnormal muscle activation, to be associated with patellofemoral pain.

In a meta-analysis analyzing risk factors for the development of patellofemoral pain syndrome, Pappas et al. [48] found lower knee extension strength to be the only predictive variable. Giles et al. [49] demonstrated atrophy of the quadriceps muscle in patients with patellofemoral pain. Hip weakness has also been reported as a predictor of patellofemoral pain [36, 50]. Decreased flexibility throughout the hip, quadriceps, hamstrings, and soleus has been associated with patellofemoral pain [36]. Coordination of muscle activation has also been studied in patellofemoral rehabilitation. Many believe there is a delay in activity of the VMO versus the vastus lateralis during both voluntary and reflexive function in patients with anterior knee pain [51]. Additionally, abnormalities in gait, most commonly excessive internal rotation of the hip during activity, have been implicated in patients with patellofemoral pain [24].

All of these factors can be altered by rehabilitation, and protocols targeting these factors have shown promise for reducing patellofemoral pain. Quadriceps strengthening has become the foundation of rehabilitation for anterior knee pain, and its benefit has been shown in multiple studies. For example, in a systematic review of seven studies, Kooiker et al. [52] found strong evidence that quadriceps strengthening improved function and reduced patellofemoral pain compared with advice and information or placebo. In a novel study in which young healthy female healthy subjects underwent motor branch block to the VMO during dynamic MRI, Sheehan et al. [53] reproduced similar kinematics to patients with patellofemoral pain, including patellofemoral lateral shift.

Recent studies have shown the importance of hip strengthening. In a randomized clinical trial involving 33 female patients with patellofemoral pain syndrome, Dolak et al. [54] compared initial hip strengthening versus initial quadriceps strengthening and found earlier pain relief in the initial hip strengthening group. Recent evidence from Hamstra-Wright et al. [3] also shows the ability of hip and knee strengthening to improve long-term (>6 months) patient-reported outcomes for patellofemoral pain. A Cochrane review of 31 trials (including 25 randomized controlled trials) involving patients with patellofemoral pain found that exercise therapy was more effective than no treatment or placebo in terms of improvement in pain and functional ability in the short and long term (16–52 weeks) [55].

One controversy in rehabilitation for patellofemoral pain has been whether open or closed kinetic chain exercises should be used. In a randomized prospective study, Witrvrouw et al. [56] found no difference between them in terms of long-term functional outcome. However, Bakhtiary and Fatemi [57] found closed kinetic chain exercises to be more effective than open kinetic chain exercises when considering chondromalacia specifically.

Alternative modalities are often incorporated into the nonoperative treatment of anterior knee pain. These include nonsteroidal anti-inflammatory drugs, corticosteroid injections, glycosaminoglycan polysulfate (GAGPS) injections, hyaluronic acid (HA) injections, patellar taping, iontophoresis, and orthotics. We will briefly describe each of these and their roles in treating patellofemoral pain.

Nonsteroidal anti-inflammatory drugs and corticosteroid injections are first-line treatments for osteoarthritis of the knee, including patellofemoral arthritis; however, their utility in treating patellofemoral pain syndrome is unclear. A Cochrane review of pharmacotherapy for treating patellofemoral pain syndrome found aspirin to be no different than placebo; however, naproxen was superior to placebo in terms of short-term pain reduction [58].

GAGPS is similar to the more commonly used HA; however, the mechanism of action is different. GAGPS has been shown to decrease cartilage-degrading enzymes such as hyaluronidase, beta-glucuronidase, and acid phosphatase, as well as to promote the synthesis of HA. In contrast, HA injections simply add more of the fully synthesized lubricating substance to the injected joint [59]. A Cochrane review showed moderate effectiveness of GAGPS intramuscular and intra-articular injections. In one study, GAGPS injection outperformed lidocaine injection in terms of improvement in function after 6 weeks [60].

No comparative studies have been conducted concerning the efficacy of HA in treating patellofemoral pain; however, a recent study by Clarke et al. [61] investigated the use of HA for treating osteoarthritis of the patellofemoral joint. They demonstrated improvements in global pain rating and pain on stair climbing in 43 patients as long as 26 weeks after a 3-injection series of HA (Synvisc; Genzyme, Cambridge, MA). However, substantial evidence exists concerning the use of HA for general and tibiofemoral knee osteoarthritis. Although studies show significant benefits with viscosupplementation vs. controls, effect sizes are small, and the clinical significance of these findings has been questioned [62, 63]. On the basis of these and other factors, the American Academy of Orthopedic Surgeons clinical practice guidelines do not recommend the use of HA for osteoarthritis of the knee [64].

Iontophoresis is a process that uses electrical currents to move ionic compounds through the skin and into the connective tissue. Because much of the pain in patellofemoral pain syndrome is generated within the soft tissues (e.g., retinaculum, patellar tendon), corticosteroid iontophoresis is typically tried as a first-line treatment before intra-articular injection, which is more helpful in conditions with a subchondral or osseous source of pain. Iontophoresis has been shown to penetrate up to 30 mm below the skin in humans, which is more than enough depth to reach the patellofemoral structures involved [65].

Patellar taping is a main component of multimodal physical therapy for patellofemoral pain. The goal of taping is to apply medially directed forces to the patella to address lateral pathoanatomy and to ultimately reduce pain. Substantial research has been conducted concerning the effectiveness of patellar taping. A systematic review and meta-analysis by Barton et al. [66] identified 20 studies and found patellar taping to provide immediate pain reduction and, when combined with exercise, to be superior to exercise alone for pain reduction for up to 4 weeks. They make a distinction between tailored taping as described by Gilleard et al. [67], which addresses patient-specific patellar glide, tilt, and spin versus untailored taping that attempts only to apply a medially directed force. They found tailored taping to result in greater reduction in pain versus the untailored method [66].

There is little evidence of the efficacy of knee bracing for patellofemoral pain. However, a dynamic MRI study demonstrated that a patellofemoral brace could reduce lateral translation of the patella and patellar tilt near full extension. The study also showed a patellar sleeve to reduce lateral translation, although less so than the brace. The sleeve had no effect on patellar tilt [68]. In their systematic review of orthotic devices and bracing for patellofemoral pain, Swart et al. [69] determined that none of the braces they evaluated provided significant improvement in pain compared with exercise alone. However, the authors allowed for the possibility that certain well-designed braces, which have shown promise in some studies [70, 71], may aid in relieving symptoms.

Foot orthotics have also become an area of interest in managing patellofemoral pain. In a prospective study, Thijs et al. [26] found an association between patellofemoral pain and foot function during gait, including a less pronated heel strike and more pressure over the lateral side of the foot in patients with patellofemoral pain. The theorized connection between this foot function and patellofemoral pain is twofold. First, less pronation of the foot at heel strike allows for less shock absorption when the foot strikes the ground, leading to stress on the more proximal joints. Second, less tibial internal rotation results from less pronation of the foot throughout rollover, leading to a dynamically lateralized tibial tuberosity and a larger Q-angle [26]. A prospective study by Sutlive et al. [25] supports this theory. However, others believe excessive pronation to be the culprit [72]. Regardless, foot function has become a target for managing patellofemoral pain because pronation and rollover are modifiable with orthotics. A randomized controlled trial by Collins et al. [73] found that orthotics provided better pain relief than did flat shoe inserts at 6 weeks. However, the authors found no difference between combined physical therapy plus orthoses versus physical therapy alone. They concluded that orthoses are best reserved for hastening recovery in some patients.

The remainder of our discussion focuses on specific diagnoses around the knee that manifest as anterior and lateral knee pain. These include iliotibial band syndrome (ITBS), lateral patellofemoral compression (LPFC), patellar and quadriceps tendinopathy, plica syndrome, and chondral pathology. We will discuss each of these conditions and their diagnosis and treatment.

Iliotibial Band Syndrome

ITBS is common in young, active patients with anterolateral knee pain. It has been cited as the most common cause of lateral knee pain in runners, as well as cyclists [74]. As first described by Lieutenant Commander James Renne [75] in US Marine Corps second lieutenants, ITBS is believed to be caused by rubbing of the iliotibial band over the prominence of the lateral femoral epicondyle during cyclical flexion and extension, as occurs during running. This explanation is still highly regarded today, although some believe the condition to be more of a stretching of the distal iliotibial band or an underlying iliotibial band bursitis [76, 77].

Regardless of cause, diagnosis and treatment are similar. Patients' descriptions of ITBS are fairly consistent. They report pain over the lateral aspect of the knee just distal to the lateral femoral condyle and proximal to Gerdy's tubercle. This pain is aggravated by running, especially on hilly terrain and at a slower pace [78]. Physical examination commonly reveals tenderness at the site of the lateral femoral epicondyle. The Ober test is the classical examination for ITBS. In 1936, Ober described the test as follows: "The patient lies on his side, with the thigh next to the table and flexed enough to obliterate any lumbar lordosis. The upper leg is flexed at a right angle at the knee. The examiner grasps the ankle lightly with one hand and steadies the patient's hip with the other. The upper leg is abducted widely and extended so that the thigh is in line with the body. If there is an abduction contracture, the leg will remain more or less passively abducted, depending upon the shortening of the iliotibial band" [37][p. 107–108] (Fig. 2.4).

In refractory cases or when the diagnosis is unclear, MRI may be used to identify high signal in and around the iliotibial band, as well as to rule out other pathology [76]. Nonsurgical management, including activity modification and physical therapy, is the mainstay of treatment for ITBS. Runners should be encouraged to undergo a period of rest followed by gradual return to activity. An iliotibial band-specific stretching program can be initiated and often includes the use of a foam roller. Strengthening of the hip abductors and core musculature is also beneficial. Surgical lengthening of the iliotibial band is rarely necessary because most patients achieve pain relief and return to activities within 6–8 weeks [74].

Lateral Patellofemoral Compression

Lateral patellofemoral compression (LPFC) can be thought of in a similar manner to patellofemoral pain syndrome in terms of causes and treatments. A tight lateral retinaculum is present in LPFC, resulting in increased lateral patellar tilt that leads to increased contact pressures in the lateral patellofemoral joint. In the presence of LPFC and increased patellar tilt, it is critical to confirm that no patellar

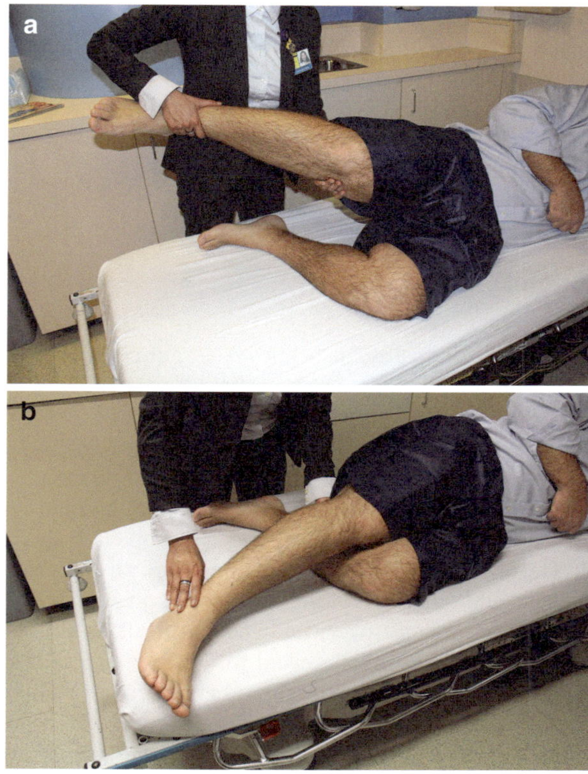

Fig. 2.4 Ober's test showing (**a**) extension and abduction of the hip in the test position and (**b**) a negative test with passive adduction of the hip

instability is present. As in the previous discussion of anterior knee pain, the exact pain generator in LPFC is unknown and is likely a combination of factors, including abnormal or hypersensitive nerves within the lateral retinaculum, sensitivity of the subchondral bone to increased lateral patellofemoral loading, and chondromalacia.

Patients with LPFC present with anterolateral knee pain with repetitive knee flexion and when sitting for long periods [27]. Physical examination demonstrates excessive lateral patellar tilt with a tight lateral retinaculum that limits eversion of the patella and medial patellar mobility. AJ sign may be present, indicating unbalanced lateral tethering of the patella. VMO strengthening and iliotibial band stretching to rebalance the patellofemoral joint are the focus rehabilitation for LPFC.

LPFC is one of the conditions that, when refractory to nonoperative management, may meet the indications for lateral retinacular release or lengthening, although this is uncommon. As stated by Fulkerson, "lateral release is most appropriate for patients with a tight lateral retinaculum associated with rotational (tilt) malalignment of the patella. This mechanical configuration is often associated with an excessive lateral pressure syndrome" [79][p. 452] (Fig. 2.5). However, clinicians should be cautioned that this is performed only in refractory cases with true lateral compression and that iatrogenic medial instability can be a complication of this procedure.

Patellar Tendinopathy

Patellar tendinopathy, also known as jumper's knee, can be a persistent, painful condition for young, active patients, especially athletes. A Norwegian cross-sectional study reported a prevalence of 14% in all athletes and up to 32% and 45% in basketball and volleyball players, respectively [80]. Tendinopathy is considered to be an overuse phenomenon. The three major explanations behind the development of tendinopathy are the mechanical, vascular, and neural theories, with the mechanical theory being most widely accepted [81].

The mechanical theory describes cyclical microtrauma as a cause of cellular changes and alteration of the mechanical properties of the tendon [82]. This microtrauma accumulates over time and can result in substantial tissue damage without any identifiable traumatic event [81]. The vascular theory is offered less often for patellar tendinopathy than for other vascular "vulnerable" tendons such as the Achilles, supraspinatus, and tibialis posterior [82]; however, the idea is that tendons possess a poor blood supply, leaving them susceptible to vascular compromise, poor healing, and degeneration. Much like the neural theory of general patellofemoral pain, the neural theory of tendinopathy points to cellular changes within the nerves leading to release of substance P and pain-generating neurotransmitters [81].

Many clues from the patient history and physical examination aid in the diagnosis of patellar tendinopathy. Like with most patients with anterior knee pain, patients with patellar tendinopathy report pain that occurs instantly when the tendon is stressed, such as during squatting and stair climbing [83]. Tenderness at the inferior pole of the patella is the key physical examination finding [84], and this often correlates with findings on MRI (Fig. 2.6). Nonoperative treatment consists of activity modification, anti-inflammatory medications [85], and a guided strengthening program, including eccentric exercises [86, 87]. However, there has been much interest in other modalities, including extracorporeal shock-wave therapy (ESWT) and platelet-rich plasma (PRP) injection. A systematic review of ESWT for patellar tendinopathy found it to be beneficial in the short and long term; however, the authors cautioned that the evidence is limited. The literature contains conflicting results. In a randomized controlled trial, Zwerver et al. [88] found ESWT to be no better than placebo for treating actively competing athletes with patellar tendinopathy. Yet Taunton et al. [89] found ESWT to produce significant improvement in short-term outcome scores over placebo. It is similar for evidence regarding PRP injections. A recent systematic review of PRP injection in patellar tendinopathy found significant

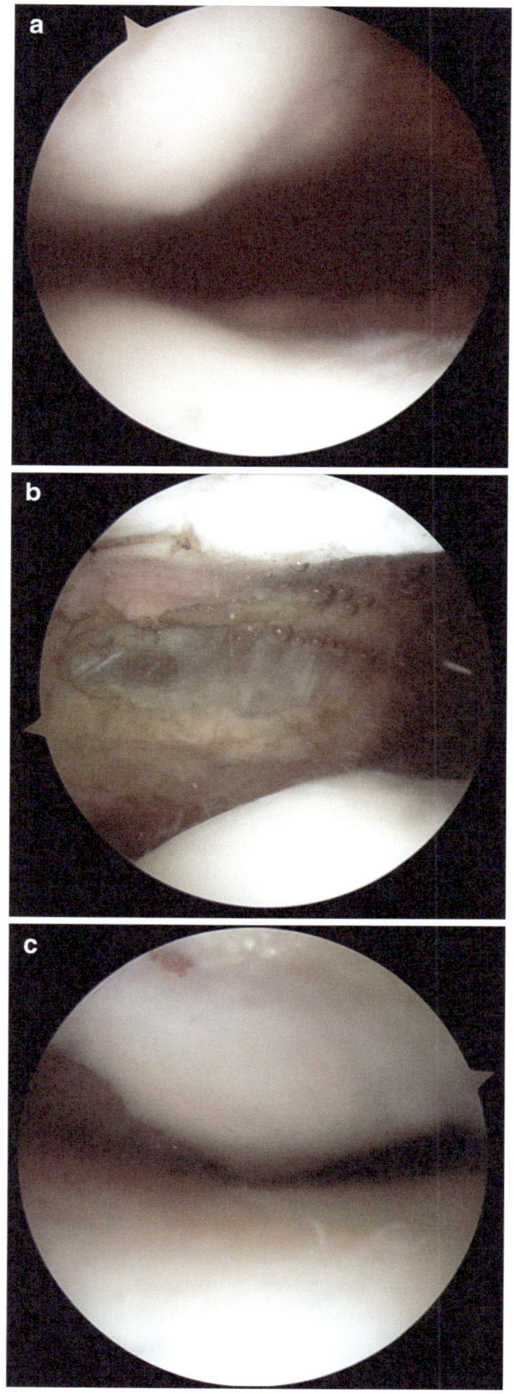

Fig. 2.5 Arthroscopic images of the correction of lateral patellar tilt with a lateral retinacular release procedure showing (**a**) increased patellar tilt, (**b**) release of the lateral patellar retinaculum, and (**c**) correct alignment of the patellofemoral joint after lateral release

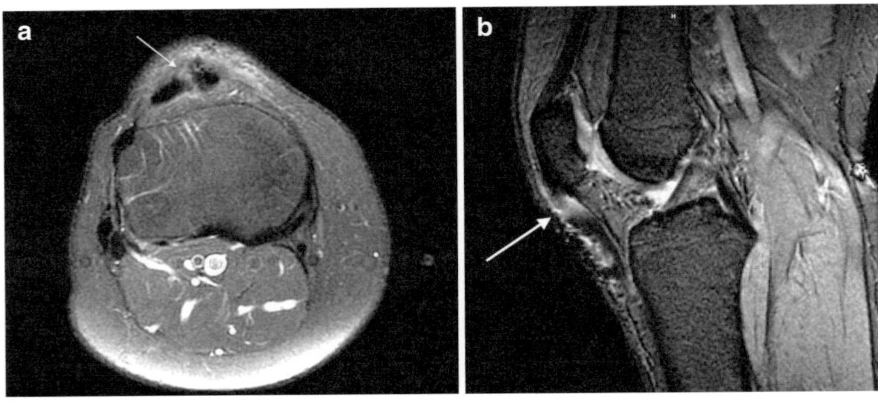

Fig. 2.6 (**a**) Axial proton density fat-suppressed magnetic resonance images and (**b**) sagittal T2-weighted images show tendinopathy within the central portion of the proximal patellar tendon (arrow)

improvements in pain and function after injection in noncomparative studies but inconsistent results in comparative studies, leading the authors to conclude that it has not been proven to be superior to standard physical therapy regimens [90].

Up to 14% of patients with patellar tendinopathy will develop a chronic case of the condition [80], and approximately 10% of nonoperatively treated patients eventually undergo surgical intervention, consisting primarily of arthroscopic or open debridement at the inferior pole of the patella [91]. This involves excision of the section of persistent tendinopathy, with repair of the tendon if a substantial portion of the tendon is debrided. A systematic review of surgical treatment of patellar tendinopathy found arthroscopic treatment to be as effective as open surgery in terms of pain reduction and patient satisfaction while providing faster recovery and faster return to sport activities [92].

Medial Patellar Plica Syndrome

Synovial bands, or plicae, within the knee began to garner increased attention with the advent of knee arthroscopy. These bands are thought to be formed when bordering synovial tissue fails to resorb and when synovial compartments are fused in the knee during fetal development [93]. Plicae are believed to become symptomatic when they undergo inherent structural changes, including fibrosis caused by an inflammatory process that leads to internal derangement within the knee. This process can be any transient or chronic synovitis, synovial hematoma caused by trauma, or hemarthrosis caused by intra-articular pathology, such as a torn meniscus [94].

The medial patellar plica (MPP) is most associated with symptoms [95]. It is believed to impinge upon the medial trochlea or medial edge of the medial femoral condyle in midflexion, causing synovial irritation and degeneration of the corresponding cartilage over the medial femoral condyle [95]. Patients present with dull, aching pain at the superior portion of the knee that increases with activity [96]. Up

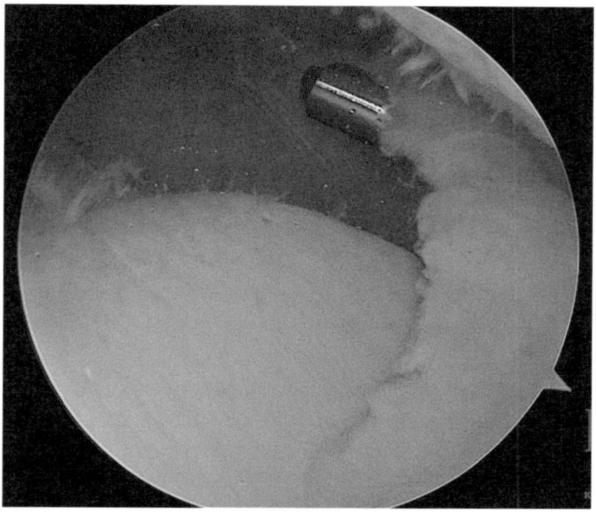

Fig. 2.7 Arthroscopic image of a medial plica

to 50% of patients have a history of injury and hemarthrosis [95]. Medial tenderness proximal to the joint line is seen frequently on examination. The MPP test is also very helpful in making the diagnosis. It is performed by applying a force to the inferomedial pole of the patella while flexing the knee to 90° from full extension. The test is considered positive if the patient experiences pain with the knee in extension and relief of pain with the knee flexed to 90 °. A recent meta-analysis by Stubbings and Smith [97] demonstrated the importance of physical examination in relation to advanced imaging. They found the MPP test to have a sensitivity of 90% and a specificity of 89% for detecting MPP syndrome. Ultrasonography was similar, with a sensitivity of 90% and a specificity of 83% [98]. MRI was less sensitive (77%) and less specific (58%) than the MPP test or ultrasonography [97].

Treatment begins with activity modification and rest followed by hamstring stretching and quadriceps strengthening [99]. Surgical treatment is reserved for recalcitrant cases in which stretching, strengthening, nonsteroidal anti-inflammatory medications, and corticosteroid injections have failed. Surgical treatment has changed little since the classic report by Muse et al. [100] of 53 arthroscopic plica resections in 1985. A systematic review of 23 studies involving 969 patients found plica resection to yield complete relief from or significant improvement in pain in 90% of patients at more than 2 years of follow-up (Fig. 2.7) [95].

Chondral Pathology

Although it does not always lead to symptoms, chondral pathology can be a contributing source of anterior knee pain. Among patients undergoing arthroscopy for anterior knee pain, approximately 45% will have patellar chondral lesions [101]. Among patients undergoing knee arthroscopy for any reason, 21–23% will have localized, full-thickness cartilage defects of the patella, and 8–15% will have lesions of the trochlea [102, 103]. Cartilage defects are common after certain injuries, including patellar dislocation (57%) and anterior cruciate ligament ruptures (29%) [102].

Because there are many potential causes of anterior knee pain and patellar cartilage defects are common, it is sometimes difficult to declare a cartilage defect as symptomatic and as the primary cause of a patient's knee pain. Therefore, some have suggested that chondral defects should be considered a "diagnosis of exclusion" for anterior knee pain [101]. However, for many patients, patellar cartilage lesions are symptomatic and require treatment, particularly if they cause mechanical symptoms (Fig. 2.8). Patients with symptomatic patellar chondral lesions report pain with activities that load the patellofemoral joint, including ascending and descending stairs. A history of a knee effusion can indicate the presence of a symptomatic chondral defect. Clinical suspicion is elevated if the patient has a history of patellar dislocation [104]. Much of the recent research involving patellar cartilage defects has focused on surgical treatments, including microfracture, autologous chondrocyte implantation (ACI), particulated juvenile cartilage allograft, osteochondral autograft transfer, and patellofemoral realignment. Despite some reports of good long-term results with microfracture [105, 106], improvements in pain and outcome scores for microfracture of patellofemoral lesions appear to be short-lived (<18 months) [107, 108]. These findings are unsurprising because microfracture results in fibrocartilage that has inferior mechanical properties to native hyaline cartilage [109]. ACI has shown favorable outcomes for the patellofemoral joint with long-term follow-up of up to 20 years [110]. However, a recent randomized controlled trial comparing ACI versus microfracture for femoral condylar lesions showed no differences at long-term follow-up [111]. Particulated juvenile cartilage allografts are a relatively new option for treating patellofemoral cartilage lesions. In the short term (mean, 8 months), improvements have been shown in outcome scores and pain relief [112]. Osteochondral autograft transfer is attractive for treating cartilage lesions because it restores a stable articular surface with hyaline cartilage

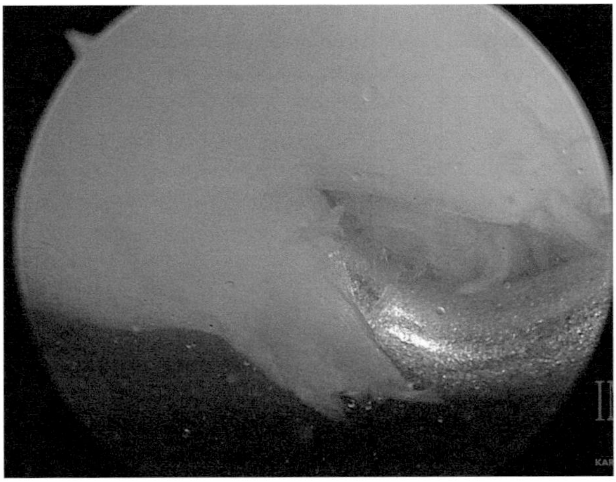

Fig. 2.8 Arthroscopic image of a displaced patellar chondral flap causing mechanical symptoms in the patellofemoral joint

[113]. A recent study by Astur et al. [113] found significant improvement in pain 2 years after surgery in all 33 patients with patellar cartilage injuries <2.5 cm treated with autologous patellar chondral transplantation. Regardless of the technique used to address these cartilage lesions, if an underlying biomechanical abnormality led to the development of the defect, this abnormality should be considered in the treatment plan. For this reason, patellar realignment surgery is performed routinely in isolation or in conjunction with any of the previously mentioned procedures as treatment for symptomatic patellofemoral cartilage defects. For example, evidence supports concomitant extensor realignment with ACI versus ACI alone in select patients [114]. We have a good understanding of which patellar articular lesions may benefit from anteromedial tibial tuberosity osteotomy (TTO) procedures. Pidoriano et al. [115] correlated patient results after TTO with location of patellar lesion. They found that type-I lesions at the inferior pole and type-II lesions at the lateral facet of the patella responded well to TTO, with good/excellent results in >85% of patients. Type-III lesions of the medial facet and diffuse or proximal type-IV lesions responded poorly, with good and excellent results in 56% and 20% of patients, respectively [115].

Conclusion

Patellofemoral pain is multifactorial and complex; however, an understanding of the leading theories of patellofemoral pain, familiarity with the principles of diagnosis and treatment, and knowledge of the specific patellar pain-generating conditions give the clinician a firm foundation from which to help patients presenting with this common condition. As the body of patellofemoral research continues to grow, so will our understanding of anterior knee pain. The theories and principles presented here will evolve, and this review can serve as a starting point for future research.

Acknowledgment The authors thank Gail Richter-Nelson for her assistance with the figures for this article.

References

1. DeHaven KE, Lintner DM. Athletic injuries: comparison by age, sport, and gender. Am J Sports Med. 1986;14:218–24.
2. Wood L, Muller S, Peat G. The epidemiology of patellofemoral disorders in adulthood: a review of routine general practice morbidity recording. Prim Health Care Res Dev. 2011;12:157–64. https://doi.org/10.1017/s1463423610000460.
3. Hamstra-Wright KL, Aydemir B, Earl-Boehm J, Bolgla L, Emery C, Ferber R. Patient-reported outcomes remain improved 6-months post patellofemoral pain rehabilitation. J Sport Rehabil. 2017;26:223–33. https://doi.org/10.1123/jsr.2015-0176.
4. Devereaux MD, Lachmann SM. Patello-femoral arthralgia in athletes attending a sports injury clinic. Br J Sports Med. 1984;18:18–21.

5. Boling M, Padua D, Marshall S, Guskiewicz K, Pyne S, Beutler A. Gender differences in the incidence and prevalence of patellofemoral pain syndrome. Scand J Med Sci Sports. 2010;20:725–30. https://doi.org/10.1111/j.1600-0838.2009.00996.x.
6. Sanchis-Alfonso V, Rosello-Sastre E. Immunohistochemical analysis for neural markers of the lateral retinaculum in patients with isolated symptomatic patellofemoral malalignment. A neuroanatomic basis for anterior knee pain in the active young patient. Am J Sports Med. 2000;28:725–31.
7. Fulkerson JP, Tennant R, Jaivin JS, Grunnet M. Histologic evidence of retinacular nerve injury associated with patellofemoral malalignment. Clin Orthop. 1985;197:196–205.
8. Jerosch J, Prymka M. Knee joint proprioception in patients with posttraumatic recurrent patella dislocation. Knee Surg, Sports Traumatol, Arthros : Off J ESSKA. 1996;4:14–8.
9. Sanchis-Alfonso V, Rosello-Sastre E, Revert F, Garcia A. Histologic retinacular changes associated with ischemia in painful patellofemoral malalignment. Orthopedics. 2005;28:593–9.
10. Insall JN, Aglietti P, Tria AJ Jr. Patellar pain and incongruence. II: Clinical application. Clin Orthop Relat Res. 1983;176:225–32.
11. Leslie IJ, Bentley G. Arthroscopy in the diagnosis of chondromalacia patellae. Ann Rheum Dis. 1978;37:540–7.
12. Royle SG, Noble J, Davies DR, Kay PR. The significance of chondromalacic changes on the patella. Arthrosc : J Arthrosc Relat Surg : Off Publication of the Arthrosc Assoc North Am Int Arthrosc Assoc. 1991;7:158–60.
13. Ficat RP, Hungerford DS. Disorders of the Patello-femoral joint. Baltimore: Williams & Wilkins; 1977.
14. Fulkerson JP. The etiology of patellofemoral pain in young, active patients: a prospective study. Clin Orthop. 1983;179:129–33.
15. Dye SF, Staubli HU, Biedert RM, Vaupel GL. The mosaic of pathophysiology causing patellofemoral pain: therapeutic implications. Oper Tech Sports Med. 1999;7:46–54.
16. Dye SF. The knee as a biologic transmission with an envelope of function: a theory. Clin Orthop. 1996;325:10–8.
17. Witvrouw E, Bellemans J, Lysens R, Danneels L, Cambier D. Intrinsic risk factors for the development of patellar tendinitis in an athletic population. A two-year prospective study. Am J Sports Med. 2001;29:190–5.
18. Domenech J, Sanchis-Alfonso V, Lopez L, Espejo B. Influence of kinesiophobia and catastrophizing on pain and disability in anterior knee pain patients. Knee Surg, Sports Traumatol, Arthrosc : Off J ESSKA. 2013;21:1562–8. https://doi.org/10.1007/s00167-012-2238-5.
19. Gracely RH, Geisser ME, Giesecke T, Grant MA, Petzke F, Williams DA, Clauw DJ. Pain catastrophizing and neural responses to pain among persons with fibromyalgia. Brain :J Neurol. 2004;127:835–43. https://doi.org/10.1093/brain/awh098.
20. Hungerford DS, Barry M. Biomechanics of the patellofemoral joint. Clin Orthop Relat Res. 1979;144:9–15.
21. Yard E, Comstock D. Injury patterns by body mass index in US high school athletes. J Phys Act Health. 2011;8:182–91.
22. Zhai G, Cicuttini F, Ding C, Scott F, Garnero P, Jones G. Correlates of knee pain in younger subjects. Clin Rheumatol. 2007;26:75–80. https://doi.org/10.1007/s10067-006-0248-8.
23. Barber Foss KD, Hornsby M, Edwards NM, Myer GD, Hewett TE. Is body composition associated with an increased risk of developing anterior knee pain in adolescent female athletes? Phys Sports Med. 2012;40:13–9. https://doi.org/10.3810/psm.2012.02.1947.
24. Souza RB, Powers CM. Predictors of hip internal rotation during running: an evaluation of hip strength and femoral structure in women with and without patellofemoral pain. Am J Sports Med. 2009;37:579–87. https://doi.org/10.1177/0363546508326711.
25. Sutlive TG, Mitchell SD, Maxfield SN, McLean CL, Neumann JC, Swiecki CR, Hall RC, Bare AC, Flynn TW. Identification of individuals with patellofemoral pain whose symptoms improved after a combined program of foot orthosis use and modified activity: a preliminary investigation. Phys Ther. 2004;84:49–61.

26. Thijs Y, Van Tiggelen D, Roosen P, De Clercq D, Witvrouw E. A prospective study on gait-related intrinsic risk factors for patellofemoral pain. Clin J Sport Med : Off J Can Acad Sport Med. 2007;17:437–45. https://doi.org/10.1097/JSM.0b013e31815ac44f.
27. Larson RL, Cabaud HE, Slocum DB, James SL, Keenan T, Hutchinson T. The patellar compression syndrome: surgical treatment by lateral retinacular release. Clin Orthop Relat Res. 1978;134:158–67.
28. Eckhoff DG, Montgomery WK, Kilcoyne RF, Stamm ER. Femoral morphometry and anterior knee pain. Clin Orthop. 1994;302:64–8.
29. Post WR. Current concepts. clinical evaluation of patients with patellofemoral disorders. Arthroscopy. 1999;15:841–51.
30. Huberti HH, Hayes WC. Patellofemoral contact pressures. The influence of q-angle and tendofemoral contact. J Bone Joint Surg Am. 1984;66:715–24.
31. Sendur OF, Gurer G, Yildirim T, Ozturk E, Aydeniz A. Relationship of Q angle and joint hypermobility and Q angle values in different positions. Clin Rheumatol. 2006;25:304–8. https://doi.org/10.1007/s10067-005-0003-6.
32. Aglietti P, Insall JN, Cerulli G. Patellar pain and incongruence. I: Measurements of incongruence. Clin Orthop Relat Res. 1983;176:217–24.
33. Horton MG, Hall TL. Quadriceps femoris muscle angle: normal values and relationships with gender and selected skeletal measures. Phys Ther. 1989;69:897–901.
34. Park SK, Stefanyshyn DJ. Greater Q angle may not be a risk factor of patellofemoral pain syndrome. Clin Biomech (Bristol, Avon). 2011;26:392–6. https://doi.org/10.1016/j.clinbiomech.2010.11.015.
35. Baldon Rde M, Nakagawa TH, Muniz TB, Amorim CF, Maciel CD, Serrao FV. Eccentric hip muscle function in females with and without patellofemoral pain syndrome. J Athl Train. 2009;44:490–6. https://doi.org/10.4085/1062-6050-44.5.490.
36. Piva SR, Goodnite EA, Childs JD. Strength around the hip and flexibility of soft tissues in individuals with and without patellofemoral pain syndrome. J Orthop Sports Phys Ther. 2005;35:793–801. https://doi.org/10.2519/jospt.2005.35.12.793.
37. Ober FR. The role of the iliotibial band and fascia lata as a factor in the causation of low-back disabilities and sciatica. J Bone Joint Surg Am. 1936;18:105–10.
38. al-Rawi Z, Nessan AH. Joint hypermobility in patients with chondromalacia patellae. Br J Rheumatol. 1997;36:1324–7.
39. Beighton P, Solomon L, Soskolne CL. Articular mobility in an African population. Ann Rheum Dis. 1973;32:413–8.
40. Cook C, Mabry L, Reiman MP, Hegedus EJ. Best tests/clinical findings for screening and diagnosis of patellofemoral pain syndrome: a systematic review. Physiotherapy. 2012;98:93–100. https://doi.org/10.1016/j.physio.2011.09.001.
41. Laurin CA, Levesque HP, Dussault R, Labelle H, Peides JP. The abnormal lateral patellofemoral angle: a diagnostic roentgenographic sign of recurrent patellar subluxation. J Bone Joint Surg Am. 1978;60:55–60.
42. Macnab I. Recurrent dislocation of the patella. J Bone Joint Surg Am. 1952;34 a:957–67. passim.
43. Merchant AC, Mercer RL, Jacobsen RH, Cool CR. Roentgenographic analysis of patellofemoral congruence. J Bone Joint Surg Am. 1974;56:1391–6.
44. Subhawong TK, Eng J, Carrino JA, Chhabra A. Superolateral Hoffa's fat pad edema: association with patellofemoral maltracking and impingement. AJR Am J Roentgenol. 2010;195:1367–73. https://doi.org/10.2214/ajr.10.4668.
45. McNally EG, Ostlere SJ, Pal C, Phillips A, Reid H, Dodd C. Assessment of patellar maltracking using combined static and dynamic MRI. Eur Radiol. 2000;10:1051–5.
46. Muhle C, Brossmann J, Heller M. Kinematic CT and MR imaging of the patellofemoral joint. Eur Radiol. 1999;9:508–18.
47. Dupuy DE, Hangen DH, Zachazewski JE, Boland AL, Palmer W. Kinematic CT of the patellofemoral joint. AJR Am J Roentgenol. 1997;169:211–5. https://doi.org/10.2214/ajr.169.1.9207527.

48. Pappas E, Wong-Tom WM. Prospective predictors of patellofemoral pain syndrome: a systematic review with meta-analysis. Sports Health. 2012;4:115–20. https://doi.org/10.1177/1941738111432097.
49. Giles LS, Webster KE, McClelland JA, Cook J. Does quadriceps atrophy exist in individuals with patellofemoral pain? A systematic literature review with meta-analysis. J Orthop Sports Phys Ther. 2013;43:766–76. https://doi.org/10.2519/jospt.2013.4833.
50. Bolgla LA, Malone TR, Umberger BR, Uhl TL. Hip strength and hip and knee kinematics during stair descent in females with and without patellofemoral pain syndrome. J Orthop Sports Phys Ther. 2008;38:12–8. https://doi.org/10.2519/jospt.2008.2462.
51. Chester R, Smith TO, Sweeting D, Dixon J, Wood S, Song F. The relative timing of VMO and VL in the aetiology of anterior knee pain: a systematic review and meta-analysis. BMC Musculoskelet Disord. 2008;9:64. https://doi.org/10.1186/1471-2474-9-64.
52. Kooiker L, Van De Port IG, Weir A, Moen MH. Effects of physical therapist-guided quadriceps-strengthening exercises for the treatment of patellofemoral pain syndrome: a systematic review. J Orthop Sports Phys Ther. 2014;44:391–b391. https://doi.org/10.2519/jospt.2014.4127.
53. Sheehan FT, Borotikar BS, Behnam AJ, Alter KE. Alterations in in vivo knee joint kinematics following a femoral nerve branch block of the vastus medialis: implications for patellofemoral pain syndrome. Clin Biomech (Bristol, Avon). 2012;27:525–31. https://doi.org/10.1016/j.clinbiomech.2011.12.012.
54. Dolak KL, Silkman C, Medina McKeon J, Hosey RG, Lattermann C, Uhl TL. Hip strengthening prior to functional exercises reduces pain sooner than quadriceps strengthening in females with patellofemoral pain syndrome: a randomized clinical trial. J Orthop Sports Phys Ther. 2011;41:560–70. https://doi.org/10.2519/jospt.2011.3499.
55. Van Der Heijden RA, Lankhorst NE, Van Linschoten R, Bierma-Zeinstra SM, Van Middelkoop M. Exercise for treating patellofemoral pain syndrome: an abridged version of Cochrane systematic review. Eur J Phys Rehabil Med. 2016;52:110–33.
56. Witvrouw E, Danneels L, Van Tiggelen D, Willems TM, Cambier D. Open versus closed kinetic chain exercises in patellofemoral pain: a 5-year prospective randomized study. Am J Sports Med. 2004;32:1122–30. https://doi.org/10.1177/0363546503262187.
57. Bakhtiary AH, Fatemi E. Open versus closed kinetic chain exercises for patellar chondromalacia. Br J Sports Med. 2008;42:99–102.; discussion 102. https://doi.org/10.1136/bjsm.2007.038109.
58. Heintjes E, Berger MY, Bierma-Zeinstra SM, Bernsen RM, Verhaar JA, Koes BW. Pharmacotherapy for patellofemoral pain syndrome. Cochrane Database Syst Rev. 2004;3:Cd003470. https://doi.org/10.1002/14651858.CD003470.pub2.
59. Nethery A, Giles I, Jenkins K, Jackson C, Brooks P, Burkhardt D, Ghosh P, Whitelock J, O'Grady RL, Welgus HG, et al. The chondroprotective drugs, Arteparon and sodium pentosan polysulphate, increase collagenase activity and inhibit stromelysin activity in vitro. Biochem Pharmacol. 1992;44:1549–53.
60. Kannus P, Natri A, Paakkala T, Jarvinen M. An outcome study of chronic patellofemoral pain syndrome. Seven-year follow-up of patients in a randomized, controlled trial. J Bone Joint Surg Am. 1999;81:355–63.
61. Clarke S, Lock V, Duddy J, Sharif M, Newman JH, Kirwan JR. Intra-articular hylan G-F 20 (Synvisc) in the management of patellofemoral osteoarthritis of the knee (POAK). Knee. 2005;12:57–62. https://doi.org/10.1016/j.knee.2004.03.002.
62. Lohmander LS, Dalen N, Englund G, Hamalainen M, Jensen EM, Karlsson K, Odensten M, Ryd L, Sernbo I, Suomalainen O, Tegnander A. Intra-articular hyaluronan injections in the treatment of osteoarthritis of the knee: a randomised, double blind, placebo controlled multicentre trial. Hyaluronan multicentre trial group. Ann Rheum Dis. 1996;55:424–31.
63. Petrella RJ, Petrella M. A prospective, randomized, double-blind, placebo controlled study to evaluate the efficacy of intraarticular hyaluronic acid for osteoarthritis of the knee. J Rheumatol. 2006;33:951–6.

64. American Academy of Orthopedic Surgeons (2018) Treatment of osteoarthritis of the knee: evidence-based guideline. 2nd edition. Available at https://www.aaos.org/research/guidelines/TreatmentofOsteoarthritisoftheKneeGuideline.pdf. Accessed on May 31.
65. Gurney B, Wascher D, Eaton L, Benesh E, Lucak J. The effect of skin thickness and time in the absorption of dexamethasone in human tendons using iontophoresis. J Orthop Sports Phys Ther. 2008;38:238–45. https://doi.org/10.2519/jospt.2008.2648.
66. Barton C, Balachandar V, Lack S, Morrissey D. Patellar taping for patellofemoral pain: a systematic review and meta-analysis to evaluate clinical outcomes and biomechanical mechanisms. Br J Sports Med. 2014;48:417–24. https://doi.org/10.1136/bjsports-2013-092437.
67. Gilleard W, McConnell J, Parsons D. The effect of patellar taping on the onset of vastus medialis obliquus and vastus lateralis muscle activity in persons with patellofemoral pain. Phys Ther. 1998;78:25–32.
68. Draper CE, Besier TF, Santos JM, Jennings F, Fredericson M, Gold GE, Beaupre GS, Delp SL. Using real-time MRI to quantify altered joint kinematics in subjects with patellofemoral pain and to evaluate the effects of a patellar brace or sleeve on joint motion. J Orthop Res. 2009;27:571–7. https://doi.org/10.1002/jor.20790.
69. Swart NM, van Linschoten R, Bierma-Zeinstra SM, van Middelkoop M. The additional effect of orthotic devices on exercise therapy for patients with patellofemoral pain syndrome: a systematic review. Br J Sports Med. 2012;46:570–7. https://doi.org/10.1136/bjsm.2010.080218.
70. Denton J, Willson JD, Ballantyne BT, Davis IS. The addition of the Protonics brace system to a rehabilitation protocol to address patellofemoral joint syndrome. J Orthop Sports Phys Ther. 2005;35:210–9. https://doi.org/10.2519/jospt.2005.35.4.210.
71. Schneider F, Labs K, Wagner S. Chronic patellofemoral pain syndrome: alternatives for cases of therapy resistance. Knee Surg, Sports Traumatol, Arthrosc : Off J ESSKA. 2001;9:290–5. https://doi.org/10.1007/s001670100219.
72. Tiberio D. The effect of excessive subtalar joint pronation on patellofemoral mechanics: a theoretical model. J Orthop Sports Phys Ther. 1987;9:160–5.
73. Collins N, Crossley K, Beller E, Darnell R, McPoil T, Vicenzino B. Foot orthoses and physiotherapy in the treatment of patellofemoral pain syndrome: randomised clinical trial. BMJ (Clin Res ed). 2008;337:a1735. https://doi.org/10.1136/bmj.a1735.
74. Strauss EJ, Kim S, Calcei JG, Park D. Iliotibial band syndrome: evaluation and management. J Am Acad Orthop Surg. 2011;19:728–36.
75. Renne JW. The iliotibial band friction syndrome. J Bone Joint Surg Am. 1975;57:1110–1.
76. Ekman EF, Pope T, Martin DF, Curl WW. Magnetic resonance imaging of iliotibial band syndrome. Am J Sports Med. 1994;22:851–4.
77. Fairclough J, Hayashi K, Toumi H, Lyons K, Bydder G, Phillips N, Best TM, Benjamin M. The functional anatomy of the iliotibial band during flexion and extension of the knee: implications for understanding iliotibial band syndrome. J Anat. 2006;208:309–16. https://doi.org/10.1111/j.1469-7580.2006.00531.x.
78. Orchard JW, Fricker PA, Abud AT, Mason BR. Biomechanics of iliotibial band friction syndrome in runners. Am J Sports Med. 1996;24:375–9.
79. Fulkerson JP. Diagnosis and treatment of patients with patellofemoral pain. Am J Sports Med. 2002;30:447–56.
80. Lian OB, Engebretsen L, Bahr R. Prevalence of jumper's knee among elite athletes from different sports: a cross-sectional study. Am J Sports Med. 2005;33:561–7. https://doi.org/10.1177/0363546504270454.
81. Rees JD, Maffulli N, Cook J. Management of tendinopathy. Am J Sports Med. 2009;37:1855–67. https://doi.org/10.1177/0363546508324283.
82. Ker RF. The implications of the adaptable fatigue quality of tendons for their construction, repair and function. Comp Biochem Physiol A Mol Integr Physiol. 2002;133:987–1000.
83. Rio E, Moseley L, Purdam C, Samiric T, Kidgell D, Pearce AJ, Jaberzadeh S, Cook J. The pain of tendinopathy: physiological or pathophysiological? Sports Med (Auckland, NZ). 2014;44:9–23. https://doi.org/10.1007/s40279-013-0096-z.

84. Cook JL, Khan KM, Kiss ZS, Purdam CR, Griffiths L. Reproducibility and clinical utility of tendon palpation to detect patellar tendinopathy in young basketball players. Victorian Institute of Sport tendon study group. Br J Sports Med. 2001;35:65–9.
85. Almekinders LC, Temple JD. Etiology, diagnosis, and treatment of tendonitis: an analysis of the literature. Med Sci Sports Exerc. 1998;30:1183–90.
86. Mafi N, Lorentzon R, Alfredson H. Superior short-term results with eccentric calf muscle training compared to concentric training in a randomized prospective multicenter study on patients with chronic Achilles tendinosis. Knee Surg, Sports Traumatol, Arthrosc : Off J ESSKA. 2001;9:42–7. https://doi.org/10.1007/s001670000148.
87. Purdam CR, Jonsson P, Alfredson H, Lorentzon R, Cook JL, Khan KM. A pilot study of the eccentric decline squat in the management of painful chronic patellar tendinopathy. Br J Sports Med. 2004;38:395–7. https://doi.org/10.1136/bjsm.2003.000053.
88. Zwerver J, Hartgens F, Verhagen E, van der Worp H, van den Akker-Scheek I, Diercks RL. No effect of extracorporeal shockwave therapy on patellar tendinopathy in jumping athletes during the competitive season: a randomized clinical trial. Am J Sports Med. 2011;39:1191–9. https://doi.org/10.1177/0363546510395492.
89. Taunton JE, Taunton KM, Khan KM. Treatment of patellar tendinopathy with extracorporeal shock wave therapy. B C Med J. 2003;45:1–7.
90. Liddle AD, Rodriguez-Merchan EC. Platelet-rich plasma in the treatment of patellar tendinopathy: a systematic review. Am J Sports Med. 2015;43:2583–90. https://doi.org/10.1177/0363546514560726.
91. Ferretti A, Puddu G, Mariani PP, Neri M. The natural history of jumper's knee. Patellar or quadriceps tendonitis. Int Orthop. 1985;8:239–42.
92. Brockmeyer M, Diehl N, Schmitt C, Kohn DM, Lorbach O. Results of surgical treatment of chronic patellar tendinosis (Jumper's knee): a systematic review of the literature. Arthrosc : J Arthrosc Relat Surg: Off Publication Arthrosc Assoc North Am Int Arthrosc Assoc. 2015;31:2424–2429.e2423. https://doi.org/10.1016/j.arthro.2015.06.010.
93. Ogata S, Uhthoff HK. The development of synovial plicae in human knee joints: an embryologic study. Arthrosc: J Arthrosc Relat Surg: Off Publication Arthrosc Assoc North Am Int Arthrosc Assoc. 1990;6:315–21.
94. Munzinger U, Ruckstuhl J, Scherrer H, Gschwend N. Internal derangement of the knee joint due to pathologic synovial folds: the mediopatellar plica syndrome. Clin Orthop. 1981;155:59–64.
95. Schindler OS. 'The sneaky Plica' revisited: morphology, pathophysiology and treatment of synovial plicae of the knee. Knee Surg Sports Traumatol Arthrosc. 2014;22:247–62. https://doi.org/10.1007/s00167-013-2368-4.
96. Hardaker WT, Whipple TL, Bassett FH 3rd. Diagnosis and treatment of the plica syndrome of the knee. J Bone Joint Surg Am. 1980;62:221–5.
97. Stubbings N, Smith T. Diagnostic test accuracy of clinical and radiological assessments for medial patella plica syndrome: a systematic review and meta-analysis. Knee. 2014;21:486–90. https://doi.org/10.1016/j.knee.2013.11.001.
98. Paczesny L, Kruczynski J. Medial plica syndrome of the knee: diagnosis with dynamic sonography. Radiology. 2009;251:439–46. https://doi.org/10.1148/radiol.2512081652.
99. Blackburn TA, Eiland G, Bandy WD. An introduction to the plica. J Orthop Sports Phys Ther. 1982;3:171–7. https://doi.org/10.2519/jospt.1982.3.4.171.
100. Muse GL, Grana WA, Hollingsworth S. Arthroscopic treatment of medial shelf syndrome. Arthrosc : J Arthrosc Relat Surg: Off Publication Arthrosc Assoc North Am Int Arthrosc Assoc. 1985;1:63–7.
101. Pihlajamaki HK, Kuikka PI, Leppanen VV, Kiuru MJ, Mattila VM. Reliability of clinical findings and magnetic resonance imaging for the diagnosis of chondromalacia patellae. J Bone Joint Surg Am. 2010;92:927–34. https://doi.org/10.2106/jbjs.h.01527.
102. Aroen A, Loken S, Heir S, Alvik E, Ekeland A, Granlund OG, Engebretsen L. Articular cartilage lesions in 993 consecutive knee arthroscopies. Am J Sports Med. 2004;32:211–5.

103. Curl WW, Krome J, Gordon ES, Rushing J, Smith BP, Poehling GG. Cartilage injuries: a review of 31,516 knee arthroscopies. Arthroscopy. 1997;13:456–60.
104. Nomura E, Inoue M, Kurimura M. Chondral and osteochondral injuries associated with acute patellar dislocation. Arthroscopy. 2003;19:717–21.
105. Knutsen G, Engebretsen L, Ludvigsen TC, Drogset JO, Grontvedt T, Solheim E, Strand T, Roberts S, Isaksen V, Johansen O. Autologous chondrocyte implantation compared with microfracture in the knee. A randomized trial. J Bone Joint Surg Am. 2004;86-a:455–64.
106. Steadman JR, Briggs KK, Rodrigo JJ, Kocher MS, Gill TJ, Rodkey WG. Outcomes of microfracture for traumatic chondral defects of the knee: average 11-year follow-up. Arthroscopy. 2003;19:477–84. https://doi.org/10.1053/jars.2003.50112.
107. Kreuz PC, Steinwachs MR, Erggelet C, Krause SJ, Konrad G, Uhl M, Sudkamp N. Results after microfracture of full-thickness chondral defects in different compartments in the knee. Osteoarthr Cartil. 2006;14:1119–25. https://doi.org/10.1016/j.joca.2006.05.003.
108. Mithoefer K, McAdams T, Williams RJ, Kreuz PC, Mandelbaum BR. Clinical efficacy of the microfracture technique for articular cartilage repair in the knee: an evidence-based systematic analysis. Am J Sports Med. 2009;37:2053–63. https://doi.org/10.1177/0363546508328414.
109. Furukawa T, Eyre DR, Koide S, Glimcher MJ. Biochemical studies on repair cartilage resurfacing experimental defects in the rabbit knee. J Bone Joint Surg Am. 1980;62:79–89.
110. Peterson L, Vasiliadis HS, Brittberg M, Lindahl A. Autologous chondrocyte implantation: a long-term follow-up. Am J Sports Med. 2010;38:1117–24. https://doi.org/10.1177/0363546509357915.
111. Knutsen G, Drogset JO, Engebretsen L, Grontvedt T, Ludvigsen TC, Loken S, Solheim E, Strand T, Johansen C. A randomized multicenter trial comparing autologous chondrocyte implantation with microfracture: long-term follow-up at 14 to 15 years. J Bone Joint Surg Am. 2016;98:1332–9. https://doi.org/10.2106/jbjs.15.01208.
112. Buckwalter JA, Bowman GN, Albright JP, Wolf BR, Bollier M. Clinical outcomes of patellar chondral lesions treated with juvenile particulated cartilage allografts. Iowa Orthop J. 2014;34:44–9.
113. Astur DC, Arliani GG, Binz M, Astur N, Kaleka CC, Amaro JT, Pochini A, Cohen M. Autologous osteochondral transplantation for treating patellar chondral injuries: evaluation, treatment, and outcomes of a two-year follow-up study. J Bone Joint Surg Am. 2014;96:816–23. https://doi.org/10.2106/jbjs.m.00312.
114. Henderson IJ, Lavigne P. Periosteal autologous chondrocyte implantation for patellar chondral defect in patients with normal and abnormal patellar tracking. Knee. 2006;13:274–9. https://doi.org/10.1016/j.knee.2006.04.006.
115. Pidoriano AJ, Weinstein RN, Buuck DA, Fulkerson JP. Correlation of patellar articular lesions with results from anteromedial tibial tubercle transfer. Am J Sports Med. 1997;25:533–7.

Chapter 3
Malalignment and Overload Syndromes

Brandon J. Erickson and Andreas H. Gomoll

Introduction

Anterior knee pain is a common complaint that many orthopedic surgeons evaluate on a daily basis [1, 2]. There are many conditions that can cause anterior knee pain including an imbalance between the quadriceps and hamstrings, patellofemoral instability, chondral wear on patella or trochlea, and lateral retinacular tightness [3–8]. Specifically, fixed lateral patellar tilt due to excessive lateral retinacular tightness can result in overload of the lateral patellofemoral joint, leading to chondral degeneration and pain [9]. While nonsurgical treatment can frequently alleviate symptoms in the short term, patients presenting with chondral damage secondary to overload often require surgical intervention to obtain long-lasting pain relief and functional improvement [10]. This chapter will discuss the pathogenesis, diagnosis, surgical treatment, complications, and outcomes of lateral patella and trochlea overload treated with tibial tubercle osteotomy (TTO).

Pathogenesis

A subset of patients presenting with anterior knee pain experience pain because of increased contact pressures between the lateral patella and trochlea. Patellofemoral contact pressures in the extended knee are very low, but with increasing knee flexion, there is a proportional increase in the posteriorly directed force vector from the patellar and quadriceps tendons, thereby increasing joint reaction force [11]. Furthermore, lateral retinacular tightness can lead to fixed lateral patellar tilt, a

B. J. Erickson (✉) · A. H. Gomoll
Hospital for Special Surgery, Division of Sports and Shoulder, New York, NY, USA

B. E. Shubin Stein, S. M. Strickland (eds.), *Patellofemoral Pain and Instability*,
https://doi.org/10.1007/978-3-319-97640-2_3

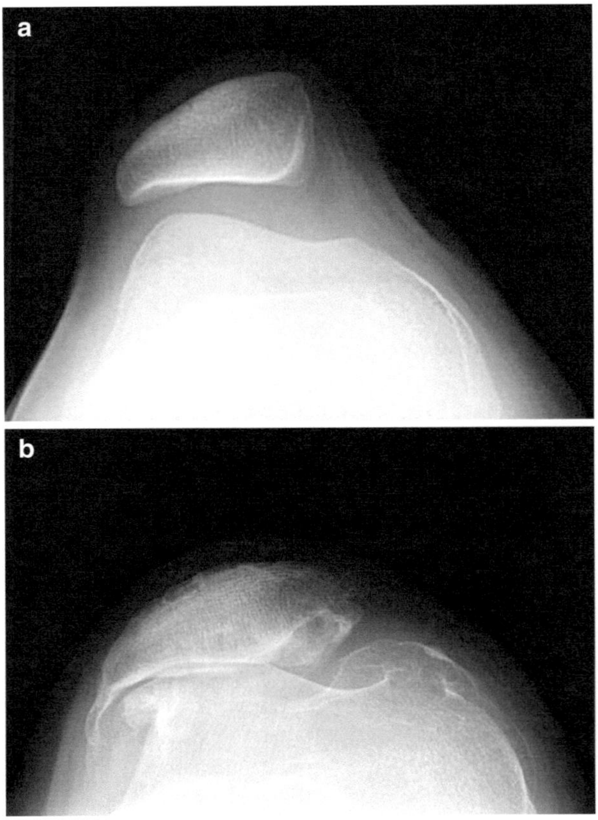

Fig. 3.1 (**a**, **b**) Merchant view radiographs demonstrating lateral patellar tilt (**a**) and significant lateral patellar facet and trochlear arthrosis (**b**)

problem that causes force overload of the lateral patella facet (Fig. 3.1a) [9, 12]. This excessive pressure can lead to accelerated wear of the chondral surfaces and increased loading of the subchondral bone, ultimately leading to persistent pain and functional disability (Fig. 3.1b).

History and Physical Exam

Patients with symptomatic lateral patellar overload will present with pain, rather than instability, as their primary complaint [10]. Their pain will be worse with bent knee activities, such as stairs and squatting, and is generally localized peripatellar in the anterior knee. It is important to investigate any potential history of instability events. Previous surgical treatments should be discussed, and operative repots should be obtained and reviewed. Following the history, a thorough physical exam should be performed. The physical exam begins by properly exposing the knee and assessing the resting alignment of the patient's knee while standing, sitting, and lying down. Although the exam will focus on the knee, it is important to examine the patient's hips, specifically for signs of excessive femoral version that could be contributing to their symptoms. Following the hip exam and inspection of the knee, the patient should be asked to flex and extend their knee while sitting both actively and passively to evaluate crepitus. Any patellofemoral crepitation during open knee extension will be noted.

The rest of the exam should be performed with the patient in the supine position. The quadriceps muscle circumference should be measured and compared to the unaffected side to determine the extent (if any) of quadriceps atrophy. Patellar mobility should be assessed, and medial and lateral glide should be recorded based on the number of quadrants the patella translates. The examiner should attempt to evert the patella to neutral. If the patella cannot be everted to neutral, a lateral release or, preferably, lateral lengthening should be added to the TTO at the time of surgery. The medial and lateral facets of the patella should be palpated to see if this causes pain. Palpation of the lateral patellar facet should elicit pain, but there should be minimal to no pain with palpation of the medial patellar facet. A patellar grind test should be performed to evaluate for chondral wear. The examiner should perform a standard knee ligamentous exam as well as a distal neurovascular exam prior to conclusion of the physical exam.

Diagnostic Imaging

All patients who present with knee pain should undergo a standard radiographic series with standing anteroposterior (AP), lateral, and merchant or sunrise views. While attention should be focused on the patellofemoral joint, it is important to evaluate the medial and lateral tibiofemoral joints for evidence of arthrosis. Patellar height should be assessed on the lateral view, and patellar tilt should be measured on the merchant view. The sulcus angle can also be assessed on the merchant view (Fig. 3.2). Following plain films, a magnetic resonance imaging (MRI) should be obtained to evaluate the chondral surfaces of the patella and trochlea. Chondral

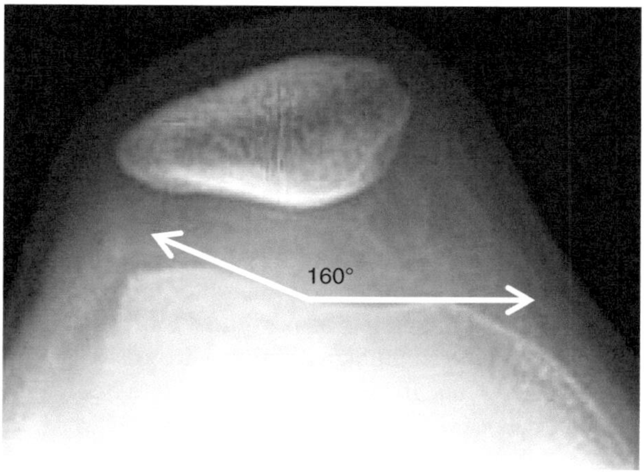

Fig. 3.2 Merchant view radiograph demonstrating the sulcus angle

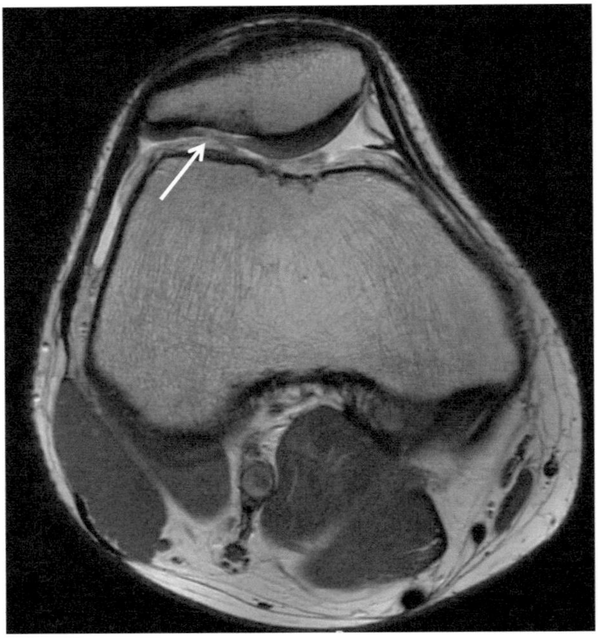

Fig. 3.3 Axial proton density magnetic resonance image demonstrating a chondral defect in the lateral patellar facet

lesions should be measured, as lesion size dictates treatment (Fig. 3.3). The examiner should also note subchondral edema within the patella or trochlea (Fig. 3.4). Close attention should be paid to the location of the chondral defect within the patella and/or trochlea, as the presence of chondral defects in the medial patella or medial trochlea is a relative contraindication to a TTO [13]. The tibial tubercle trochlear groove (TT-TG) distance should be measured, as should patellar height [10].

Treatment

Treatment of patients with lateral compression overload involves decreasing the overall contact pressure and moving the contact pressure from the symptomatic, lateral side of the patellofemoral joint to the asymptomatic medial side. When considering TTO, contact pressures on both patella and trochlea need to be taken into account [14–16]. Fulkerson et al. used five cadaveric knees to measure the contact pressure of the medial and lateral patellar facets at varying degrees of knee flexion before an AMZ and following two versions of an AMZ [15]. In the first AMZ, the tibial tubercle was moved 8.8 mm anteriorly and 8.4 mm medially. In the second AMZ, the tibial tubercle was moved 14.8 mm anteriorly and 8.4 mm medially. The authors found no significant difference in contact areas between baseline values and the first AMZ but found significantly decreased patella contact pressure between baseline values and the second AMZ. Beck et al. performed a cadaveric study to

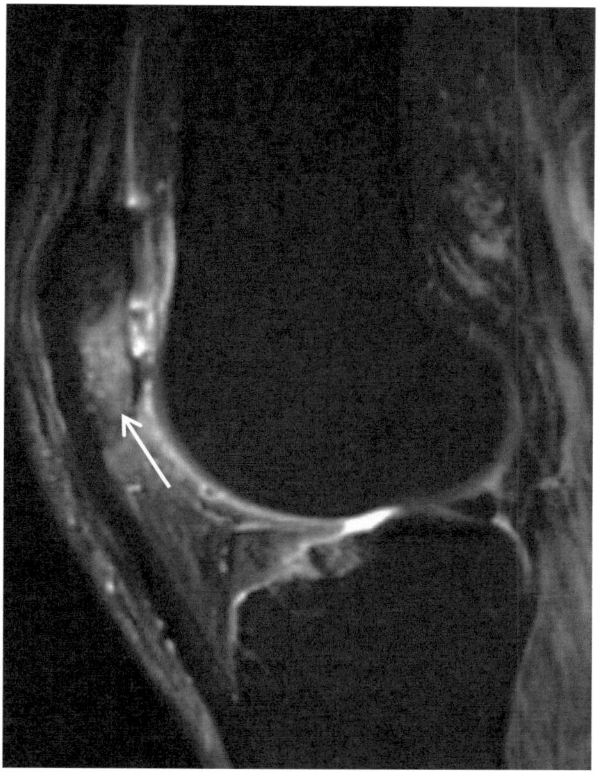

Fig. 3.4 Sagittal inversion recovery magnetic resonance image demonstrating subchondral edema within the lateral patellar facet

examine the effect of anteromedialization (AMZ) on the contact pressure across the trochlea [14]. The authors tested trochlear contact pressure in ten cadaveric knees before and after AMZ at varying degrees of knee flexion. The AMZ was performed at 30°, and the tibial tubercle was moved 15 mm anteromedially. The authors found a significant decrease in the average total contact pressure at all knee flexion angles. The authors also found significant decrease in the mean lateral and central trochlear contact pressure at all knee flexion angles and a significant increase in the average medial trochlear contact pressure at all flexion angles.

Saranathan et al. performed a similar study in ten cadaveric knees using pressure sensors to measure contact pressure across the patella at varying degrees of knee flexion before and after AMZ [16]. The authors found significantly decreased contact pressure on the lateral patella facet following the AMZ, as well as increased pressure on the medial patellar facet (although the medial pressure did not reach that of the lateral side in the pathologic state). Hence, the AMZ was effective in offloading the patellofemoral joint as a whole and shifted the contact pressure to the medial patella and trochlea. A distalization can be performed in conjunction with the AMZ if the patient has excessive patellar height, although an aggressive distalization should be avoided as this will increase joint contact pressure [17].

Patients who present with anterior knee pain secondary to lateral overload can sometimes initially be managed with rest, anti-inflammatory medications, physical therapy, and injections. While these modalities can decrease pain, they do not treat the underlying issue of lateral overload and as such often cannot provide long-term symptom relief. In patients with symptomatic lateral overload, the treatment of choice after failed conservative management is a tibial tubercle osteotomy. As shown in cadaveric studies, the osteotomy will offload the lateral, symptomatic portion of the patella and trochlea, decrease overall patellofemoral joint contact pressure, and shift the load to the medial aspect of the patella and trochlea [14, 16]. Furthermore, the TTO will protect any chondral procedures performed concomitantly to the lateral patella or lateral trochlea [18–20]. However, if a patient has medial patella/trochlea or proximal patella chondral damage, a TTO is relatively contraindicated as it will shift the stress to an already damaged part of the knee, unless there was significant lateral subluxation resulting in incongruency of the patellofemoral joint [21].

The amount of anteriorization and medialization is based on the patient's anatomy. In patients with a TT-TG of less than 10, there should be a significant amount of anteriorization and less medialization to prevent over-medialization. Making a steep step cut rather than a standard oblique osteotomy cut will allow for preferential anteriorization. In patients with an elevated TT-TG (>15 mm), a standard anteromedialization can be performed, still ensuring more anteriorization than medialization, as the patient's primary goal is to achieve pain relief through reduction in contact forces and not stability. Anteriorization of the tubercle is an effective means of decreasing pain [22, 23]. However, overly aggressive anteriorization (>2 cm), as historically performed with the Maquet procedure, should be avoided because of issues with wound breakdown. A pure medialization is not performed in this setting as a medialization is not an unloading procedure but rather is used to correct coronal plane malalignment for instability.

Surgical Technique

Patients are brought to the operating room and undergo anesthesia. A long-acting sciatic nerve block should be avoided to prevent masking of a potential compartment syndrome postoperatively. The patient is placed supine on the OR table with a bump under the hip if necessary to achieve neutral alignment of the knee. A tourniquet is placed high on the operative thigh, and the patient is prepped and draped in the usual sterile fashion. A complete exam under anesthesia is performed, and an attempt is made to evert the patella to neutral. If the patella does not evert to neutral, a lateral release or lateral lengthening should be performed later in the case. Tranexamic acid (1 g intravenous), a clot-stabilizing agent, is considered prior to incision to minimize postoperative bruising and swelling. Following time-out, a diagnostic knee arthroscopy is performed with special attention paid to the chondral surface of the patella and trochlea. Any intraarticular pathology is addressed, and if a lateral release is indicated, this can now be performed arthroscopically. The arthroscope is removed and the tourniquet is inflated to 250 mmHg. If the patient has a cartilage lesion that necessitates treatment, this is performed now through a medial or lateral parapatellar arthrotomy, and a lateral lengthening can be performed at this point as well. Cartilage repair treatment is based on defect size and condition of the subchondral bone. For purely chondral defects, matrix-associated chondrocyte implantation (MACI) is preferred for larger lesions. Juvenile particulated cartilage allograft can be considered for smaller lesions, but insurance approval is challenging (Fig. 3.5a–d). Osteochondral defects are considered for osteochondral autograft transfer for small and fresh osteochondral allograft transplantation for larger defects.

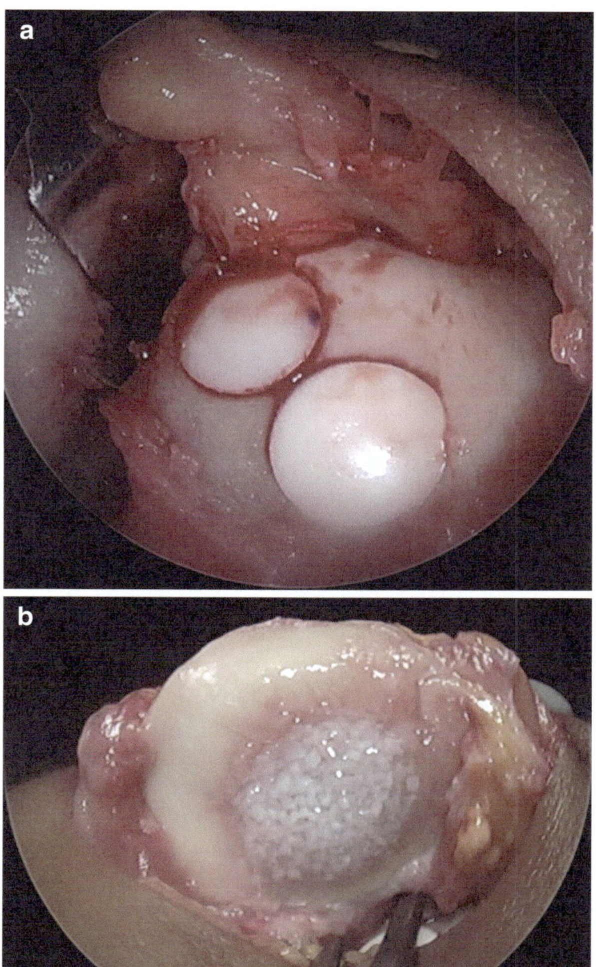

Fig. 3.5 (**a**, **b**) Intraoperative images demonstrating the completed osteochondral allograft to the trochlea (**a**) and juvenile particulated cartilage allograft to the patella (**b**). (**c**, **d**) Axial magnetic resonance images (MRI) demonstrating a patellar chondral defect before (**a**) and 6 months after (**d**) it was treated using DeNovo

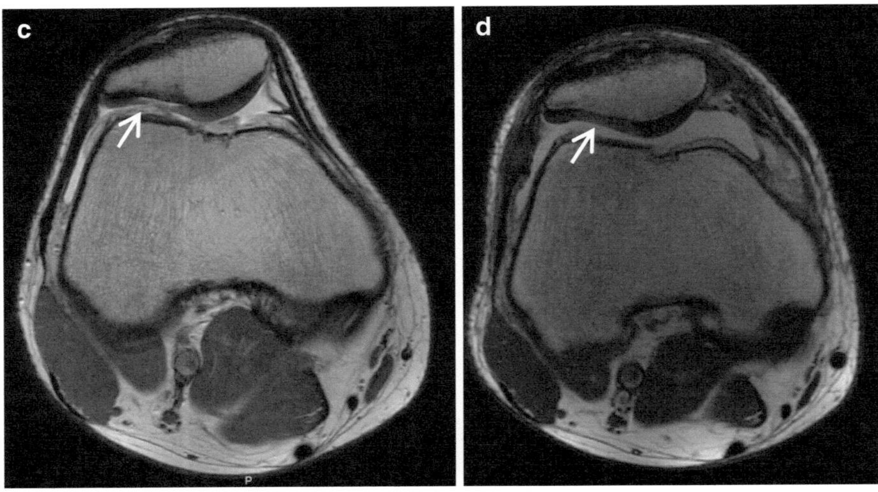

Fig. 3.5 (continued)

For the TTO, an approximately 5 cm incision is made just off the lateral edge of the tibial tubercle, and dissection is taken sharply down to fascia. The anterior compartment musculature is subperiosteally elevated off of the lateral tibia as one sleeve to minimize bleeding and trauma to the muscle. The medial and lateral aspects of the patellar tendon are exposed at the tibial tubercle, and the tendon is freed up to ensure the surgeon can place a retractor under the patellar tendon. While there are commercially available guides to perform the osteotomy, the authors prefer a freehand technique. Two k-wires are placed at the desired angle of the cut. For preferential anteriorization, a steeper angle is chosen. An oscillating saw is used to initiate the cut from the medial tibial cortex, aiming posteriorly toward, but not perforating the lateral cortex. The distal aspect of the osteotomy is left intact. The lateral cortex of the tibia is now counter-cut. A small osteotome is used to perform the proximal aspect of the osteotomy, and great care is taken to avoid damage to the patellar tendon. The osteotomy is checked to ensure it is mobile. Once it is mobile, a large flat osteotome is used to crack the distal hinge and translate the tibial tubercle anteriorly and medially. The tubercle is anteromedialized approximately 1.2–1.5 cm to decrease contact pressures (Fig. 3.6). The tibial tubercle is then secured using two 4.5 mm fully threaded screws placed in lag fashion. Meticulous attention must be paid when drilling for the screws to ensure the drill is perpendicular to the osteotomy site to allow compression across the osteotomy site. Finally, fluoroscopic images are taken to ensure proper screw length. The tourniquet is deflated and hemostasis is achieved. The authors do not typically use a drain, and a complete anterior compartment fasciotomy is not performed unless there is a concern for an impending compartment syndrome. Patients are placed into a hinged knee brace locked in extension and are kept touchdown weight bearing for 4–6 weeks. If desired, patients can be discharged home or admitted overnight for compartment checks and pain control. Range of

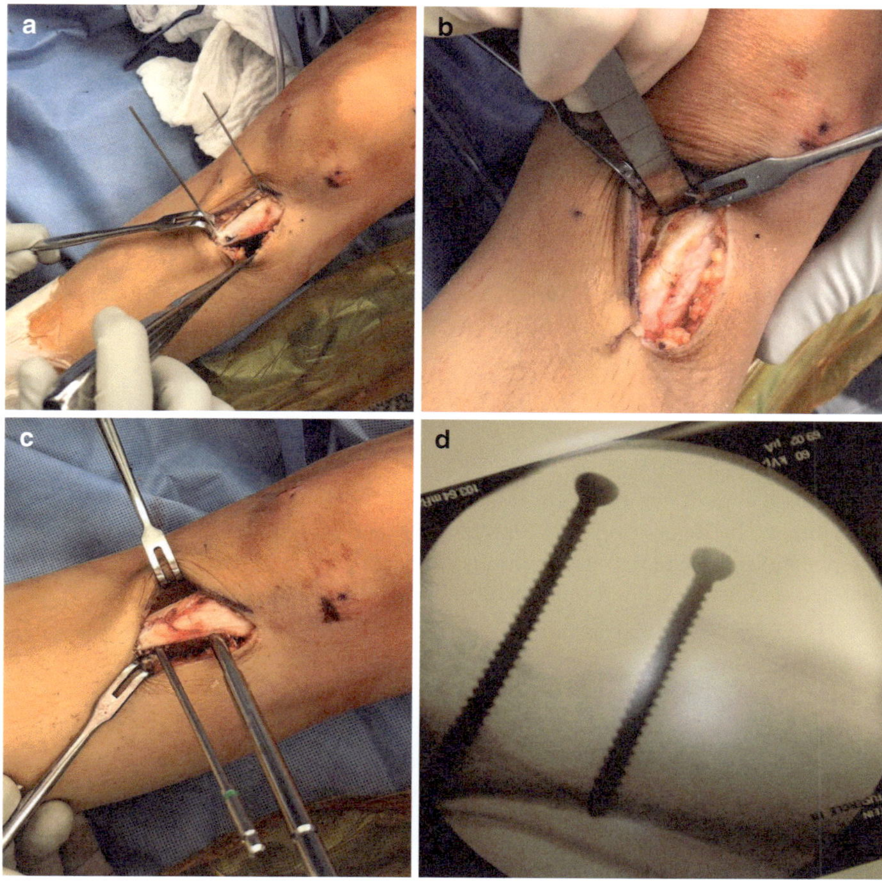

Fig. 3.6 (**a**–**d**) Intraoperative photos demonstrating the tibial tubercle osteotomy (TTO) procedure. (a) Placement of k-wires to direct the osteotomy. (**b**) Use of an osteotome to make the proximal aspect of the osteotomy once the medial to lateral cut has been made with the saw. (**c**) Placement of screws once the osteotomy has been shifted. (**d**) Intraoperative image demonstrating proper placement of the two lag screws

motion is started on the first postoperative day and progressed with a goal of achieving 90° of motion by 6 weeks. Active knee extension and straight leg raises are avoided for 6 weeks; quad isometrics are permitted as tolerated.

Results

Results following TTO as a pain relieving procedure have been encouraging [24–27]. A recent systematic review of the literature that included 976 patients from 21 studies found statistically significant improvements in Lysholm, Kujala, and visual analog scale scores following TTO. Liu et al. reported the results of 48 patients who underwent TTO for a primary diagnosis of pain and/or osteoarthritis [25]. The authors found significant improvement in average pain (4.1–1.8 ($p < 0.001$)) and Kujala (51.2–82.6 ($p < 0.0001$) scores following TTO. The authors also evaluated the ability to return to sport (RTS) following TTO and found that 83.3% of patients were able to RTS at an average of 7.8 months after surgery. Rosso et al. evaluated 69 patients who underwent TTO as treatment for patellofemoral chondral disease to determine potential negative prognostic factors [26]. While the authors found significant improvement in all outcome scores following TTO, they identified increased age, increased femoral anteversion, foot pronation, and postoperative patellofemoral crepitus as negative prognostic factors.

Complications

The most common complication following TTO is subsequent surgery to remove symptomatic hardware (reported between 16% and 50% of patients) [27, 28]. Other complications include non-union, compartment syndrome, infection, fracture, peroneal nerve injury, and deep venous thrombosis (DVT) [20, 27, 29].

Conclusion

TTO performed to offload the lateral patellofemoral compartment for a primary indication of patellofemoral pain is a useful and successful treatment option after failure of conservative management. Proper preoperative planning and meticulous surgical technique can afford patient excellent outcomes with the ability to return to sports in the majority of cases.

References

1. Blond L, Hansen L. Patellofemoral pain syndrome in athletes: a 5.7-year retrospective follow-up study of 250 athletes. Acta Orthop Belg. 1998;64(4):393–400.
2. Fairbank JC, Pynsent PB, van Poortvliet JA, Phillips H. Mechanical factors in the incidence of knee pain in adolescents and young adults. J Bone Joint Surg Br. 1984;66(5):685–93.
3. Ebert JR, Fallon M, Smith A, Janes GC, Wood DJ. Prospective clinical and radiologic evaluation of patellofemoral matrix-induced autologous chondrocyte implantation. Am J Sports Med. 2015;43(6):1362–72.
4. Erickson BJ, Mascarenhas R, Sayegh ET, et al. Does operative treatment of first-time patellar dislocations lead to increased patellofemoral stability? A systematic review of overlapping meta-analyses. Arthroscopy. 2015;31:1207–15.
5. Petersen W, Ellermann A, Gosele-Koppenburg A, et al. Patellofemoral pain syndrome. Knee Surg Sports Traumatol Arthrosc. 2014;22(10):2264–74.
6. Saper MG, Shneider DA. Diagnosis and treatment of lateral patellar compression syndrome. Arthrosc Tech. 2014;3(5):e633–8.

7. Sherman SL, Erickson BJ, Cvetanovich GL, et al. Tibial tuberosity osteotomy: indications, techniques, and outcomes. Am J Sports Med. 2014;42:2006–17.
8. van Middelkoop M, van der Heijden RA, Bierma-Zeinstra SMA. Characteristics and outcome of patellofemoral pain in adolescents: do they differ from adults? J Orthop Sports Phys Ther. 2017;47(10):801–5.
9. Fu FH, Maday MG. Arthroscopic lateral release and the lateral patellar compression syndrome. Orthop Clin North Am. 1992;23(4):601–12.
10. Grawe B, Stein BE. Tibial tubercle osteotomy: indication and techniques. J Knee Surg. 2015;28(4):279–84.
11. Hungerford DS, Barry M. Biomechanics of the patellofemoral joint. Clin Orthop Relat Res. 1979;144:9–15.
12. Paulos LE, O'Connor DL, Karistinos A. Partial lateral patellar facetectomy for treatment of arthritis due to lateral patellar compression syndrome. Arthroscopy. 2008;24(5):547–53.
13. Lewallen DG, Riegger CL, Myers ER, Hayes WC. Effects of retinacular release and tibial tubercle elevation in patellofemoral degenerative joint disease. J Orthop Res. 1990;8(6):856–62.
14. Beck PR, Thomas AL, Farr J, Lewis PB, Cole BJ. Trochlear contact pressures after anteromedialization of the tibial tubercle. Am J Sports Med. 2005;33(11):1710–5.
15. Fulkerson JP, Becker GJ, Meaney JA, Miranda M, Folcik MA. Anteromedial tibial tubercle transfer without bone graft. Am J Sports Med. 1990;18(5):490–6. discussion 496-497
16. Saranathan A, Kirkpatrick MS, Mani S, et al. The effect of tibial tuberosity realignment procedures on the patellofemoral pressure distribution. Knee Surg Sports Traumatol Arthrosc. 2012;20(10):2054–61.
17. Yang JS, Fulkerson JP, Obopilwe E, et al. Patellofemoral contact pressures after patellar distalization: a biomechanical study. Arthroscopy. 2017;33(11):2038–44.
18. Cotter EJ, Waterman BR, Kelly MP, Wang KC, Frank RM, Cole BJ. Multiple osteochondral allograft transplantation with concomitant tibial tubercle osteotomy for multifocal chondral disease of the knee. Arthrosc Tech. 2017;6(4):e1393–8.
19. von Keudell A, Han R, Bryant T, Minas T. Autologous chondrocyte implantation to isolated Patella cartilage defects. Cartilage. 2017;8(2):146–54.
20. Yanke AB, Wuerz T, Saltzman BM, Butty D, Cole BJ. Management of patellofemoral chondral injuries. Clin Sports Med. 2014;33(3):477–500.
21. Pidoriano AJ, Weinstein RN, Buuck DA, Fulkerson JP. Correlation of patellar articular lesions with results from anteromedial tibial tubercle transfer. Am J Sports Med. 1997;25(4):533–7.
22. Guillamon JL, Lord G, Marotte JH, Blanchard JP. Treatment of patello-femoral arthrosis by anterior displacement of the tibial tuberosity (Maquet procedure). Rev Chir Orthop Reparatrice Appar Mot. 1977;63(6):545–62.
23. Hirsh DM, Reddy DK. Experience with Maquet anterior tibial tubercle advancement for patellofemoral arthralgia. Clin Orthop Relat Res. 1980;148:136–9.
24. Fisher TF, Waterman BR, Orr JD, Holland CA, Bader J, Belmont PJ Jr. Tibial tubercle osteotomy for patellar chondral pathology in an active United States military population. Arthroscopy. 2016;32(11):2342–9.
25. Liu JN, Wu HH, Garcia GH, Kalbian IL, Strickland SM, Shubin Stein BE. Return to sports after tibial tubercle osteotomy for patellofemoral pain and osteoarthritis. Arthroscopy. 2018;34:1022–9.
26. Rosso F, Rossi R, Governale G, et al. Tibial tuberosity anteromedialization for patellofemoral chondral disease: prognostic factors. Am J Sports Med. 2017;45(7):1589–98.
27. Saltzman BM, Rao A, Erickson BJ, et al. A systematic review of 21 Tibial tubercle osteotomy studies and more than 1000 knees: indications, clinical outcomes, complications, and reoperations. Am J Orthop (Belle Mead NJ). 2017;46(6):E396–407.
28. Farr J. Autologous chondrocyte implantation improves patellofemoral cartilage treatment outcomes. Clin Orthop Relat Res. 2007;463:187–94.
29. Erickson BJ, Tilton A, Frank RM, Park W, Cole BJ. Rates of deep vein thrombosis occurring after osteotomy about the knee. Am J Orthop (Belle Mead NJ). 2017;46(1):E23–7.

Chapter 4
Patellofemoral Arthritis

Dean Wang, Sabrina M. Strickland, and Beth E. Shubin Stein

Etiology of Patellofemoral Arthritis

The pathogenesis of wear and damage to articular cartilage of the knee is often multifactorial. However, with isolated patellofemoral (PF) arthritis (Fig. 4.1), the pathogenesis can most commonly be attributed to mechanical causes that overload the PF cartilage or traumatic shear injuries. These include trauma, patellar instability, malalignment, and dysplasia. Disruption of the articular surface leads to loss of the cartilage fluid pressure responsible for absorbing joint loads, and the resultant high stresses can lead to breakdown of collagen fibers and propagation of chondral defects. In non-traumatic cases, any aberrant mechanics of the PF articulation causes aberrant loads on the articular cartilage, predisposing the cartilage to breakdown over time.

Traumatic injury to the PF cartilage can occur either through blunt trauma (e.g., fall on a flexed knee or direct impact from a dashboard injury) or intraarticular fracture. The most common location of the cartilage lesion from this etiology is a central bipolar lesion of both the patella and trochlea or the superomedial aspect of the patella as a result of the knee being in a flexed position at the time of injury [1]. Posttraumatic etiologies account for approximately 9% of patients with isolated PF osteoarthritis (OA) [22].

Chondral and osteochondral shear injuries are frequently observed after a patellar dislocation, which predominately affects a younger population [44]. Patellar stability relies on limb alignment, the osseous containment of the patella within the trochlea, the integrity of the static and dynamic soft tissue constraints, and general-

D. Wang (✉) · S. M. Strickland · B. E. Shubin Stein
Sports Medicine and Shoulder Service, Hospital for Special Surgery, New York, NY, USA
e-mail: Stricklandoffice@HSS.EDU; shubinsteinoffice@hss.edu

B. E. Shubin Stein, S. M. Strickland (eds.), *Patellofemoral Pain and Instability*,
https://doi.org/10.1007/978-3-319-97640-2_4

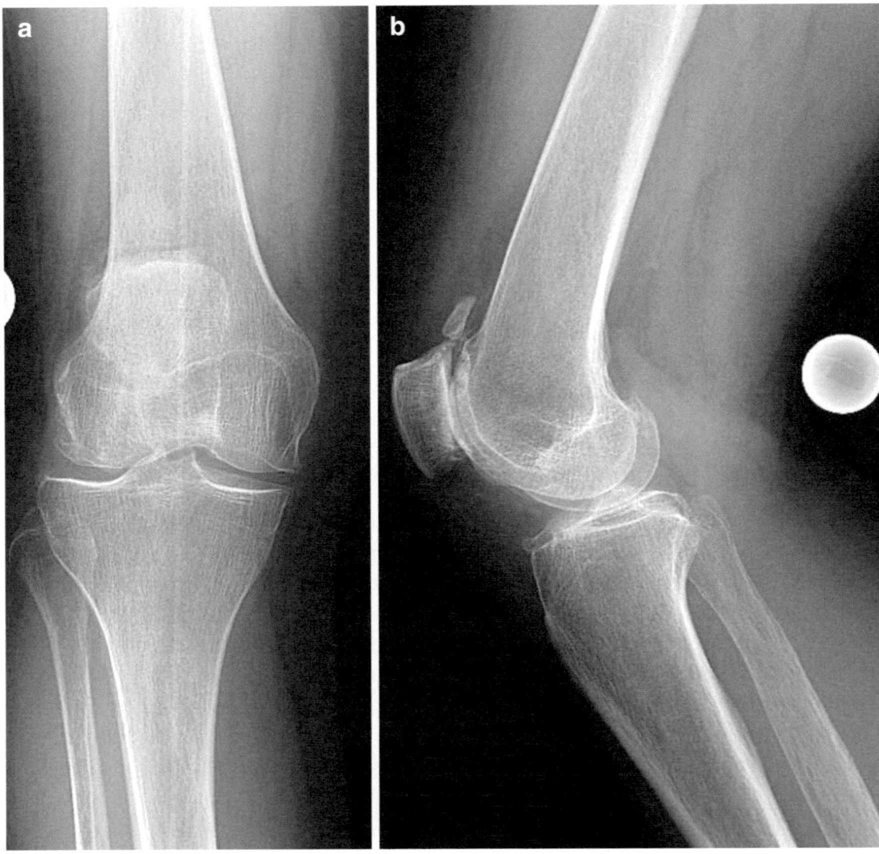

Fig. 4.1 (**a**) Anteroposterior and (**b**) lateral X-rays of a right knee with isolated patellofemoral arthritis

ized ligamentous laxity. Non-dysplastic knees require a high amount of energy to dislocate the patella from the trochlea, and therefore, the incidence of significant chondral or osteochondral injury to the medial patella facet in the setting of patellar dislocation can be up to 70–96% in these patients [12, 13, 38, 39]. On the other hand, patients with ligamentous laxity have less anatomic restraint to prevent dislocation and, as a result, have a higher rate of PF instability episodes but tend to have less severe articular cartilage damage [42]. Coexisting pathologies of trochlear dysplasia, patella alta, excessive tibial tubercle–trochlear groove (TT–TG) distance, and patholaxity of the medial patellofemoral ligament (MPFL) with recurrent patellar instability are frequently observed. Although there is evidence to suggest a strong correlation between the number of patellar dislocations and the prevalence of PF OA [17, 39], it is important to note that a history of patellar dislocation is notable in 33% of isolated PF OA patients [22].

Anatomic abnormalities including trochlear dysplasia, patella alta, and excessive TT-TG distance can be found in isolated PF OA patients without a history of patellar dislocation. In the setting of patella alta, excessive load of the distal patella can occur due to decreased engagement of the patella in the trochlea. The concentration of load on a smaller area of the cartilage results in an increase in pressure and risk of cartilage wear. Rotational malalignment in the axial plane resulting in excessive TT-TG and patellar tilt increases lateral patella facet pressures, predisposing the lateral PF joint cartilage damage. Increased TT–TG values have been shown to be proportional to the development of PF cartilage damage and OA [47]. Finally, high-grade trochlear dysplasia is present in the large majority of patients with isolated PF OA [22]. The presence of the trochlear prominences as observed in Dejour types B–D can lead to high contact loads within the PF joint during the early degrees of flexion [50].

Nonoperative Treatment

Nonoperative treatment for PF OA is focused on restoring strength, balance, and flexibility. A comprehensive rehabilitation program should first aim at restoring range of motion and flexibility, followed by gait training and a strengthening program that targets the core, pelvis, and quadriceps. Other nonoperative treatment options include nonsteroidal anti-inflammatory medications, intraarticular corticosteroid, and viscosupplementation injections, taping, and bracing. Although currently available studies on intraarticular platelet-rich plasma injections for knee OA have reported improvements in pain and knee function, the prevalence of PF OA predicts less reliable improvement in symptoms [24]. Commercial harvesting of stem cells from the bone marrow or adipose and delivery as an injection is available as another nonoperative treatment, although the data on this is currently limited. The use of McConnell taping and Kinesio taping has demonstrated equivocal results [28], but if patients experience symptomatic relief, then it may aid in allowing them to participate in their physical therapy and strengthening program.

Operative Treatment

Tibial Tubercle Osteotomy (TTO)

Tibial tubercle osteotomy (TTO) is a highly versatile operation that can be used to correct coronal plane malalignment in the setting of instability and elevated tibial tubercle to trochlear groove (TT–TG) distances, as well as to unload painful or damaged cartilage. It is often used in conjunction with cartilage restoration procedures of the patella or trochlea to unload the chondral repair site. Straight anteriorization of the tibial tubercle (Maquet procedure) by 1.3 cm can decrease inferior patellar loads by approximately 57–84% at all flexion angles [15]. Similarly, straight anteriorization of the tibial tubercle can decreased trochlear loads by approximately 20–32% at all flexion angles [43]. Anteromedialization of the tibial tubercle shifts the contact forces to the medial patella and trochlea and can significantly decrease both peak lateral and total loads across both the patella and trochlea at all flexion angles [3]. However, in the setting of physiological tracking, anteromedialization of the tibial tubercle can potentially increase the trochlea loads in patients with central or medial chondral defects. For autologous chondrocyte implantation (ACI), studies comparing results with and without TTO have confirmed that an unloading osteotomy significantly improves patient outcomes compared with ACI alone [40, 49]. Ultimately, in order to unload the cartilage repair site, the magnitude and direction of translation of the tuberosity at the time of TTO will vary depending on the patient's anatomy, etiology, and location of the chondral defect. Furthermore, in the setting of lateral PF instability, a MPFL reconstruction is recommended in conjunction with the TTO to restore patellar stability [32].

For patients with symptomatic isolated PF OA who have failed conservative treatment, treatment with TTO can improve outcomes. The outcomes of anteromedialization TTO for PF OA are correlated with the location, rather than the severity, of cartilage wear; patients with distal or lateral facet patellar lesions tend to have the best outcomes, whereas those with proximal or diffuse patellar lesions and central trochlear lesions tend to have the worst outcomes [41]. Central trochlear lesions often present with a corresponding patellar lesion, and in these patients, patellofemoral arthroplasty (PFA) may be a better option than combined TTO and cartilage restoration. Atkinson et al. examined 40 patients (50 knees) with a mean age of 29 years who underwent TTO for PF OA and reported that 94% had improved pain scores and 77% had good or excellent results at a mean follow-up of 81 months [2]. Similarly, Carofino and Fulkerson examined 17 active patients (22 knees) with a mean age of 55 years who underwent an anteromedialization TTO for PF OA and reported that 63% had good to excellent results at a mean follow-up of 77 months [8]. Liu et al. examined 57 patients (61 knees) with mean age of 30 years who underwent an anteromedialization TTO for PF OA and reported a return to sport rate of 83% at an average of 8 months postoperatively [27]. Further investigation is needed to determine the long-term complication profile and survival of primary TTO for PF OA.

Cartilage Restoration Procedures

Many of the cartilage restoration procedures available for the treatment of cartilage defects of the PF joint have been adopted from techniques successfully used for femoral condylar lesions, although the clinical outcomes of these procedures for PF

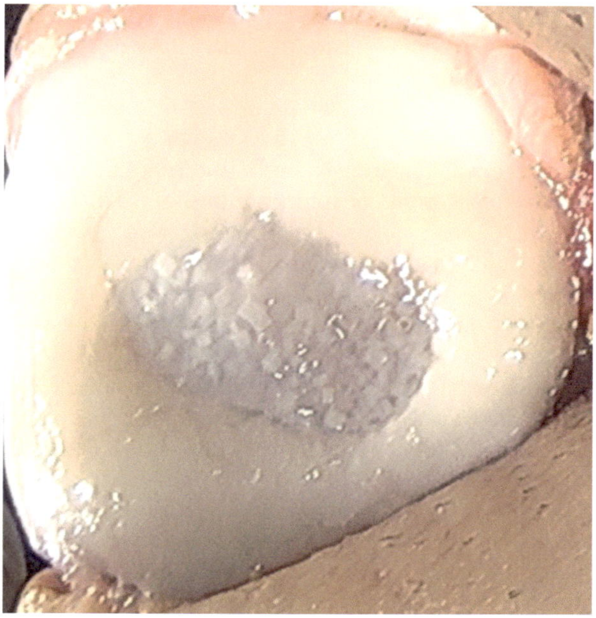

Fig. 4.2 Cartilage restoration with particulated juvenile articular cartilage for a well-shouldered lesion of the patella, which has intact cartilage margins to contain the graft

chondral lesions are often less satisfactory. Clinical outcomes are better in patients who have isolated trochlear defects than in those who have patellar defects [7, 16, 20, 45]. Cell-based techniques have become popular for treating defects of the PF joint due to the ability to contour the graft to match the surrounding articular topography. However, these techniques rely on the underlying subchondral bone to provide a stable base for the graft, as well as intact cartilage margins to contain the graft and prevent it from displacing (Fig. 4.2). Therefore, in the setting of underlying bony deformity, cystic lesions, and loss or uncontained lesions, the use of osteochondral grafts may be a more appropriate treatment option.

Microfracture

Historically, microfracture was viewed as the first-line treatment for chondral defects in the knee. For the PF joint, specialized awls were utilized to allow for perpendicular penetration of the subchondral plate of the patella and trochlea. However, multiple studies have demonstrated deterioration of the initial clinical improvement between 18 and 36 months after the procedure [25, 35]. Although microfracture provides an attractive option due to its ease of use, low cost, and ability to be performed arthroscopically, the questionable durability of the fibrocartilage tissue produced (especially in the patellofemoral joint, which sees increased shear forces) and its inability to treat larger lesions (>2 cm) have limited the use of the procedure.

Autologous Chondrocyte Implantation (ACI) and Matrix-Induced Autologous Chondrocyte Implantation (MACI)

ACI is a two-stage procedure that first involves harvesting a small amount of cartilage from the non-weight bearing region of the knee, which is then digested and the chondrocytes expanded in cell culture for approximately 3 weeks. During the second stage, the chondral defect is prepared, and a patch (previously the periosteum but now more commonly the collagen) is sewn to seal the defect. The expanded chondrocytes are then injected underneath the patch. For PF chondral defects, the advantages of ACI include the ability to treat large lesions and its ease of use in the PF joint, where the complex geometry can make contouring of other grafts difficult. Although the early results of first-generation ACI for patellar lesions were poor [5], functional outcomes and patient satisfaction were significantly improved when ACI was performed in conjunction with a TTO to offload the PF joint [40, 49]. More recent studies have demonstrated good long-term outcomes of ACI in patients with PF defects, with satisfaction rates of >80% to 90% [18, 19]. However, concerns have been raised about the implantation of chondrocytes in suspension, which may result in the uneven distribution of chondrocytes within the defect, potential for cell leakage, and loss of the normal chondrocyte phenotype. In order to overcome these concerns, matrix-induced autologous chondrocyte implantation (MACI) was introduced and seeds the patients' chondrocytes on three-dimensional porcine type I/type III collagen bilayer scaffold (Fig. 4.3). The early results of MACI in the PF joint are promising [11, 34], although long-term studies are needed to evaluate for any superiority over ACI.

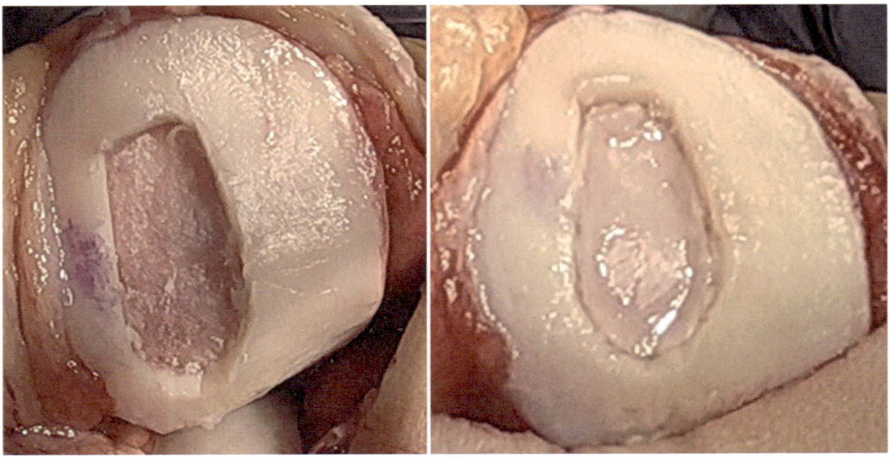

Fig. 4.3 A well-shouldered patellar chondral defect (left) treated with matrix-induced autologous chondrocyte implantation (right)

Particulated Juvenile Articular Cartilage

Another cell-based restoration procedure is particulated juvenile articular cartilage. This technique employs an off-the-shelf source of chondrocytes to resurface cartilage defects, thus providing a single-stage procedure that avoids the morbidity of cartilage harvest associated with ACI and MACI. Cartilage is obtained from deceased juvenile (neonates to 13 years of age) donors, screened, and processed. During implantation, the particulated juvenile articular cartilage is mixed with fibrin glue and is placed in the prepared lesion site (Fig. 4.4). Like ACI and MACI, the particulated graft/fibrin glue construct can be easily contoured to match the articular topography of PF joint. Although cartilage restoration with particulated juvenile articular cartilage for unshouldered patellar lesions has a higher risk of graft displacement in the setting of malalignment-related OA, this technique combined with an offloading TTO can still result in good cartilage fill (Fig. 4.5). Currently, there is limited data on the use of particulated juvenile articular cartilage for the PF joint.

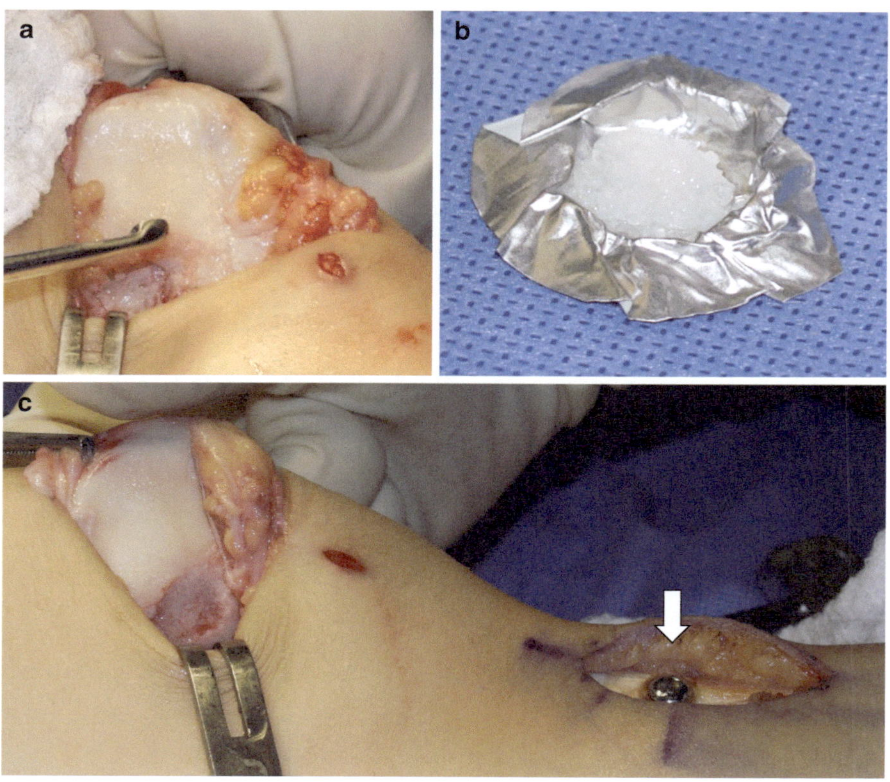

Fig. 4.4 Cartilage restoration of a patellar chondral defect using particulated juvenile articular cartilage. (**a**) Preparation of the chondral defect with a curette, leaving an intact border of healthy cartilage with stable margins. (**b**) Creation of the fibrin glue and particulated juvenile articular cartilage mixture in its foil package. (**c**) Implantation of the particulated juvenile articular cartilage into the patellar chondral defect. A concomitant anteromedialization tibial tubercle osteotomy (arrow) was performed prior to implantation

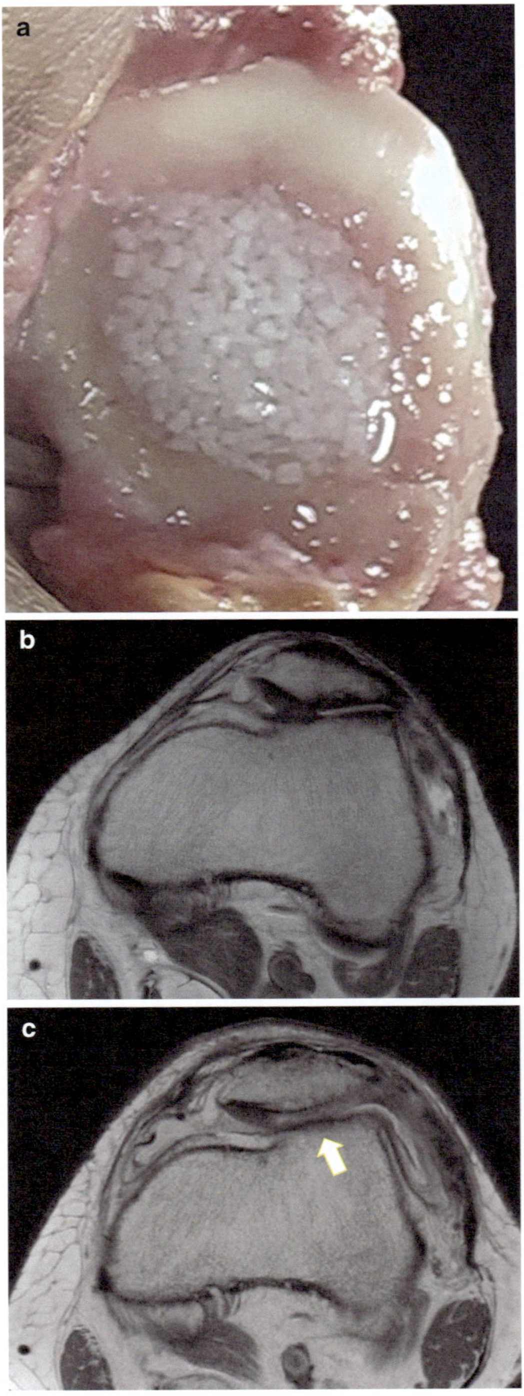

Fig. 4.5 (**a**) Cartilage restoration with particulated juvenile articular cartilage for an unshouldered lesion of the patella. In the setting of malalignment-related OA, this generally results in a higher risk of graft displacement. However, in this patient, particulated juvenile articular cartilage was performed in conjunction with an offloading tibial tubercle osteotomy, and (**b**) preoperative and (**c**) 3-month postoperative axial magnetic resonance imaging demonstrate interval fill of the patellar cartilage defect (arrow)

Two of the first studies on this procedure, which were funded by the industry developer for DeNovo (Zimmer), evaluated patients treated with particulated juvenile articular cartilage for defects of the patella and reported substantial improvements in clinical outcome scores, reduction in pain levels, and >90% fill of the cartilage defects [6, 48]. Other nonindustry-funded short-term studies have since confirmed MRI evidence of progressive graft maturation over time [21] and histologic evidence of type II collagen production in the repair tissue [14].

Osteochondral Grafts

For lesions with underlying osseous abnormalities (cystic changes) or bone loss, treatment with osteochondral grafts is advantageous due to the single-stage implantation of viable, mature, and structurally stable grafts that replace both the cartilage and the underlying abnormal bone. The biggest challenge with implantation of osteochondral grafts in the PF joint is matching the curvature of the surrounding articular surface of the patella and/or trochlea. Any mismatch in contour between graft and recipient can lead to increased contact pressures if the plug is left proud or rim loading if the plug is recessed. Additionally, the cartilage of the patella is substantially thicker, and the curvature of both patella and trochlea is unique and different than other sites in the knee. Therefore, implanted osteochondral plugs harvested from sites other than the patella can result in the cartilage portion of the graft being thin and the bony portion of the plug extending above the native surrounding subchondral plate, which may create a stress riser and lead to cyst formation and graft failure [51]. For most locations on the trochlea, the curvatures are substantially different from the convex nature of the femoral condyles, and osteochondral grafts that are harvested from the condyles will likely not reproduce the native architecture of the trochlea.

The use of osteochondral autograft transfer (OAT) for PF cartilage defects is limited for patients who have small (<2 cm^2) lesions of the patella or trochlea due to the autogenous harvesting of donor plugs. Clinical outcomes have been inconsistent and can be partially attributed to the fact that the autograft plugs can only be harvested from the periphery of the trochlea or intercondylar notch. A few studies have demonstrated significant clinical improvement and MRI evidence of good cartilage fill, complete trabecular incorporation, and fibrocartilage filling of the donor sites in patients treated with OAT of the patella and trochlea [23, 37]. In contrast, within a randomized controlled trial of 100 patients with osteochondral defects of the knee treated with either OAT or ACI, for patellar lesions, 60% of patients treated with OAT ($n = 5$) had an excellent or good result, compared to 85% of patients treated with ACI ($n = 20$). All five patients treated with patellar OAT had failed at final follow-up [4].

Osteochondral allograft transplantation (OCA) does not suffer from donor site morbidity, and size-matched allografts can be requested to optimize the ability to match the topography of the recipient PF joint. Because the limitations associated with donor site morbidity are avoided, OCA can be used to treat large lesions and is frequently used as a salvage procedure after failed cartilage repair. Graft availability (depending on size matching, donor age, and disease screening) and the narrow window of time in which the graft can be implanted remain the biggest disadvantages of this technique. Fresh osteochondral allografts have demonstrated superiority over frozen allografts, largely because chondrocyte viability has been reported to be critically important for maintaining the biochemical and biomechanical properties of OCA [10]. Chondrocyte viability steadily declines after procurement and falls below acceptable levels (<70% viable cells) by 28 days [52]. Mandatory disease screening requires approximately 14 days, resulting in a narrow window of time (approximately 14 days) for scheduling surgery and transporting tissues. For this procedure, lesions are sized and reamed to a bed of normal bone, and a corresponding dowel is taken from the allograft, contoured to match the recipient site, and gently implanted into place for press-fit fixation (Fig. 4.6). In some instances where press-fit fixation is not attainable, supplemental fixation with the use of headless compression screws or absorbable pins may be needed. Like the results of other cartilage restoration tech-

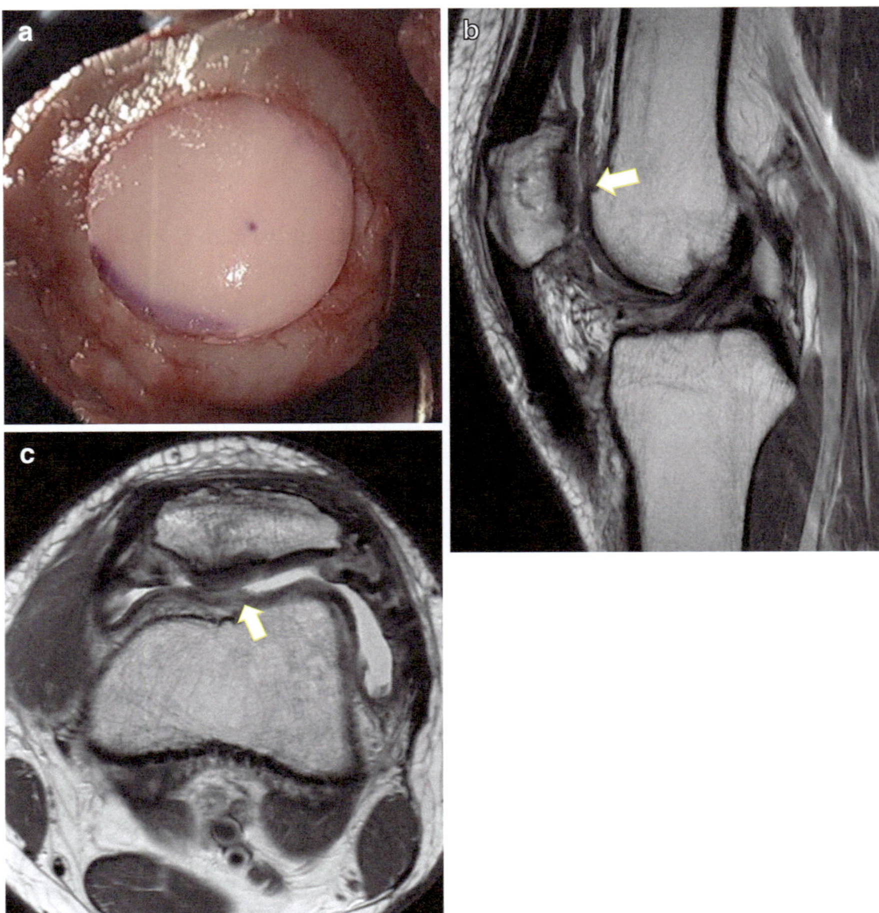

Fig. 4.6 (**a**) Cartilage restoration of a patellar chondral defect using osteochondral allograft transplantation. (**b**) Lateral and (**c**) axial magnetic resonance imaging demonstrates reconstitution of the patellar articular surface (arrow) and partial trabecular integration

niques, graft survivorship and clinical outcomes of OCA in the PF joint are generally inferior to that of the femoral condyle [9]. Bugbee and colleagues reported that in their series of patients, 10-year graft survivorship was 78% for isolated patellar defects and 92% for isolated trochlear defects, with significant improvement in clinical outcome scores in both groups of patients [7, 20]. For bipolar lesions treated with OCA, high reoperation and failure rates have been reported [33].

Patellofemoral Arthroplasty (PFA)

Since its introduction in 1955, patellofemoral arthroplasty (PFA) (Fig. 4.7) has evolved in sophistication and efficacy. PFA performed with the use of first-generation implants resulted in revision rates as high as 63% [46]. Over time, improved prosthetic design and patient selection have led to improved patient

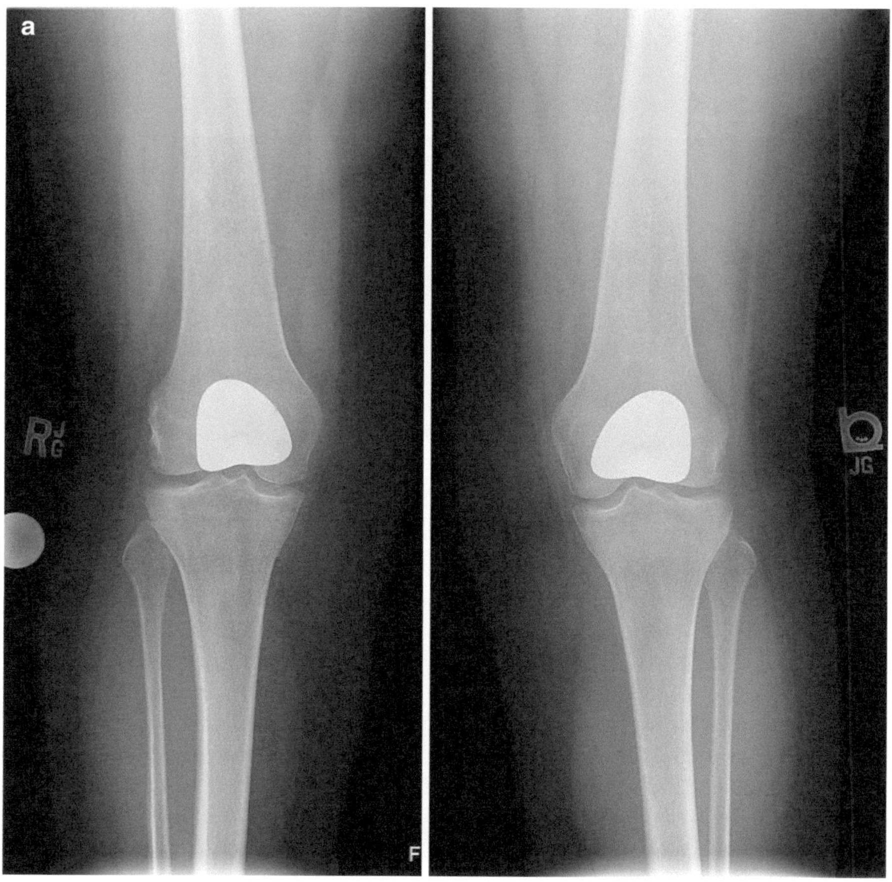

Fig. 4.7 (**a**) Anteroposterior, (**b**) lateral, and (**c**) merchant postoperative standing X-rays showing a successful patellofemoral arthroplasty

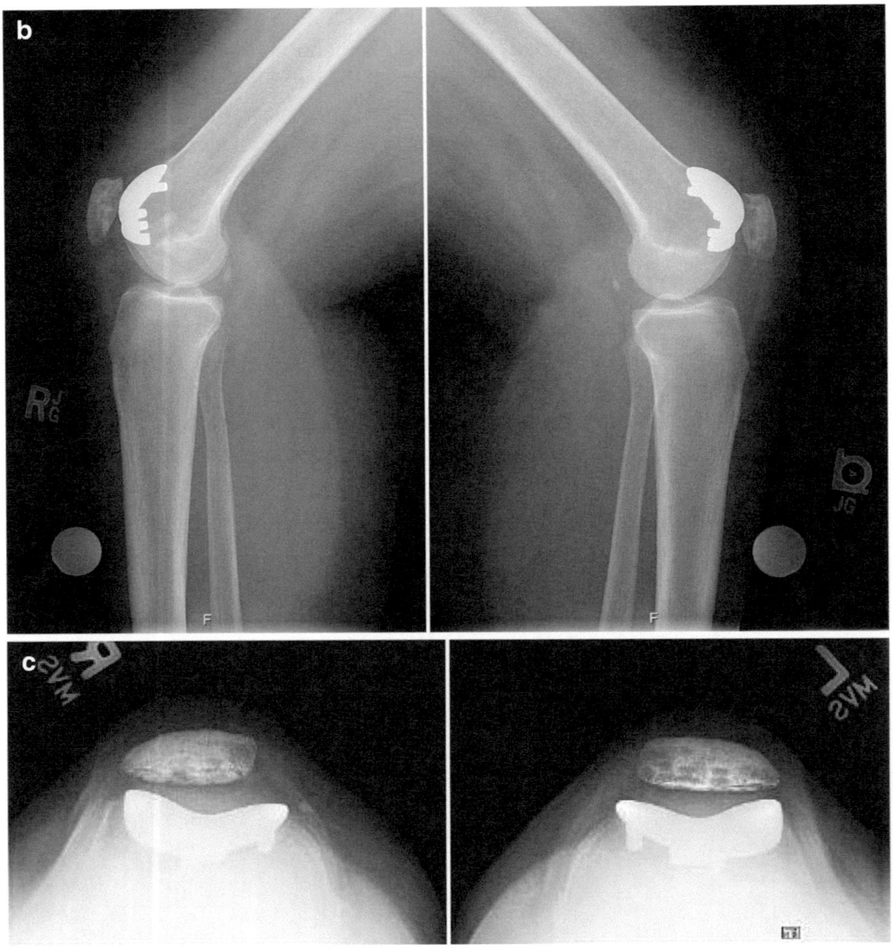

Fig. 4.7 (continued)

outcomes [29, 31]. With any PFA, there is always the risk for progressive tibiofemoral arthritis in the remainder of the knee. However, unlike its medial and lateral unicompartmental counterparts, survivorship of PFA is closely tied to the etiology of the disease, with posttraumatic, malalignment, and instability-related degenerative joint disease faring significantly better than primary osteoarthritis. The reason for the improved survivorship seen in patients with posttraumatic, malalignment, and instability-related OA is that the source of the arthritis is clear and limited to the PF joint, and therefore, the risk of progression to the uninvolved tibiofemoral compartments is less likely. In patients with primary OA of the PF joint without trochlear dysplasia or one of the above etiologies, the OA is presumed to be the initial presentation and so will commonly go on to affect the tibiofemoral joint at some point in the future. PFA is still a good option in young patients with primary OA who do not presently exhibit tibiofemoral OA on MRI; however, they should be counselled that a PFA is likely a bridging operation that will at some point require conversion to a total knee arthroplasty (TKA). Although TKA may be an effective treatment option [26, 36], PFA has many advantages over TKA for the treatment of isolated patellofemoral arthritis. It is less invasive, requires shorter tourniquet times, has less blood loss, has a faster recovery, preserves native knee kinematics, and is bone conserving [29].

Compared to first-generation PFAs, newer designs have features that optimize patellar tracking which has solved some of the earlier problems of patella catching and recurrent instability. Most notably, there is a longer proximal trochlear component and wider anterior flanges, which prevents the patella from jumping onto the trochlear component from the native femur during early knee flexion. Currently, there are two styles of PFA: inlay and onlay. The inlay-style component is set into the anterior trochlear surface, while the onlay prosthesis is implanted flush to the anterior femoral cortex (thus requiring an anterior femoral cut similar to that of a total knee arthroplasty). Though the inlay design resects less bone, it does not allow for any change in rotation of the trochlear component relative to the patients' own anatomy (which often times is pathologic in this group). Thus the inlay style has a higher tendency for patellar maltracking [30]. Both onlay and inlay components allow for creation of a trochlear groove when the native femoral trochlea is dysplastic. However, in patients with a previous or current history of patellar instability, the onlay design is preferred given the ability to increase external rotation of the trochlear implant.

Severe coronal deformity, if left uncorrected, can negatively affect patellar tracking and predispose to progression of tibiofemoral arthritis after PFA. In addition, a PFA cannot completely correct a severely malaligned or unstable patellofemoral joint. Therefore, candidates for a PFA who have an elevated TT-TG distance combined with a history of previous or present instability should be considered for a concomitant MPFL reconstruction. We prefer to use an onlay-style PFA as it allows the surgeon to change the rotation of the femoral component to some degree, which can be very helpful in cases of PF OA due to instability. Furthermore, it is important to recognize patella maltrackers early and perform PFA before significant erosion (Fig. 4.8a) and patella acetabularization (Fig. 4.8b) occur, which can result in insufficient patellar bone for implanting a patellar component. In patients with maltracking-related PF OA and fixed tilt, we use a lateral parapatellar arthrotomy combined with a lateral lengthening which allows us to address the tilt concomitantly. The lateral approach with lengthening can be done in patients with isolated maltracking OA and in those with malalignment and instability. In those cases with combined instability, we add an MPFL reconstruction in addition to the lateral lengthening (Fig. 4.9).

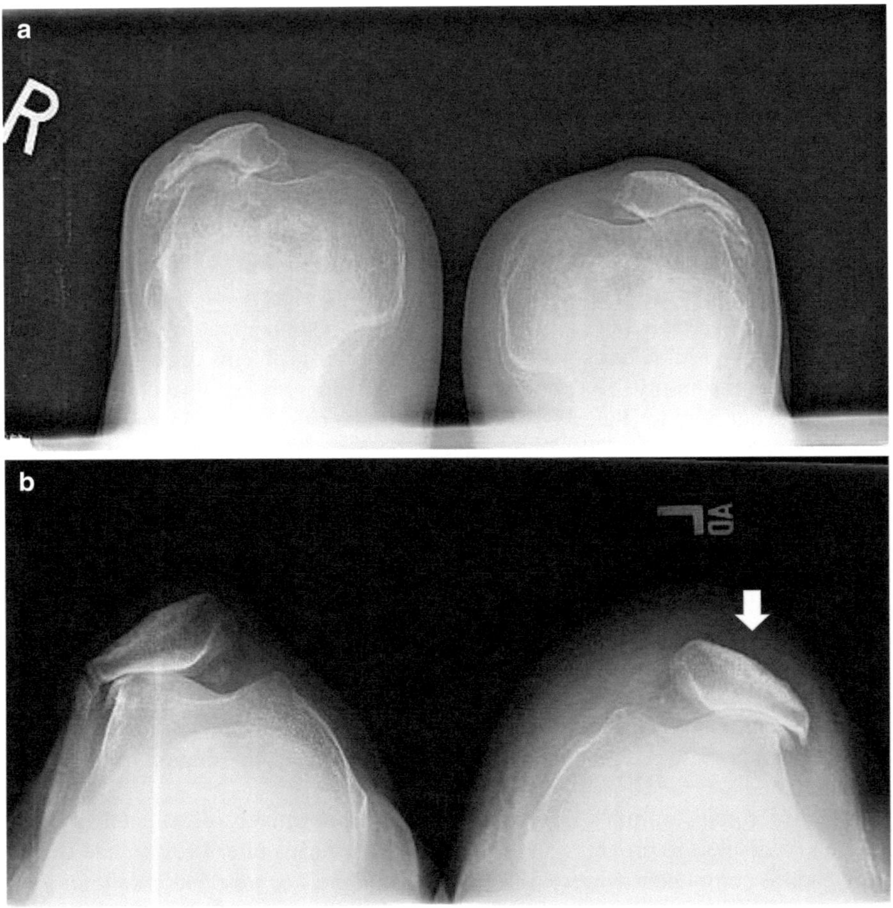

Fig. 4.8 A merchant view showing (**a**) severe patellar bone loss bilaterally and (**b**) patella acetabularization of the left knee (arrow)

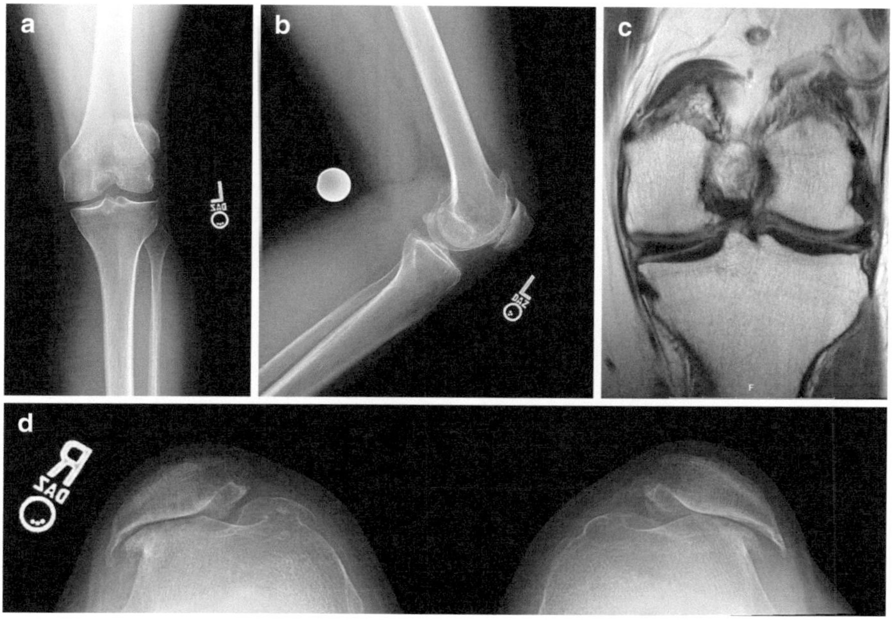

Fig. 4.9 (**a**, **b**, **d**) Preoperative posteroanterior, lateral, and merchant views of the left knee of a patient with maltracking-related patellofemoral osteoarthritis and fixed patellar tilt, (**c**) coronal magnetic resonance image demonstrates preserved tibiofemoral cartilage and joint space, (**e**–**g**) postoperative posteroanterior, lateral, and merchant views of the left knee in the same patient after combined patellofemoral arthroplasty through a lateral parapatellar arthrotomy, lateral lengthening, and medial patellofemoral ligament reconstruction

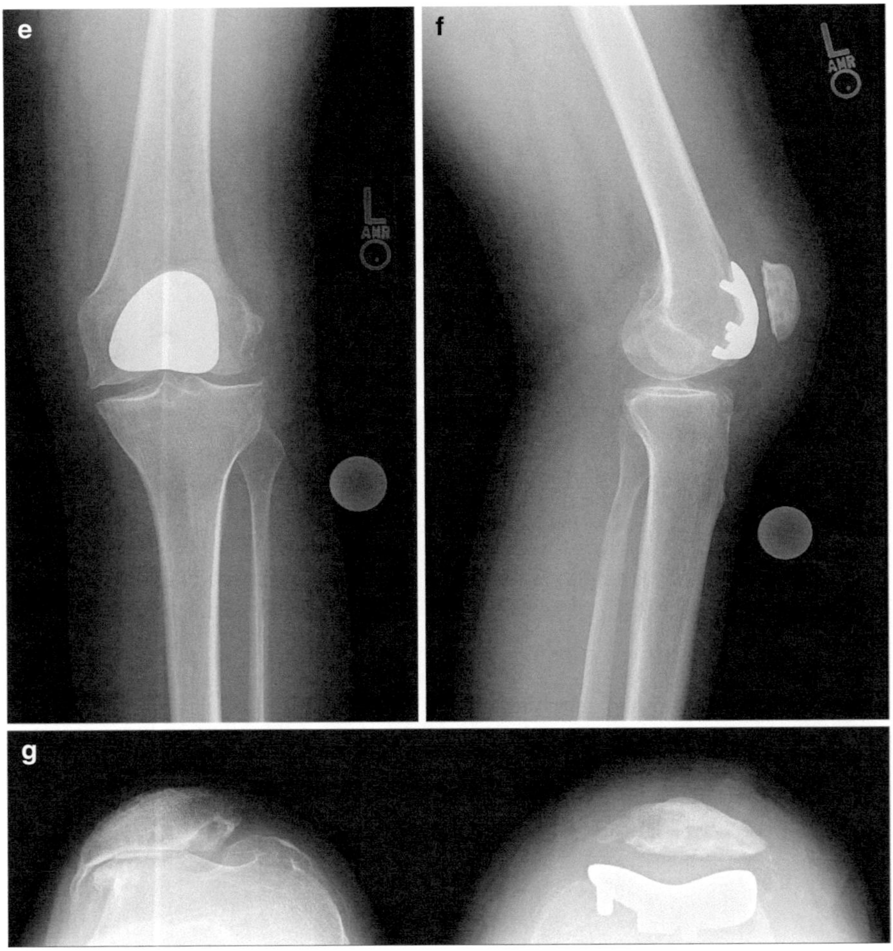

Fig. 4.9 (continued)

References

1. Arendt EA, Berruto M, Filardo G, Ronga M, Zaffagnini S, Farr J, Ferrua P, Grassi A, Condello V. Early osteoarthritis of the patellofemoral joint. Knee Surg Sports Traumatol Arthrosc. 2016;24:1836–44.
2. Atkinson HD, Bailey CA, Anand S, Johal P, Oakeshott RD. Tibial tubercle advancement osteotomy with bone allograft for patellofemoral arthritis: a retrospective cohort study of 50 knees. Arch Orthop Trauma Surg. 2012;132:437–45.
3. Beck PR, Thomas AL, Farr J, Lewis PB, Cole BJ. Trochlear contact pressures after anteromedialization of the tibial tubercle. Am J Sports Med. 2005;33:1710–5.
4. Bentley G, Biant LC, Carrington RW, Akmal M, Goldberg A, Williams AM, Skinner JA, Pringle J. A prospective, randomised comparison of autologous chondrocyte implantation versus mosaicplasty for osteochondral defects in the knee. J Bone Joint Surg Br. 2003;85:223–30.

5. Brittberg M, Lindahl A, Nilsson A, Ohlsson C, Isaksson O, Peterson L. Treatment of deep cartilage defects in the knee with autologous chondrocyte transplantation. N Engl J Med. 1994;331:889–95.
6. Buckwalter JA, Bowman GN, Albright JP, Wolf BR, Bollier M. Clinical outcomes of patellar chondral lesions treated with juvenile particulated cartilage allografts. Iowa Orthop J. 2014;34:44–9.
7. Cameron JI, Pulido PA, McCauley JC, Bugbee WD. Osteochondral allograft transplantation of the femoral trochlea. Am J Sports Med. 2016;44:633–8.
8. Carofino BC, Fulkerson JP. Anteromedialization of the tibial tubercle for patellofemoral arthritis in patients > 50 years. J Knee Surg. 2008;21:101–5.
9. Chahal J, Gross AE, Gross C, Mall N, Dwyer T, Chahal A, Whelan DB, Cole BJ. Outcomes of osteochondral allograft transplantation in the knee. Arthroscopy. 2013;29:575–88.
10. Cook JL, Stannard JP, Stoker AM, Bozynski CC, Kuroki K, Cook CR, Pfeiffer FM. Importance of donor chondrocyte viability for osteochondral allografts. Am J Sports Med. 2016;44:1260–8.
11. Ebert JR, Schneider A, Fallon M, Wood DJ, Janes GC. A comparison of 2-year outcomes in patients undergoing tibiofemoral or patellofemoral matrix-induced autologous chondrocyte implantation. Am J Sports Med. 2017;45:3243–53.
12. Elias DA, White LM, Fithian DC. Acute lateral patellar dislocation at MR imaging: injury patterns of medial patellar soft-tissue restraints and osteochondral injuries of the inferomedial patella. Radiology. 2002;225:736–43.
13. Farr J, Covell DJ, Lattermann C. Cartilage lesions in patellofemoral dislocations: incidents/locations/when to treat. Sports Med Arthrosc Rev. 2012;20:181–6.
14. Farr J, Tabet SK, Margerrison E, Cole BJ. Clinical, radiographic, and histological outcomes after cartilage repair with Particulated juvenile articular cartilage: a 2-year prospective study. Am J Sports Med. 2014;42:1417–25.
15. Ferguson AB Jr, Brown TD, Fu FH, Rutkowski R. Relief of patellofemoral contact stress by anterior displacement of the tibial tubercle. J Bone Joint Surg Am. 1979;61:159–66.
16. Filardo G, Kon E, Andriolo L, Di Martino A, Zaffagnini S, Marcacci M. Treatment of "patellofemoral" cartilage lesions with matrix-assisted autologous chondrocyte transplantation: a comparison of patellar and trochlear lesions. Am J Sports Med. 2014;42:626–34.
17. Franzone JM, Vitale MA, Shubin Stein BE, Ahmad CS. Is there an association between chronicity of patellar instability and patellofemoral cartilage lesions? An arthroscopic assessment of chondral injury. J Knee Surg. 2012;25:411–6.
18. Gillogly SD, Arnold RM. Autologous chondrocyte implantation and anteromedialization for isolated patellar articular cartilage lesions: 5- to 11-year follow-up. Am J Sports Med. 2014;42:912–20.
19. Gomoll AH, Gillogly SD, Cole BJ, Farr J, Arnold R, Hussey K, Minas T. Autologous chondrocyte implantation in the patella: a multicenter experience. Am J Sports Med. 2014;42:1074–81.
20. Gracitelli GC, Meric G, Pulido PA, Gortz S, De Young AJ, Bugbee WD. Fresh osteochondral allograft transplantation for isolated patellar cartilage injury. Am J Sports Med. 2015;43:879–84.
21. Grawe B, Burge A, Nguyen J, Strickland S, Warren R, Rodeo S, Shubin SB. Cartilage regeneration in full-thickness patellar chondral defects treated with Particulated juvenile articular allograft cartilage: an MRI analysis. Cartilage. 2017;8:374–83.
22. Grelsamer RP, Dejour D, Gould J. The pathophysiology of patellofemoral arthritis. Orthop Clin North Am. 2008;39:269–74. v
23. Hangody L, Fules P. Autologous osteochondral mosaicplasty for the treatment of full-thickness defects of weight-bearing joints: ten years of experimental and clinical experience. J Bone Joint Surg Am. 2003;85-A(Suppl 2):25–32.
24. Jang SJ, Kim JD, Cha SS. Platelet-rich plasma (PRP) injections as an effective treatment for early osteoarthritis. Eur J Orthop Surg Traumatol. 2013;23:573–80.
25. Kreuz PC, Steinwachs MR, Erggelet C, Krause SJ, Konrad G, Uhl M, Sudkamp N. Results after microfracture of full-thickness chondral defects in different compartments in the knee. Osteoarthr Cartil. 2006;14:1119–25.

26. Laskin RS, van Steijn M. Total knee replacement for patients with patellofemoral arthritis. Clin Orthop Relat Res. 1999;(367):89–95.
27. Liu JN, Wu HH, Garcia GH, Kalbian IL, Strickland SM, Shubin Stein BE. Return to Sports After Tibial Tubercle Osteotomy for Patellofemoral Pain and Osteoarthritis. *Arthroscopy*. 2018;34(4):1022–9.
28. Logan CA, Bhashyam AR, Tisosky AJ, Haber DB, Jorgensen A, Roy A, Provencher MT. Systematic review of the effect of taping techniques on patellofemoral pain syndrome. Sports Health. 2017;9:456–61.
29. Lonner JH. Patellofemoral arthroplasty. J Am Acad Orthop Surg. 2007;15:495–506.
30. Lonner JH. Patellofemoral arthroplasty: the impact of design on outcomes. Orthop Clin North Am. 2008;39:347–54. vi
31. Lonner JH, Bloomfield MR. The clinical outcome of patellofemoral arthroplasty. Orthop Clin North Am. 2013;44:271–80. vii
32. Matsushita T, Kuroda R, Oka S, Matsumoto T, Takayama K, Kurosaka M. Clinical outcomes of medial patellofemoral ligament reconstruction in patients with an increased tibial tuberosity-trochlear groove distance. Knee Surg Sports Traumatol Arthrosc. 2014;22:2438–44.
33. Meric G, Gracitelli GC, Gortz S, De Young AJ, Bugbee WD. Fresh osteochondral allograft transplantation for bipolar reciprocal osteochondral lesions of the knee. Am J Sports Med. 2015;43:709–14.
34. Meyerkort D, Ebert JR, Ackland TR, Robertson WB, Fallon M, Zheng MH, Wood DJ. Matrix-induced autologous chondrocyte implantation (MACI) for chondral defects in the patellofemoral joint. Knee Surg Sports Traumatol Arthrosc. 2014;22:2522–30.
35. Mithoefer K, McAdams T, Williams RJ, Kreuz PC, Mandelbaum BR. Clinical efficacy of the microfracture technique for articular cartilage repair in the knee: an evidence-based systematic analysis. Am J Sports Med. 2009;37:2053–63.
36. Mont MA, Haas S, Mullick T, Hungerford DS. Total knee arthroplasty for patellofemoral arthritis. J Bone Joint Surg Am. 2002;84-A:1977–81.
37. Nho SJ, Foo LF, Green DM, Shindle MK, Warren RF, Wickiewicz TL, Potter HG, Williams RJ 3rd. Magnetic resonance imaging and clinical evaluation of patellar resurfacing with press-fit osteochondral autograft plugs. Am J Sports Med. 2008;36:1101–9.
38. Nomura E, Inoue M. Cartilage lesions of the patella in recurrent patellar dislocation. Am J Sports Med. 2004;32:498–502.
39. Nomura E, Inoue M. Second-look arthroscopy of cartilage changes of the patellofemoral joint, especially the patella, following acute and recurrent patellar dislocation. Osteoarthr Cartil. 2005;13:1029–36.
40. Pascual-Garrido C, Slabaugh MA, L'Heureux DR, Friel NA, Cole BJ. Recommendations and treatment outcomes for patellofemoral articular cartilage defects with autologous chondrocyte implantation: prospective evaluation at average 4-year follow-up. Am J Sports Med. 2009;37(Suppl 1):33S–41S.
41. Pidoriano AJ, Weinstein RN, Buuck DA, Fulkerson JP. Correlation of patellar articular lesions with results from anteromedial tibial tubercle transfer. Am J Sports Med. 1997;25:533–7.
42. Redler L, Mayer G, Kalbian I, Nguyen J, Shubin Stein B, Strickland S. Does ligamentous laxity protect against chondral injury in patients with patellofemoral instability? *AOSSM 2016 Annual Meeting*. San Diego, CA: Orthop J Sports Med; 2016.
43. Rue JP, Colton A, Zare SM, Shewman E, Farr J, Bach BR Jr, Cole BJ. Trochlear contact pressures after straight anteriorization of the tibial tuberosity. Am J Sports Med. 2008;36:1953–9.
44. Stanitski CL, Paletta GA Jr. Articular cartilage injury with acute patellar dislocation in adolescents. Arthroscopic and radiographic correlation. Am J Sports Med. 1998;26:52–5.
45. Steadman JR, Briggs KK, Rodrigo JJ, Kocher MS, Gill TJ, Rodkey WG. Outcomes of microfracture for traumatic chondral defects of the knee: average 11-year follow-up. Arthroscopy. 2003;19:477–84.
46. Tauro B, Ackroyd CE, Newman JH, Shah NA. The Lubinus patellofemoral arthroplasty. A five- to ten-year prospective study. J Bone Joint Surg Br. 2001;83:696–701.

47. Thakkar RS, Del Grande F, Wadhwa V, Chalian M, Andreisek G, Carrino JA, Eng J, Chhabra A. Patellar instability: CT and MRI measurements and their correlation with internal derangement findings. Knee Surg Sports Traumatol Arthrosc. 2016;24:3021–8.
48. Tompkins M, Hamann JC, Diduch DR, Bonner KF, Hart JM, Gwathmey FW, Milewski MD, Gaskin CM. Preliminary results of a novel single-stage cartilage restoration technique: particulated juvenile articular cartilage allograft for chondral defects of the patella. Arthroscopy. 2013;29:1661–70.
49. Trinh TQ, Harris JD, Siston RA, Flanigan DC. Improved outcomes with combined autologous chondrocyte implantation and patellofemoral osteotomy versus isolated autologous chondrocyte implantation. Arthroscopy. 2013;29:566–74.
50. Van Haver A, De Roo K, De Beule M, Labey L, De Baets P, Dejour D, Claessens T, Verdonk P. The effect of trochlear dysplasia on patellofemoral biomechanics: a cadaveric study with simulated trochlear deformities. Am J Sports Med. 2015;43:1354–61.
51. von Rechenberg B, Akens MK, Nadler D, Bittmann P, Zlinszky K, Kutter A, Poole AR, Auer JA. Changes in subchondral bone in cartilage resurfacing--an experimental study in sheep using different types of osteochondral grafts. Osteoarthr Cartil. 2003;11:265–77.
52. Williams SK, Amiel D, Ball ST, Allen RT, Wong VW, Chen AC, Sah RL, Bugbee WD. Prolonged storage effects on the articular cartilage of fresh human osteochondral allografts. J Bone Joint Surg Am. 2003;85-A:2111–20.

Chapter 5
Imaging in Patellofemoral Pain

Vivek Kalia and Douglas N. Mintz

Anatomy and Biomechanics of the Patellofemoral Joint

Osseous Anatomy

The osseous structures which make up the patellofemoral joint are the *patella* and distal *femur*, specifically the trochlea.

The patella is divided by an eccentric longitudinal *median ridge* on the articular side (often miscalled the *apex)* and is thought of as having two major articulating facets: the *medial facet* and *lateral facet* (though a total of seven total facets exist). The lateral facet is typically longer and less acutely sloped (from the horizontal) compared to the medial facet (Fig. 5.1). The position of the median ridge delineates four different types of patellar morphology [59] (Fig. 5.2). Importantly, the articular surface of the patella constitutes only the superior 2/3 of the patella, as the distal pole serves only as the patellar tendon insertion [49].

The *trochlear groove* (TG) is the articulating surface of the distal femur with the patella. The normal TG depth is about 5.2 mm [43]. The lateral wall of the trochlear groove (i.e., the lateral femoral condyle) serves as the primary osseous restraint to lateral patellar subluxation and dislocation.

V. Kalia (✉) · D. N. Mintz
Hospital for Special Surgery, New York, NY, USA
e-mail: MintzD@hss.edu

B. E. Shubin Stein, S. M. Strickland (eds.), *Patellofemoral Pain and Instability*,
https://doi.org/10.1007/978-3-319-97640-2_5

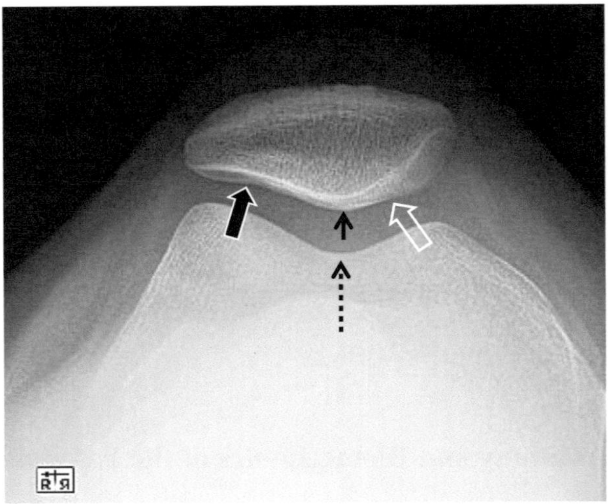

Fig. 5.1 Axial radiograph demonstrating normal anatomy of the patellofemoral joint. The lateral patellar facet (*black block arrow*) is typically longer and less acutely sloped (from the horizontal) compared to the medial patellar facet (*open block arrow*). The position of the median ridge (*solid thin arrow*) delineates four different types of patellar morphology. The trochlear sulcus is depicted by the *dashed arrow*

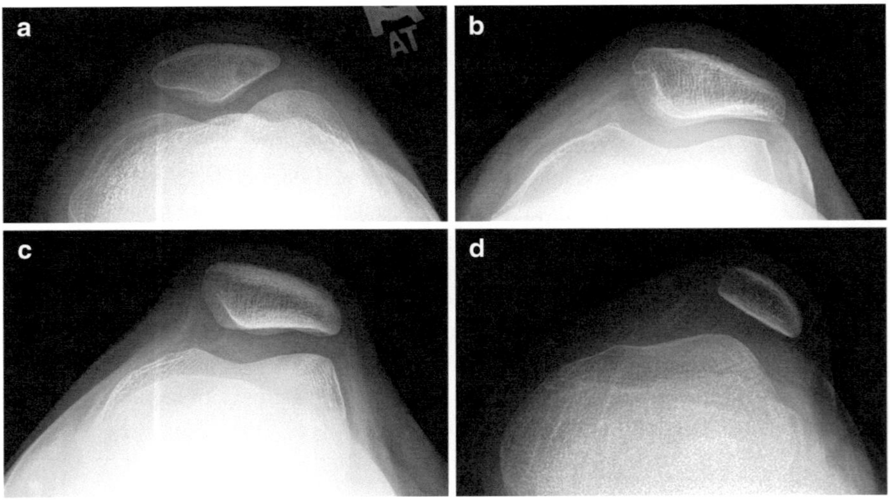

Fig. 5.2 Four axial radiographs demonstrate the four categories of patellar morphology. In *type I*, the median ridge is near the midline of a measurement of the medial-to-lateral distance of the patella. In *type II*, the median ridge resides in the normal position slightly off midline, creating an elongated lateral patellar facet and a relatively shorter medial patellar facet. In *type III*, the median ridge is more medialized, resulting in a very short medial patellar facet and a longer lateral patellar facet. In *type IV*, the median ridge is further medialized, leaving a nearly flat laterally sloped

Soft Tissue Anatomy

The *extensor mechanism* of the knee is a vital dynamic/active stabilizer of the patellofemoral joint. The *quadriceps tendon* is a confluence of four individual muscle tendons, the rectus femoris, the vastus lateralis, the vastus intermedius, and the vastus medialis muscles. The patella is a sesamoid bone within the quadriceps tendon. The portion of the patellar tendon distal to the patella is the *patellar tendon*. It runs from the inferior pole of the patella and inserts on the tibial tubercle. The average length of the patellar tendon is 4.6 cm (3.5–5.5 cm) [45].

The medial patellar stabilizers about the knee include the *medial patellofemoral ligament* (MPFL), *medial retinaculum*, *medial patellotibial ligament*, and the *vastus medialis oblique* (VMO), a portion of the vastus medialis muscle. The MPFL serves as the primary passive restraint to lateral patellar translation, particularly in early knee flexion. Laxity of the MPFL (whether congenital, traumatic, or iatrogenic) predisposes to patellar instability [1]. Together, the medial retinaculum and MPFL are the most important ligamentous stabilizers of the patellofemoral joint. The VMO muscle is the primary dynamic muscular restraint to lateral patellar tracking [21].

The primary lateral patellar soft tissue stabilizer is the *lateral retinaculum*, which comprises multiple (superficial and deep) layers. Tightness of the lateral retinaculum may result in lateral patellar tilt and lateral patellofemoral compartment overload.

Biomechanics

Anatomic function of the patellofemoral compartment requires congruency and synergy of its osseous and soft tissue components. In full extension, the patella sits in a slightly lateralized position relative to the trochlea. Throughout the normal motion arc, different components play critical roles depending on the degree of flexion of the knee. From 0° (full extension) to 30° flexion, the MPFL plays the primary role in preventing lateral patellar maltracking and a slight medial patellar shift occurs as the patella begins to engage with the trochlear groove. At about 20–30° of flexion, the patella engages in the trochlea, providing an additional (bony) stabilizer against lateral patellar maltracking. Up to about 60° of flexion, the surface area of contact between the trochlea and patella increases, increasing stability. As flexion angle increases further, the force vectors conveyed by the quadriceps and patellar tendons converge into an axially oriented patellofemoral joint reaction force (PFJRF), further increasing patellofemoral joint stability [49].

Anatomic Variants Not Typically Associated with Pain

A *bipartite patella* (Fig. 5.3) results from failed fusion of a secondary ossification center with the body of the patella during development. It is usually asymptomatic and can be bilateral in up to 40% of cases. It is nine times more common in males than females. Of importance, the associated patellar articular cartilage in a bipartite patella remains intact. In the setting of trauma or overuse, the synchondrosis at the failed fusion site may be disrupted and allow for abnormal motion or friction, which may result in pain and associated imaging findings of bone marrow edema on MRI [27].

The *dorsal defect of the patella* or *central patellar defect* (Fig. 5.4) is an anatomic variant represented by a benign well-defined subchondral lesion in the superolateral aspect of the patella. The overlying cartilage is nearly always intact, and on MRI, the overlying cartilage may appear thickened to fill the subchondral defect. It may be part of the spectrum of a bipartite patella but further along in evolution to normal.

Anatomic Variants Commonly Associated with Pain and/or Instability

Patients with *trochlear dysplasia* have trochlear grooves which are significantly shallower than normal. Trochlear dysplasia alters the contact forces of the patellofemoral joint and increases the risk of osteoarthritis. There is loss of bony restraint of the patella within the trochlear groove. Measurements of trochlear depth are best made on midsagittal MR images about 3 cm above the femorotibial joint space [43]. The Dejour classification [11–13] of trochlear dysplasia [30] (Fig. 5.5) is commonly referenced and is actually two slightly different classification schemes developed by two different French orthopedic surgeons Henri Dejour and his son David Henri Dejour.

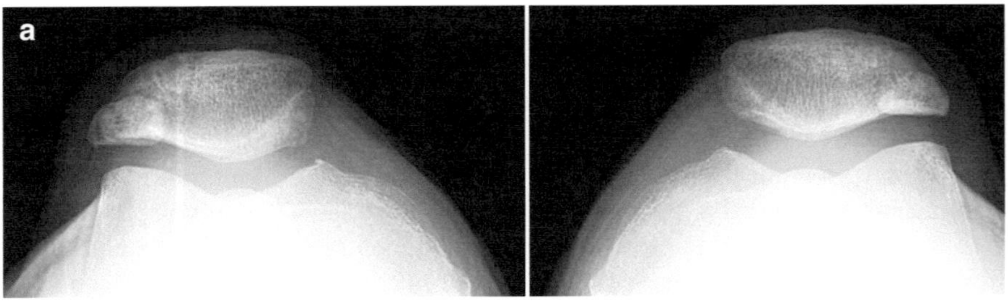

Fig. 5.3 Axial radiograph and single AP radiograph of a patient with bilateral bipartite patellae

Fig. 5.3 (continued)

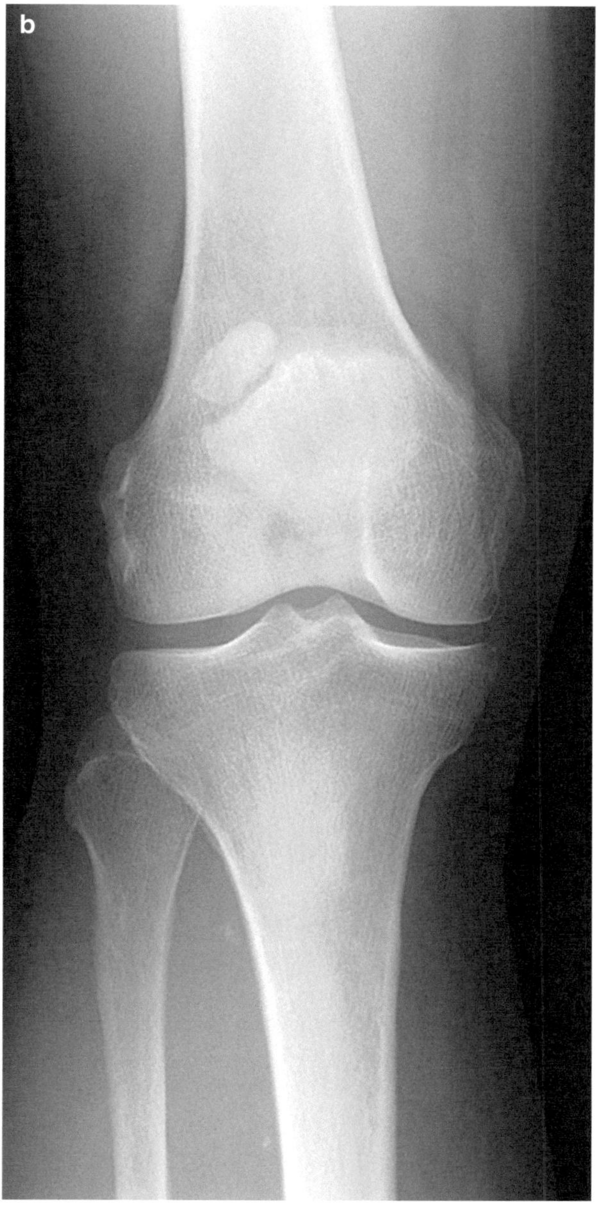

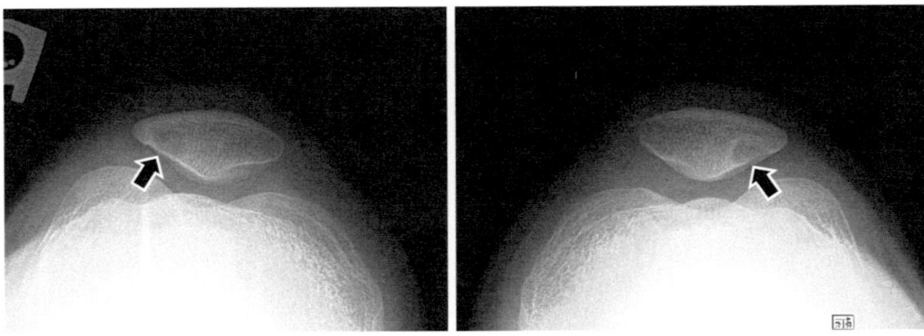

Fig. 5.4 Axial radiograph of both knees demonstrates bilateral findings of rounded radiolucencies (*black block arrows*) with vague sclerotic margins in the lateral aspect of the patellae, consistent with bilateral dorsal defects of the patella, which are normal anatomic variants and represent "do not touch" lesions

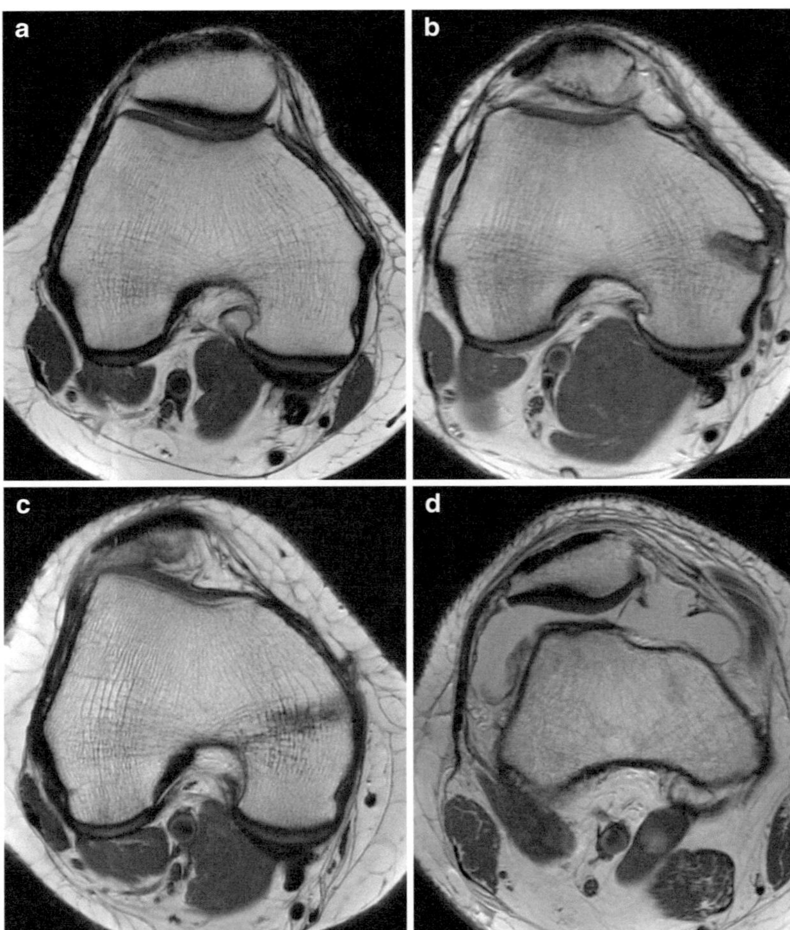

Fig. 5.5 Dejour classification system for trochlear dysplasia, types A, B, C, and D (panels **a–d**, respectively)

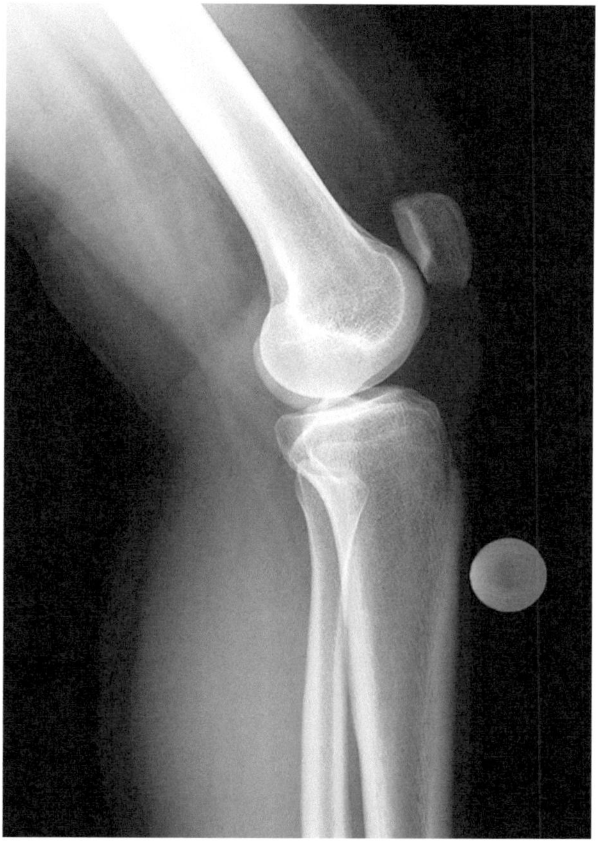

Fig. 5.6 Lateral radiograph demonstrates a high-riding patella, consistent with patella alta

Patella alta (Fig. 5.6) results from high positioning of the patella relative to the trochlea and an elongated patellar tendon. This anatomic alignment of the patella and femur requires higher flexion at the knee for the patella to become engaged in the trochlear groove, allowing for a larger arc along which patients are predisposed to abnormal patellar translation such as subluxation or dislocation [47]. Patella alta (and its opposite, *patella baja*, a low-riding patella [Fig. 5.7]) is defined by various measurements (detailed below). Patella alta increases the contact forces on the distal patella and can contribute to patellofemoral joint pain.

Imaging of the Patellofemoral Joint

Radiography

The patellofemoral joint is optimally imaged using a combination of radiographs and cross-sectional imaging. A *radiographic series* including axial views is the best initial evaluation of the joint space, patellar position, and patellar alignment

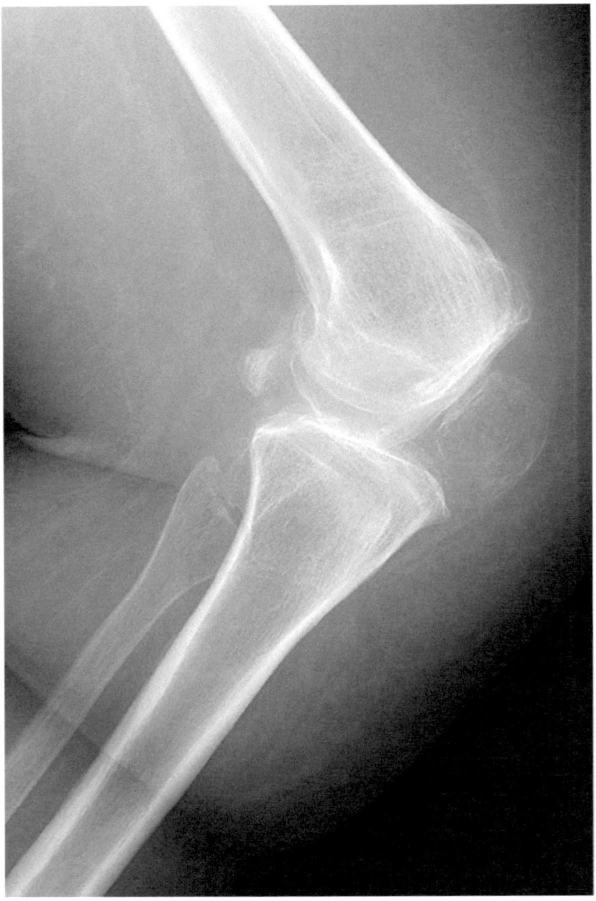

Fig. 5.7 Lateral radiograph of patient with known history of polio demonstrates a low-lying patella, consistent with patella baja. Incidental note is also made of a fabella, bony demineralization, and a dysplastic proximal tibia

(Fig. 5.8). Axial images can be obtained either with or without a device to hold position. The Merchant view [36] uses a device and can be set at various angles of knee flexion (usually 30 or 45 degrees) [40]. Multiple named slightly different views (Laurin, Settegast, Hughston, Knutsson views [31]) do not use devices. As a group they are referred to as sunrise or skyline views. A sample traditional Merchant view of the knee is depicted in Fig. 5.9. Proper positioning is illustrated in textbooks on radiographic technique.

Patellar alignment or *tilt* (Fig. 5.10) may be assessed on standardized axial radiographs using any of several available methods: (1) drawing two parallel lines, one along the lateral patellar facet and one along the anterior condylar margins and assessing visually for tilt, or (2) measuring the angle between a line drawn parallel to the posterior femoral condyles and a line drawn from the median ridge through the edge of the lateral patellar facet (Fig. 5.11). Normal patellar tilt is 2°, whereas >5° tilt is considered abnormal. Commonly measured patellofemoral indices of

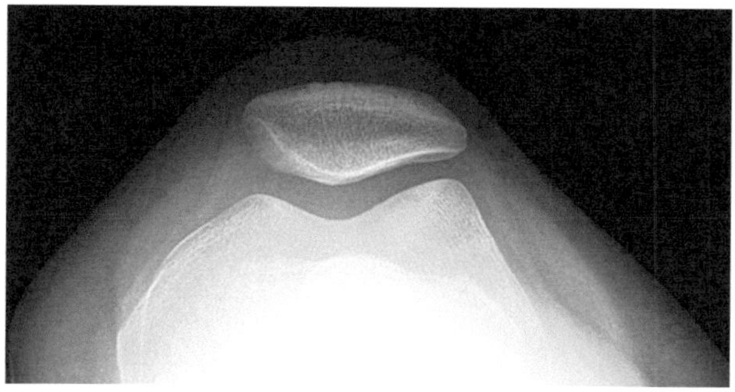

Fig. 5.8 An axial view of the knee, which is the best initial radiographic evaluation of the joint space, patellar position, and patellar alignment

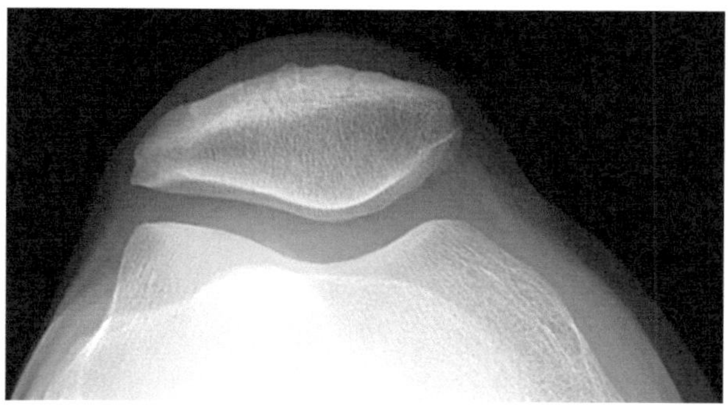

Fig. 5.9 Normal sunrise view of the knee highlighting the patellofemoral joint

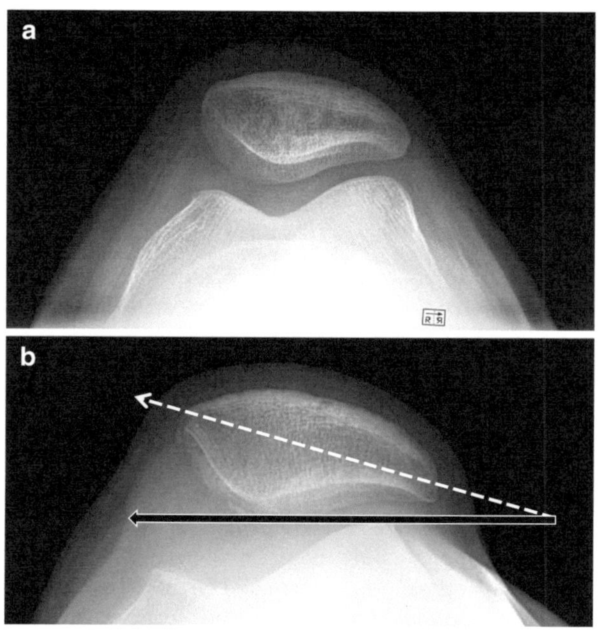

Fig. 5.10 Panel **a** is an axial radiograph showing mild lateral patellar tilt without patellar subluxation. Panel **b** is an axial radiograph showing moderate patellar tilt with patellar subluxation. Patellar tilt here is measured as the angle between two lines: (1) a horizontal line extending from the anterior edge of the lateral trochlear facet (*black block arrow*) and (2) a line extending from that same point parallel to the long axis of the patella (*dashed white arrow*)

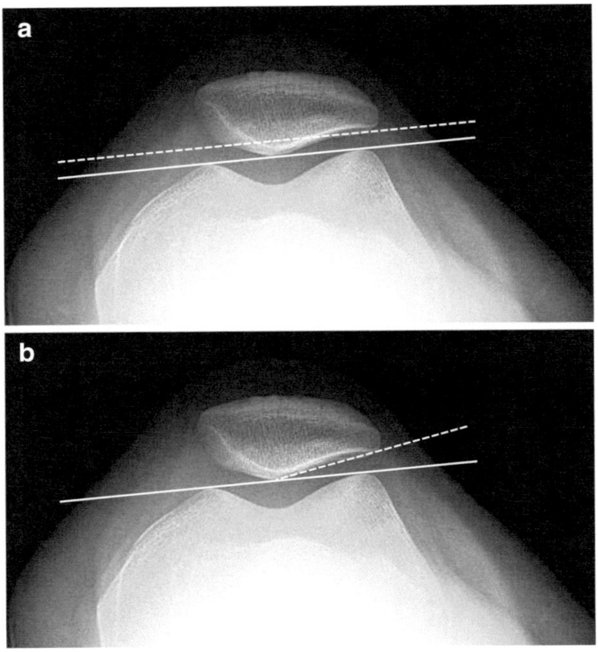

Fig. 5.11 Two axial radiographs demonstrating alternative ways to measure patellar tilt. Panel **a** draws two lines, one along the lateral patellar facet (*dashed white line*) and one along the anterior condylar margins (*solid white line*), and assesses visually for tilt. When there is no patellar tilt, the two lines should be parallel, as depicted in panel (a), with normal patellofemoral alignment and without patellar tilt. Panel **b** shows another method of patellar tilt measurement: measure the angle between a line drawn along the anterior condylar margins (*solid white line*) and a line drawn from the median ridge to the edge of the lateral patellar facet (*dashed white line*)

patellofemoral kinematics include patellar tilt angle, lateral patellofemoral angle, lateral subluxation distance, lateral patellar displacement, and congruence angle [29].

The lateral radiograph is best evaluation of patellar height. Methods of evaluating patellar height on radiograph include Insall-Salvati [26], Caton-Deschamps, and Blackburne-Peel (Fig. 5.12). These methods have been adapted for cross-sectional imaging. The Caton-Deschamps measurement method is preferred because it remains accurate regardless of degree of knee flexion [5]. In addition, the Caton-Deschamps measurement (as well as the Blackburne-Peel) references the articular length of the patella relative to the proximal tibia. Thus, these measures of patella height will change if a patient has undergone a distalizing procedure (i.e., for severe patella alta), whereas the Insall-Salvati will remain the same because it references the length of the patella tendon which does not change when a distalizing procedure is done through moving the tibial tubercle.

Trochlear dysplasia is evaluated on lateral and axial radiographs, but more easily on cross-sectional imaging. Imaging features of trochlear dysplasia are found in

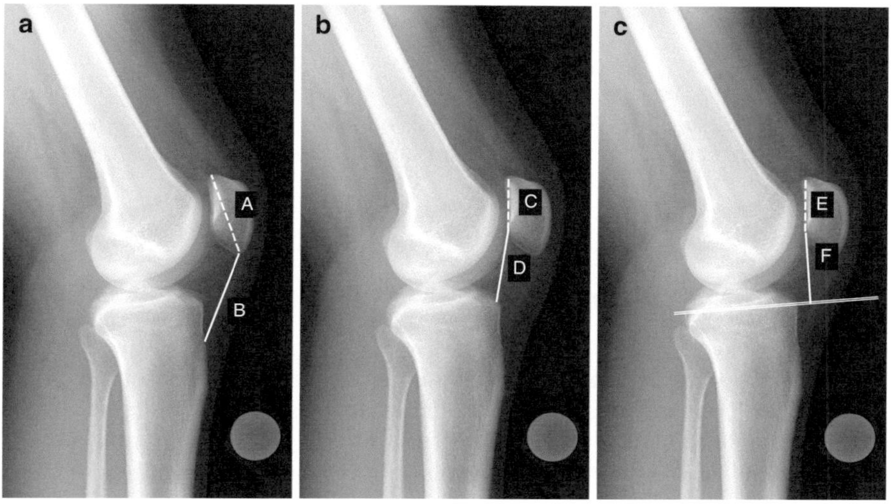

Fig. 5.12 Three methods of evaluating patellar height on lateral knee radiograph including Insall-Salvati ratio (panel **a**), Caton-Deschamps index (panel **b**), and Blackburne-Peel ratio (panel **c**)

more than 85% of patients with patellar dislocation [10]. On perfect lateral radiographic views, a trochlear depth of <5 mm suggests a risk of patellar instability [18]. Lateral radiographic views can be used to assess for Dejour A–D types of trochlear dysplasia by assessing for the crossing sign, a supratrochlear spur, and the double contour sign [30]. On axial radiographs, a sulcus angle of 145° or greater indicates a dysplastic trochlea [11]. The medial and lateral trochlear inclination can also be helpful to assess the severity of trochlear dysplasia [2].

Computed Tomography (CT)

Computed tomography is an imaging technique that uses ionizing radiation (like x-ray) to produce images. These images are tomographic and can be reconstructed in any plane. All of the measurements made on radiograph can also be made on CT, which provides a more detailed look at trochlear and patellar shape. CT scans can also be made into three-dimensional models. CT provides exquisite bone detail. It is faster than and less confining than MRI, better allowing for kinematic imaging.

To evaluate patellofemoral tracking, CT scans can be repeated at various degrees of flexion (0°, 30°, 45°, 60°) to see how the patella engages in the trochlea. Real-time imaging of knee motion is currently being developed and has been used predominantly for research applications. Although these advantages exist, for the purpose of evaluating patellofemoral disease, CT is usually reserved for evaluating union of tibial tubercle osteotomies or to obtain 3D imaging in patients with a contraindication to MR imaging (e.g., pacemaker).

Ultrasound

Ultrasound is a noninvasive imaging technique that uses sound waves to produce images. It is valuable in looking at superficial soft tissue structures such as the quadriceps/patellar tendons but also at muscles and, in experienced hands, retinacular structures.

Magnetic Resonance Imaging

Magnetic resonance imaging (MRI) offers excellent soft tissue contrast and allows detailed patellofemoral joint imaging in multiple planes. MRI can image bone and soft tissue, including articular cartilage. Various methods for imaging cartilage exist (see *Cartilage Imaging* section). The authors prefer morphologic imaging using an intermediate-echo-time 2D non fat-suppressed fast/turbo spin echo sequence at high resolution which allows evaluation of cartilage zonal anatomy [50]. Other techniques allow for quantitative evaluation of cartilage composition and health.

Like CT, MR is a tomographic technique on which all the measurements from radiographs can be readily performed and morphologic evaluation of patellar and trochlear shape is straight forward.

Patellofemoral Disorders/Specific Causes of Patellofemoral Pain

Specific causes of patellofemoral pain can be broadly split into three categories: (1) acute trauma, (2) overuse injuries ± anatomic issues, and (3) arthritis. Which imaging findings directly correlate and predict pain are unclear [55], but cartilage lesions and bone marrow edema appear to correlate to pain [51].

Acute traumatic causes of anterior knee pain, or specifically patellofemoral pain, include patellar fractures, quadriceps or patellar tendon rupture (Fig. 5.13), and patellar maltracking or patellofemoral instability (*see* Chap. 10: Imaging in Patellofemoral Instability), which may result in the clinical entity of patellofemoral pain syndrome. There may be an association of pain with a valgus knee or lateralized weight-bearing axis.

Patellofemoral maltracking is discussed in detail in Chap. 10: Imaging in Patellofemoral Instability and is a common cause of patellofemoral pain.

Common *overuse injuries* that may lead to patellofemoral pain include tendinosis of the quadriceps and patellar tendons, prepatellar bursitis, fat pad impingement, and patellofemoral overload. Other traction-related causes of patellofemoral or

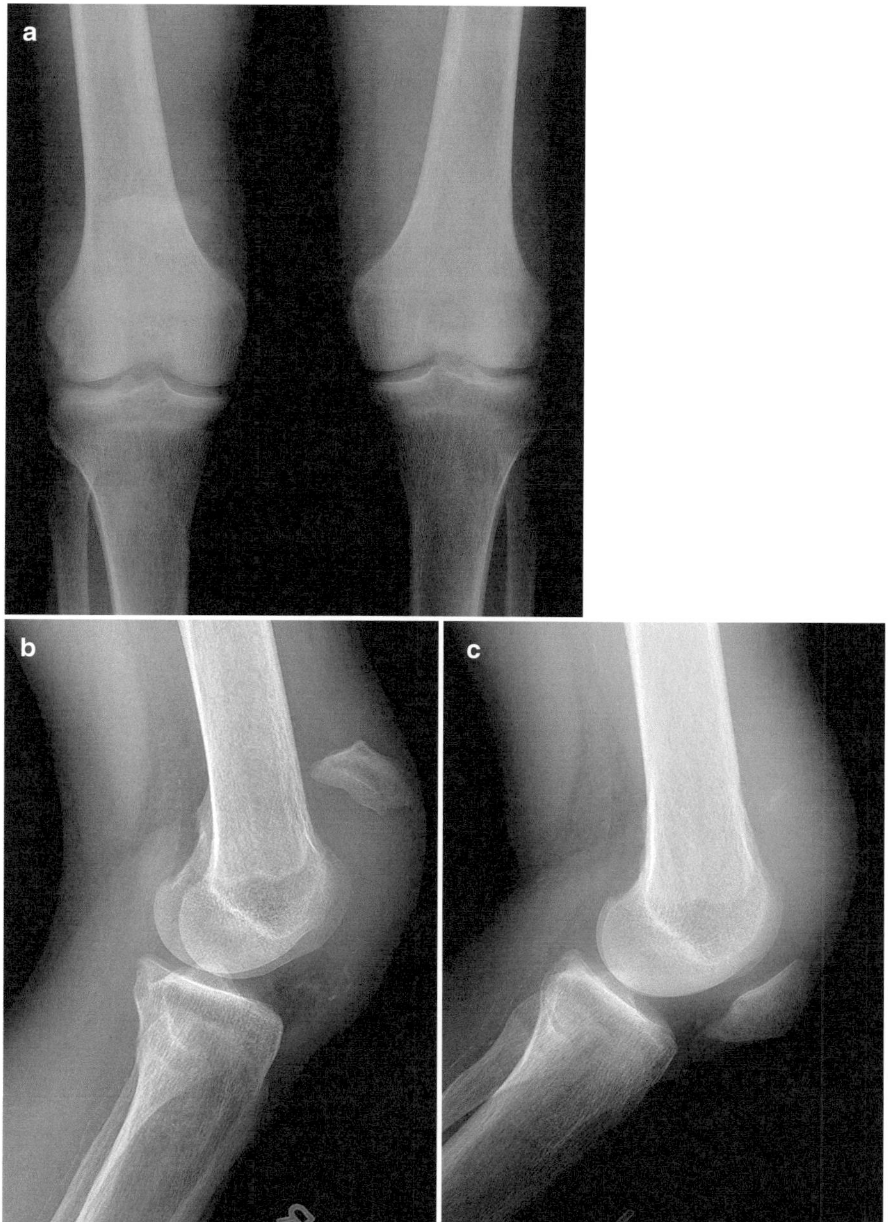

Fig. 5.13 AP (panel **a**) and lateral weight-bearing radiographs of both knees in a patient who is status-post fall. Images demonstrate right-sided patellar tendon rupture with resultant traumatic patella alta (panel **b**) and left-sided quadriceps tendon rupture with resultant traumatic patella baja (panel **c**)

anterior knee pain include *Osgood-Schlatter syndrome* (Fig. 5.14) at the patellar tendon insertion on the tibial tuberosity and *Sinding-Larsen-Johansson syndrome*, a traction apophysitis of the inferior pole of the patella. Medial *plicae* (Fig. 5.15), remnants of embryologic tissue in the knee, may cause medial patellofemoral pain or mechanical clicking or snapping.

Quadriceps and *patellar tendinopathy* consist of structural degeneration of the involved tendons and resultant decreased tensile resistive strength. The extensor mechanism of the knee can be imaged using ultrasound and MRI (Fig. 5.16) better than on radiograph.

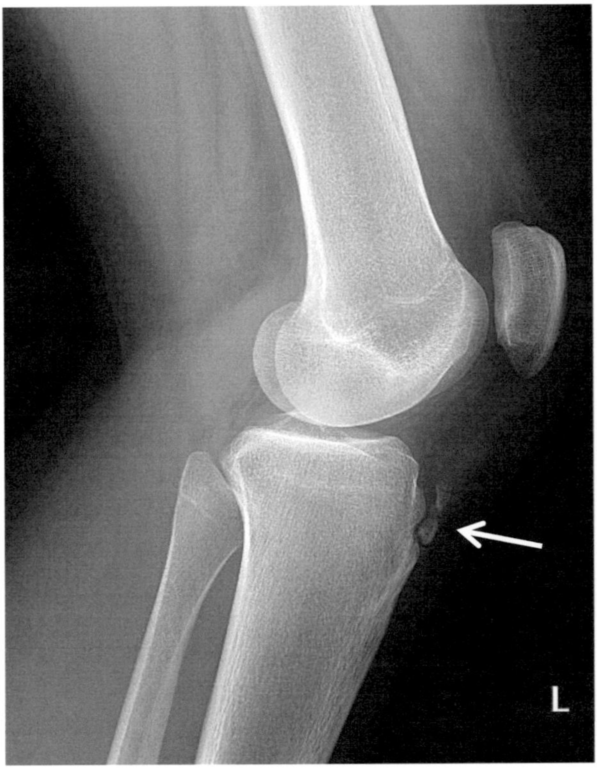

Fig. 5.14 Lateral radiograph of the knee demonstrates patella alta and findings of Osgood-Schlatter disease, including bony fragmentation (*white arrow*) at the tibial tuberosity at the insertion site of the patellar tendon

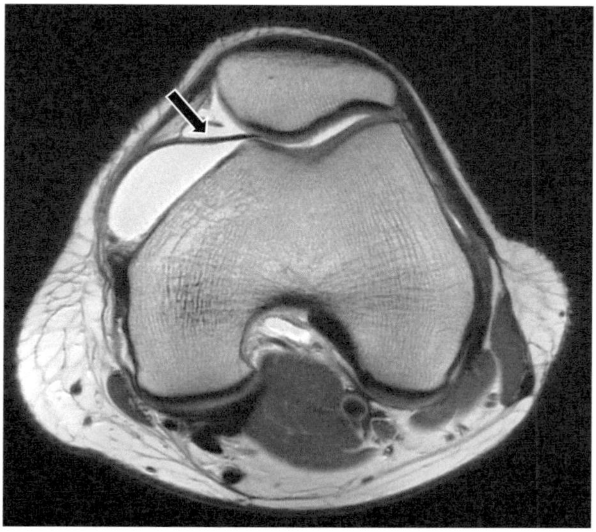

Fig. 5.15 Axial proton density-weighted MR image of the knee shows a medial parapatellar plica insinuating itself into the patellofemoral joint (*black block arrow*)

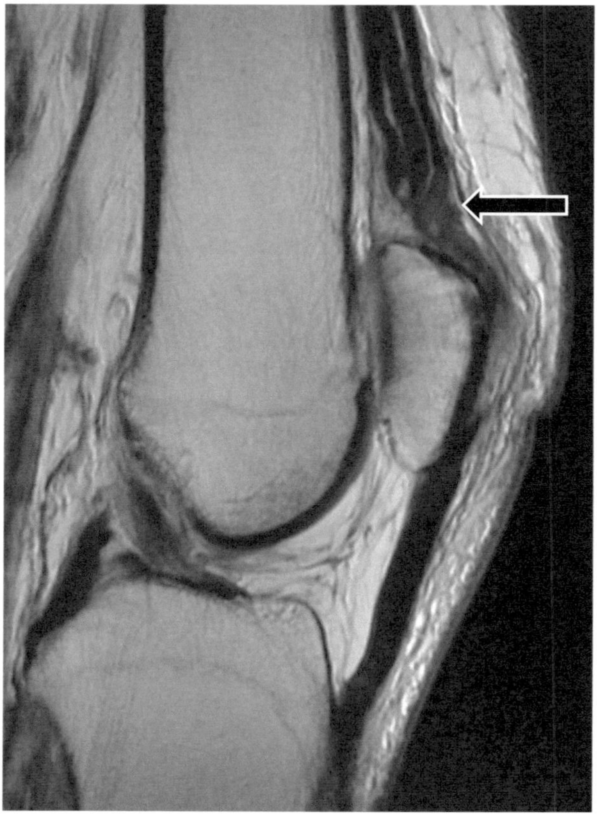

Fig. 5.16 Sagittal proton density-weighted MR image of the knee demonstrates a thickened distal quadriceps tendon with intermediate intrasubstance signal, indicating tendinosis (*black block arrow*)

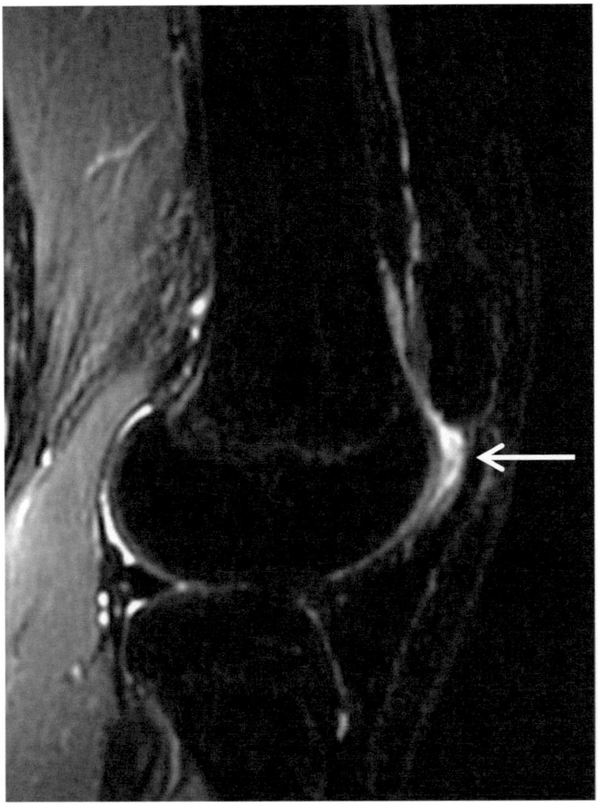

Fig. 5.17 Sagittal fluid-sensitive MR image demonstrates typical findings of fat pad impingement, including high signal intensity in the posterosuperior aspect of Hoffa's infrapatellar fat pad (*white arrow*)

Fat pad impingement is a more recently recognized cause of anterior knee pain [24]. Fat pad impingement is often associated with at least some degree of patellofemoral dysplasia and usually presents with anterior knee pain. It is best diagnosed on MRI (Fig. 5.17), where any of the three fat pads including the anterior suprapatellar, posterior suprapatellar, and infrapatellar fat pads may demonstrate increased signal intensity on fluid-sensitive sequences. The infrapatellar fat laterally is most commonly affected. Potential etiologies for fat pad impingement include patellofemoral instability, repetitive microtrauma, or direct trauma, all of which can cause injury to the knee fat pads and lead to hemorrhage, inflammation and pain, and fibrosis [19, 46].

Iliotibial band friction syndrome (Fig. 5.18) and certain forms of fat pad impingement may be different manifestations of a recently recognized entity known as *lat-*

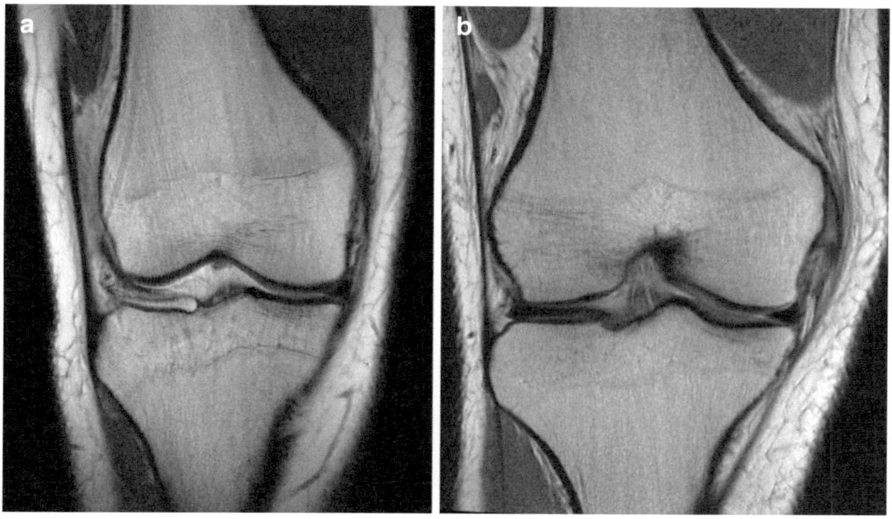

Fig. 5.18 Coronal proton density-weighted MR images in a symptomatic runner with iliotibial band friction syndrome (Panel **a**) and in a comparison asymptomatic patient (Panel **b**). Panel **a** shows increased soft tissue edema and infiltration deep to the iliotibial band and adjacent to the lateral femoral condyle

eral patellofemoral overload syndrome [53]. This overload occurs in patients with activity-related symptoms who demonstrate findings of superolateral fat pad impingement and/or iliotibial band syndrome on MRI. When imaged after a provocative activity such as running, features of both iliotibial band and lateral patellofemoral overload syndromes are often seen.

Even with normal anatomy and biomechanics, the forces that the patellofemoral joint experiences are very high: 2–5 times body weight with normal activities and 7–8 times body weight with squatting in high flexion [58]. Abnormal patellar tilt and tight retinacular support structures can lead to abnormal forces across the patellofemoral joint which can predispose to focal chondral degeneration [20]. This entity is known as *patellofemoral overload* (Fig. 5.19).

Articular cartilage abnormalities, ranging from focal defects (Fig. 5.20) to patellofemoral joint arthritis, can cause anterior knee pain. Osteochondral abnormalities include fractures, osteochondritis dissecans (a specific type of fracture), and chondral delaminating injuries that include a portion of the subchondral bone. Abnormalities isolated to cartilage are both structural (fibrillation, flaps, fissures,

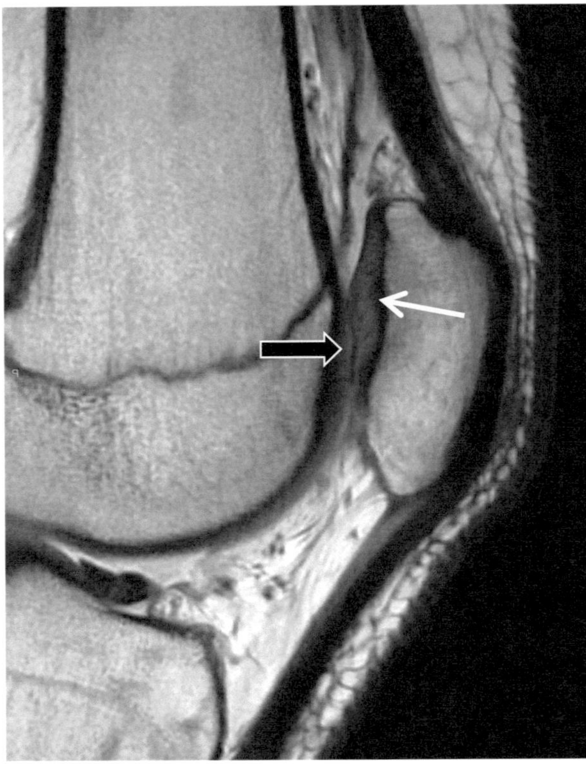

Fig. 5.19 Sagittal proton density-weighted MR image shows findings suggestive of patellofemoral overload with mild deformity and altered signal (hyperintensity) in the patellar (*white arrow*) and trochlear (*black block arrow*) cartilage

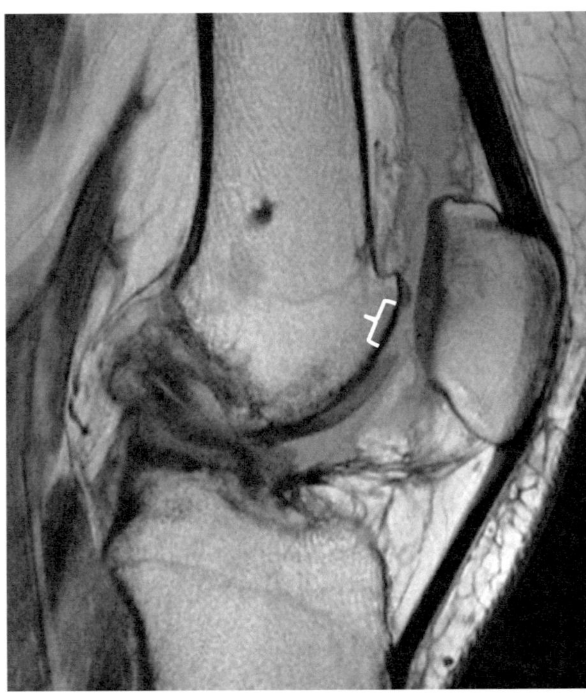

Fig. 5.20 Sagittal proton density-weighted MR image shows a focal full-thickness chondral defect in the trochlear cartilage (*white bracket*). Incidental note is made of a suprapatellar knee joint effusion

defects of various depths) and ultrastructural (softening). A classification system for cartilage abnormalities was developed in 1997 by the International Cartilage Repair Society (ICRS) based on the Outerbridge arthroscopic classification system which divides lesions into four grades based on depth [38]. The ICRS classification system uses the same four grades and describes the corresponding MRI findings [50, 3] (Table 5.1).

Isolated patellofemoral *osteoarthritis* (Fig. 5.21) is uncommon when compared to medial and/or lateral femorotibial compartments or combined patellofemoral and femorotibial arthritis. Incidence of isolated patellofemoral osteoarthritis has been reported as approximately 13–15% in symptomatic knees in patients older than 60 [9] and in about 19% of asymptomatic men and 34% of asymptomatic women [34]. Specific risk factors for patellofemoral joint osteoarthritis include patella alta, trochlear dysplasia, patellofemoral joint malalignment, and calcium pyrophosphate deposition disease [52]. Interestingly, the same group of investigators, using a 7-year follow-up longitudinal study design, found that most knees which ended up with multi-compartmental osteoarthritis started with damage isolated to the patellofemoral joint.

Table 5.1 Classification of cartilage injury by MRI, based on the International Cartilage Repair Society Classification System

MRI grade	Description of findings on MRI	Representative images
0	Normal cartilage Normal grayscale stratification	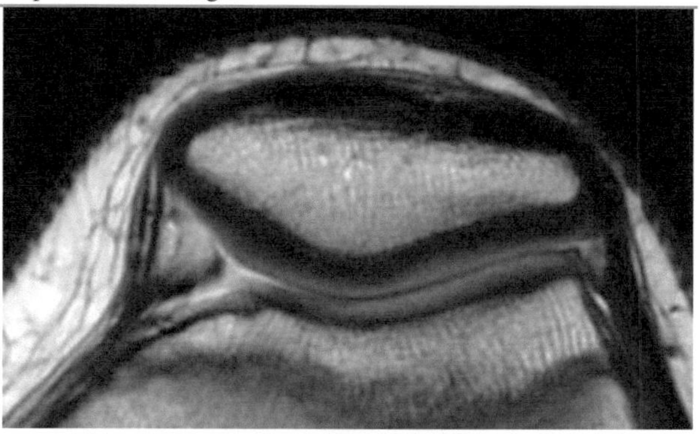
1	Chondral signal hyperintensity without focal defect	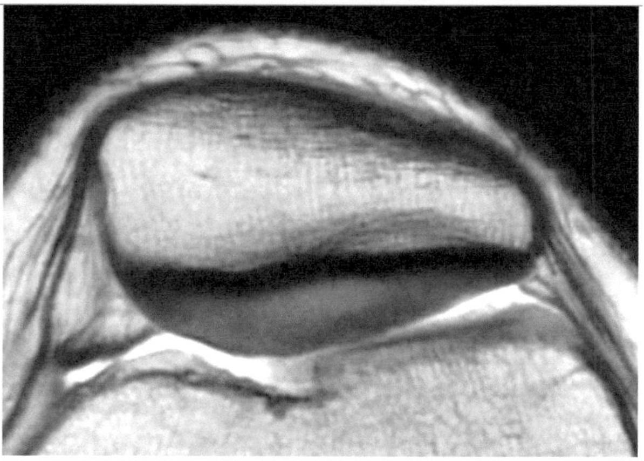

(continued)

Table 5.1 (continued)

MRI grade	Description of findings on MRI	Representative images
2	Fissures or fibrillation Involving less than 50% of the articular cartilage thickness	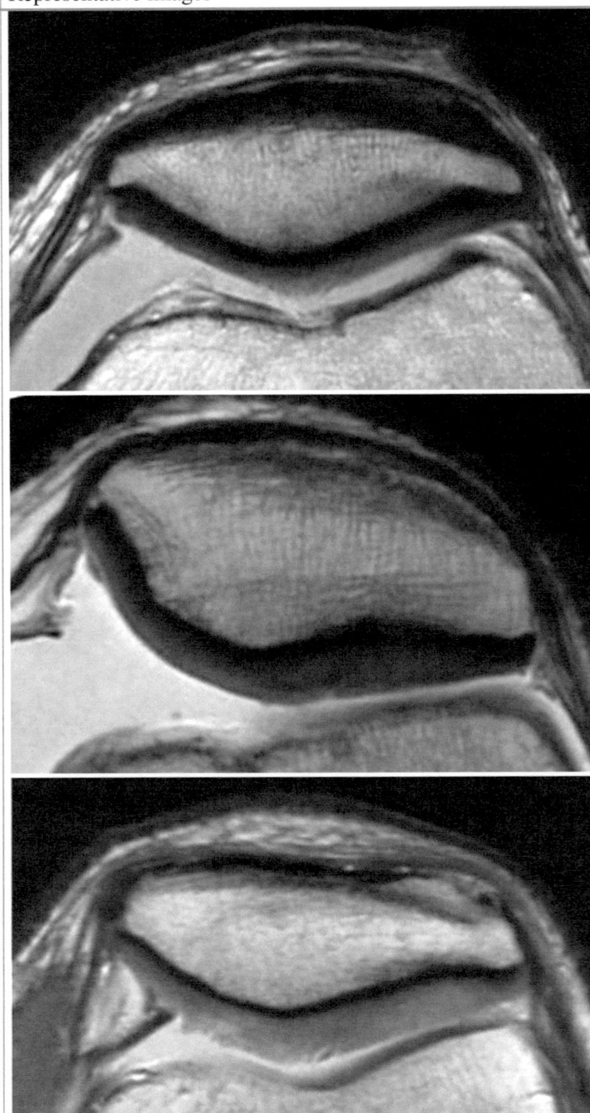

Table 5.1 (continued)

MRI grade	Description of findings on MRI	Representative images
3	Fissures or fibrillation or blistering Involving more than 50% of the articular cartilage thickness	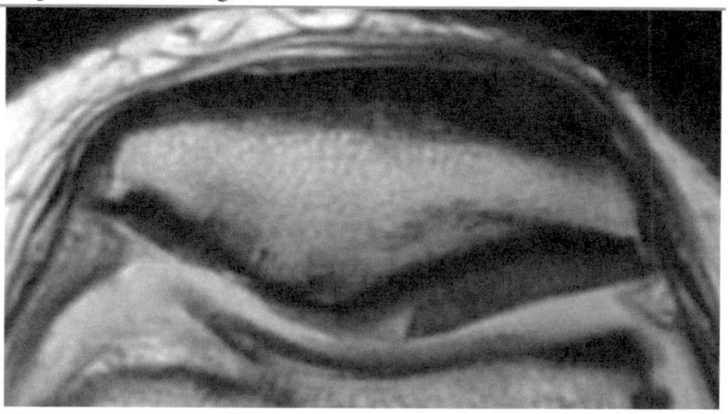
4	Complete, full-thickness cartilage loss Exposed subchondral bone	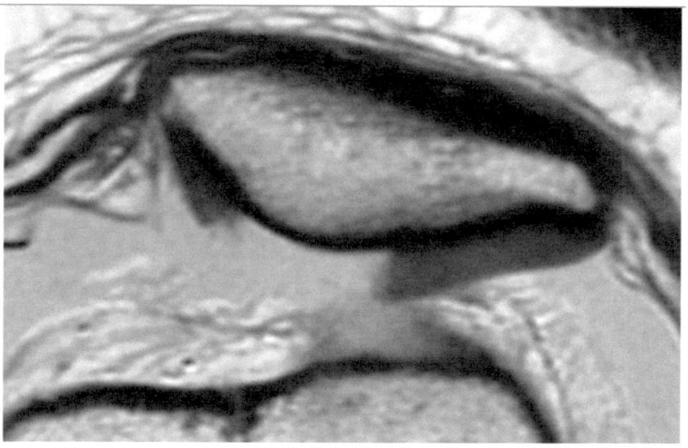

Patellofemoral Joint Replacement

Isolated patellofemoral joint replacements (Figs. 5.22 and 5.23) are becoming a more common treatment for isolated end-stage patellofemoral arthritis with pain. On imaging, they have aligned metal components with little, if any, interface between the components and the underlying bone. Like total joint arthroplasties, they cause artifact on CT and MRI, though the artifact tends to be less problematic for interpretation compared with total knee arthroplasties [23]. These artifacts can be partially overcome by adjusting scanning parameters.

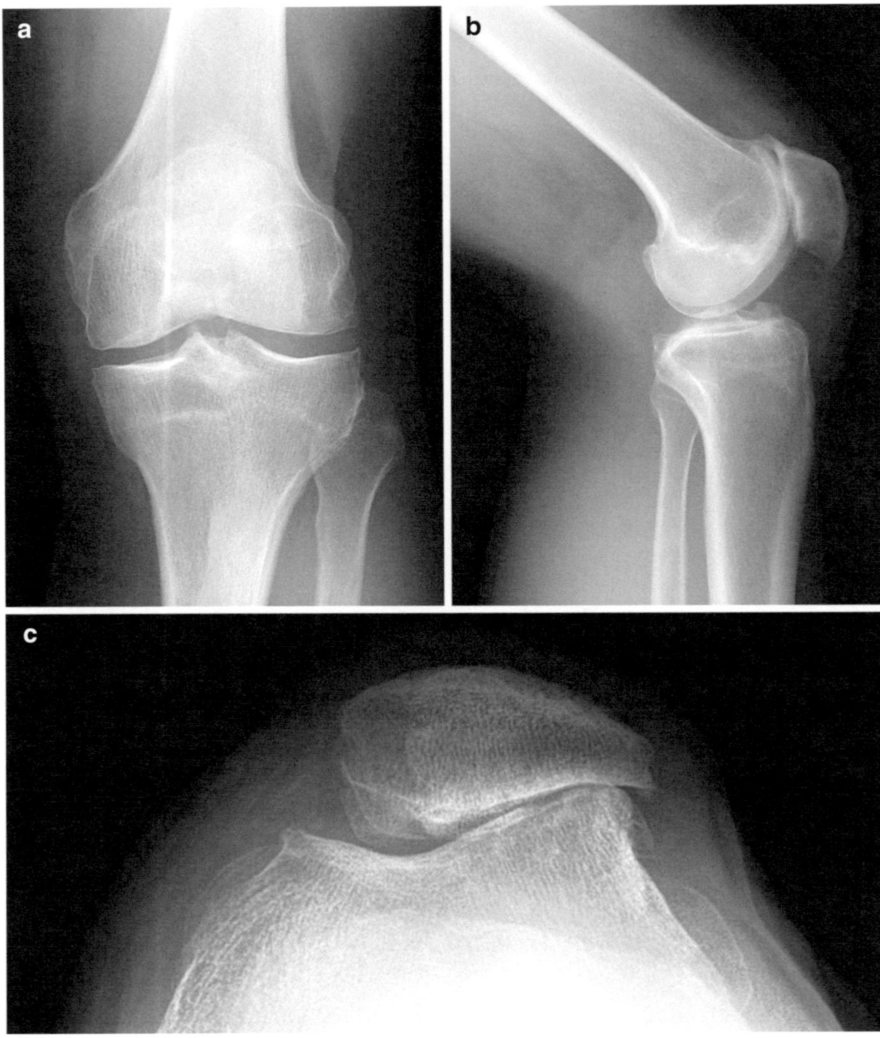

Fig. 5.21 AP, lateral, and axial radiographic views and corresponding axial proton density-weighted MR image of the knee demonstrate findings of osteoarthritis preferential to the patellofemoral joint. There is relative sparing of the medial and lateral femorotibial compartment, with small marginal osteophytes noted and spurring of the tibial spines. There is severe joint space narrowing, subchondral bone plate irregularity, and full-thickness cartilage loss (*white bracket*) on both sides of the joint in the lateral aspect of the patellofemoral compartment

Fig. 5.21 (continued)

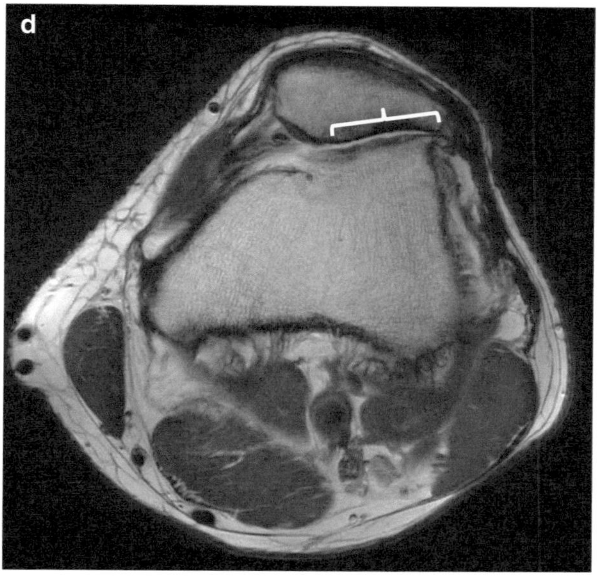

Cartilage Imaging

Imaging of cartilage is best performed with MRI. Various pulse sequences have been studied to define both morphologic and ultrastructural properties of cartilage (those not visible on routine imaging). Though institutional variations in imaging sequence preferences exist for cartilage, for morphologic imaging, the authors use a high-resolution sequence which optimizes evaluation of articular cartilage for surface delamination, fissures, and clefts, as well as overall morphology. Commonly, proton density-weighted fast spin echo sequences are employed to image cartilage [17]. Such sequences have high in-plane resolution [17] and have been shown to have high sensitivity (87%), specificity (94%), and accuracy (92%) for detection of chondral lesions in the knee joint [44]. Though isotropic 3D MRI acquisitions may be employed in the future in combination with radial and conventional three-plane reformatted images for evaluation of knee cartilage [22], 2D imaging remains the standard at present in terms of balancing clinical efficacy and efficiency.

Other protocols may include gradient recalled echo (GRE) or fat-suppressed sequences.

Traumatic chondral lesions are often graded using semiquantitative scoring systems such as the Whole-Organ Magnetic Resonance Imaging Score (WORMS) [41]

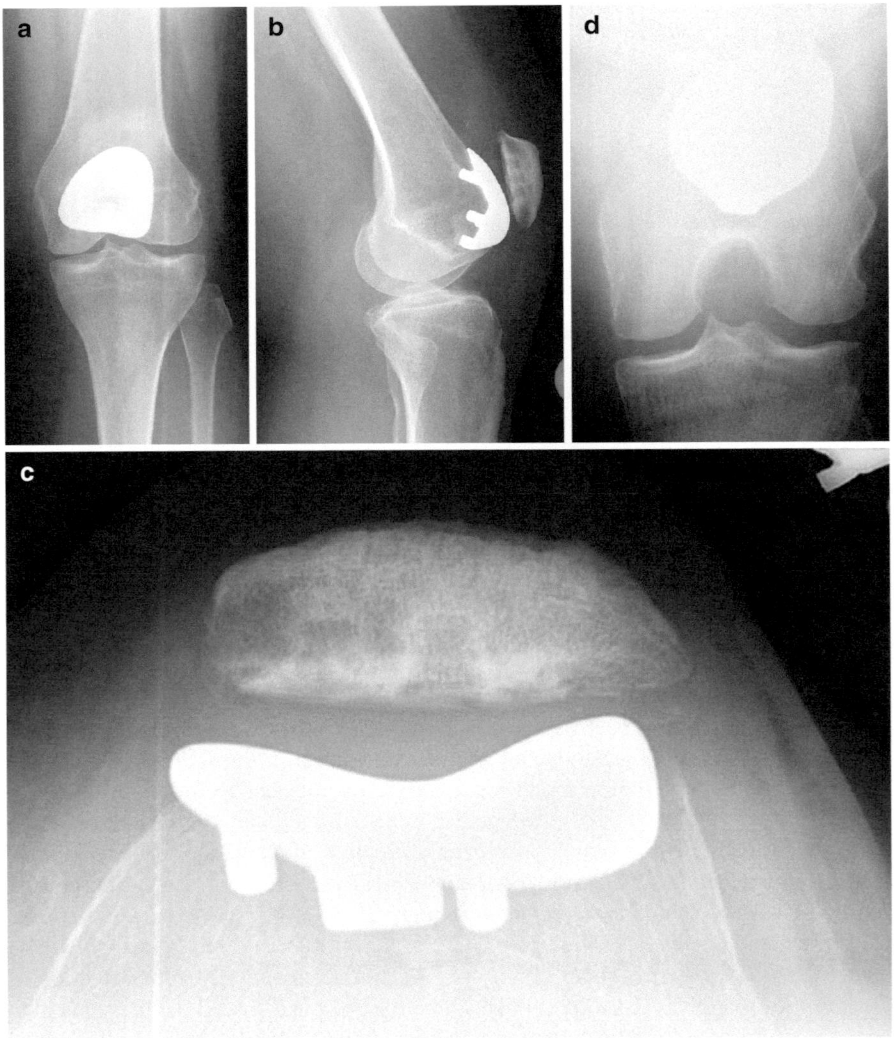

Fig. 5.22 AP, lateral, Merchant, and tunnel views of a patient who has undergone isolated patellofemoral joint replacement

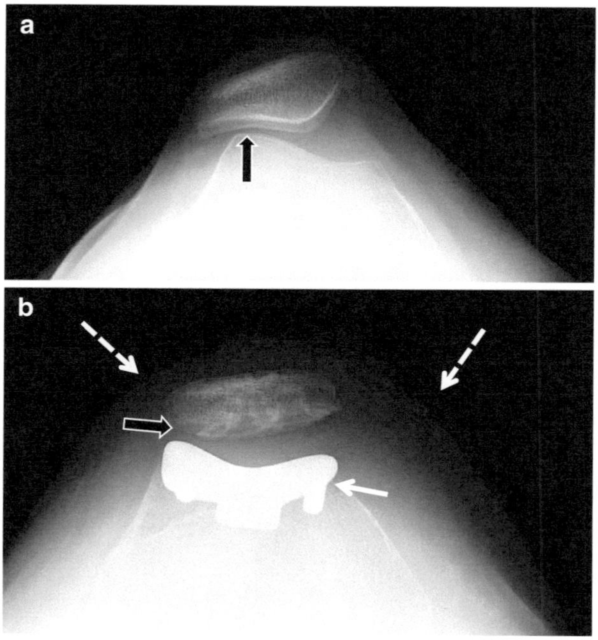

Fig. 5.23 Preoperative and postoperative axial radiographs of a patient with symptomatic isolated patellofemoral osteoarthritis, predominantly laterally (panel **a**) who underwent isolated PF joint replacement. Postoperative image (panel **b**) shows patellar surfacing (*black block arrow*), trochlear arthroplasty component (*white arrow*), and reactive soft tissue edema (*dashed white arrow*)

and the MRI Osteoarthritis Knee Score (MOAKS) [25], which contain subscales specifically for cartilage [48]. The WORMS grading protocol uses an 8-point scale to score cartilage morphology and evaluates for subarticular cysts, bone attrition, and osteophytes [17]. The MOAKS grading protocol, in addition to cartilage assessment, evaluates bone marrow lesions and meniscal abnormalities. Generally, high-grade chondral lesions are considered to be those which affect >50% of the cartilage thickness on either the patella or trochlea.

Osteochondritis dissecans (OCD) lesions, though more commonly encountered in the femorotibial compartment, can also occur along either the patella [7] or trochlea [4] (Fig. 5.24). OCD lesions involve partial or complete separation of the articular cartilage and subchondral bone from an articular surface [37, 42]. When they are found in the patellofemoral compartment, they most often present with symptoms associated with running or jumping. Patellofemoral OCD lesions more often go undetected on x-ray imaging and therefore remain undiagnosed for a longer period of time compared to lesions in the femorotibial compartment, which are often more conspicuous on radiography [35]. In some cases, small osseous fragments may accompany the sheared cartilage fragment and may be visible on radiographs (Fig. 5.25). When OCD lesions involve the femoral sulcus, they are best seen on Merchant views [4] and characteristically occur where the lateral femoral condyle contacts the lateral facet of the patella [6]. The location of lesions involving the patellar cartilage is more variable; however, they were most commonly seen along the central lateral facet, central medial facet, or inferior medial facet in 72.2% of patients in one series [7].

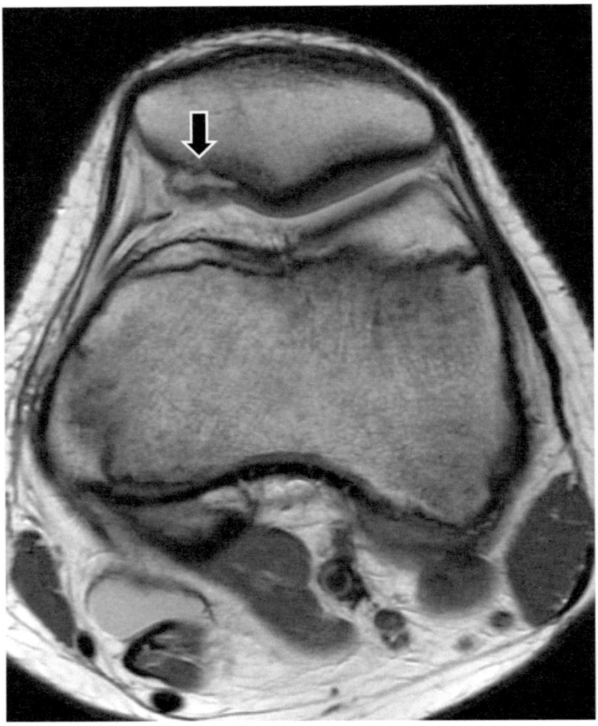

Fig. 5.24 Axial proton density-weighted image of the knee demonstrates an osteochondritis dissecans (OCD) lesion on the medial patellar facet (*black block arrow*), with partial stripping of the fragment from the underlying bone and associated high signal intensity cleft at the site of the lesion

The presence and size of chondral defects and cartilaginous loose bodies have important prognostic implications and assist in treatment planning [14] for knee OCD lesions. An unstable OCD lesion is best recognized by a high signal intensity cleft between the osteochondritic fragment and the underlying bone [14, 15, 28] (Fig. 5.26). Other MR criteria commonly used to signify OCD instability include surrounding cysts, a high T2 signal intensity cartilage fracture line, or a fluid-filled OCD defect [15].

In addition to structural/morphologic abnormalities, MRI techniques can evaluate cartilage ultrastructure using T1 rho, T2 mapping, and dGEMRIC (delayed gadolinium-enhanced magnetic resonance imaging of cartilage) most commonly. These techniques, usually presented as color maps overlying an anatomic image, show compositional changes of cartilage that represent a shift in the major elements of cartilage (water, proteoglycan, and collagen). These biochemical techniques are not routine in clinical imaging and are currently used for research purposes and for follow-up in patients who have undergone chondral repair procedures or in patients in whom suspected early chondral abnormalities are being investigated. Whether

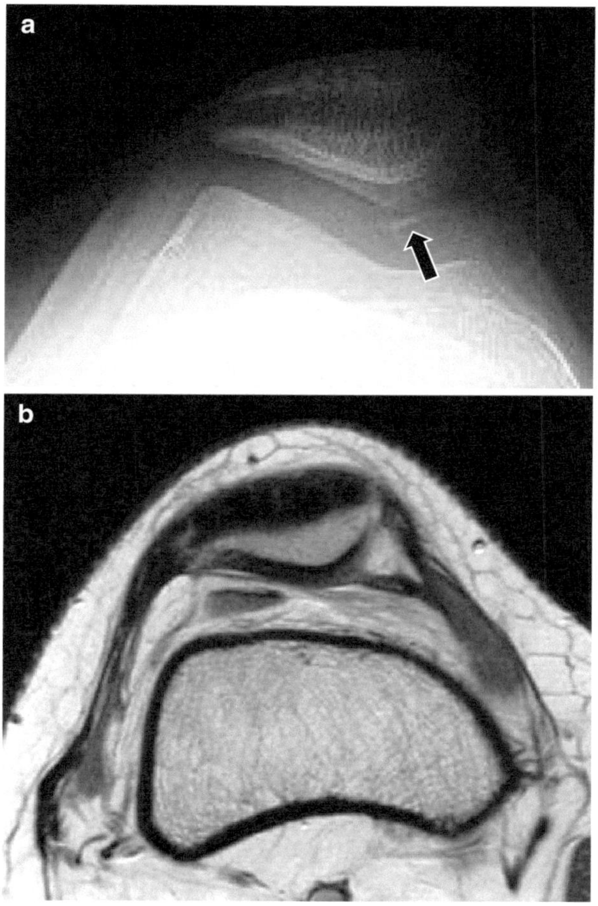

Fig. 5.25 Merchant radiograph (panel **a**) and axial proton density-weighted MR image (panel **b**) demonstrate a curvilinear osseous fragment (*black block arrow*) attached to a sheared chondral fragment. The bony fragment is seen to better effect on the radiograph

one or a combination of these biochemical techniques is used is often a matter of institutional preference.

T1 rho imaging [8, 57] is used to map proteoglycan loss from the extracellular matrix of cartilage, which is directly related to cartilage health and robustness [56], and is a very sensitive sign of early osteoarthritis [54]. Patients with osteoarthritis have elevated cartilage T1rho values compared with healthy patients [32, 39] (Fig. 5.28).

T2 mapping assesses the degree of organization or order of collagen network in cartilage and helps to identify sites of early degeneration, which appear as high signal or areas with high T2 values relative to normal cartilage [16] (Fig. 5.27). In normal cartilage, ordered collagen adjacent to the subchondral bone shows lower signal intensity, while the middle transitional zone has more randomly ordered col-

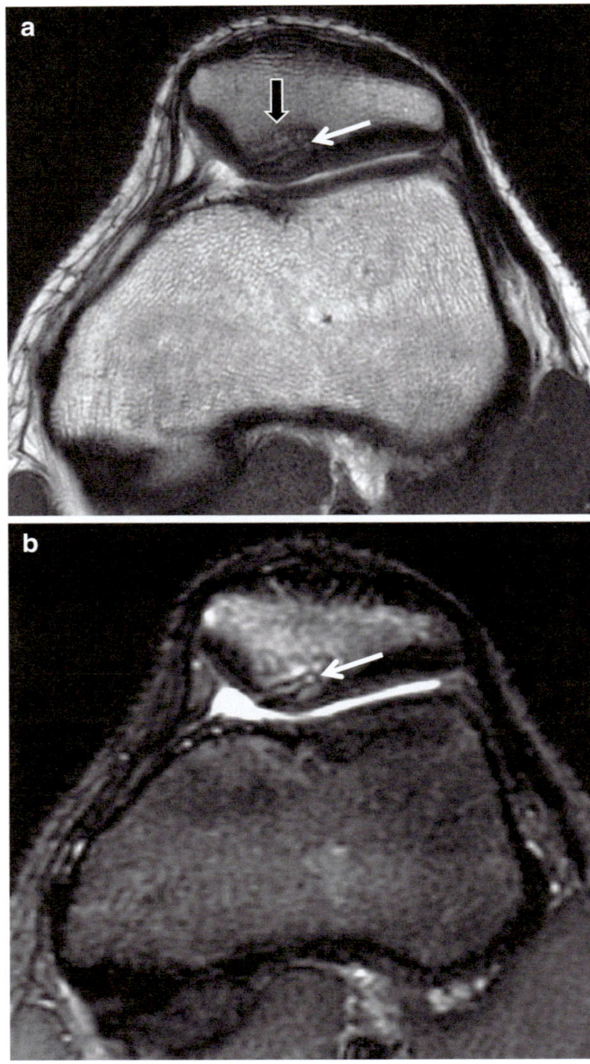

Fig. 5.26 Axial proton density-weighted (panel **a**) and inversion recovery (panel **b**) images of the knee demonstrate an unstable OCD lesion on the lateral patellar facet (*black block arrow*), with a high signal intensity cleft (*white arrow*) separating the in situ fragment from the underlying bone, better depicted on the inversion recovery sequence

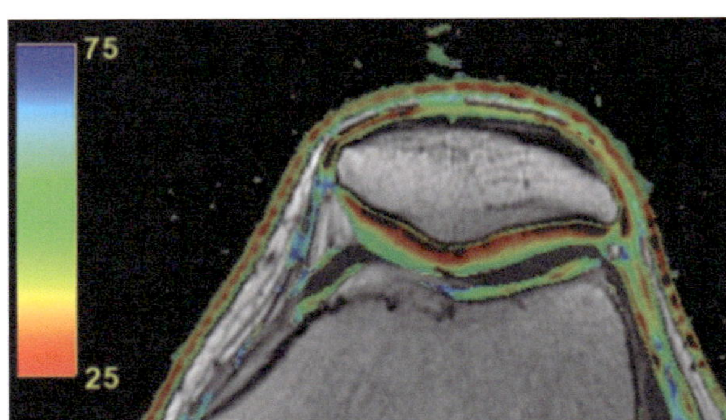

Fig. 5.27 Axial T2 color map demonstrating normal proteoglycan content of articular cartilage in the patellofemoral joint. In diseased cartilage, lower proteoglycan content would cause a shift

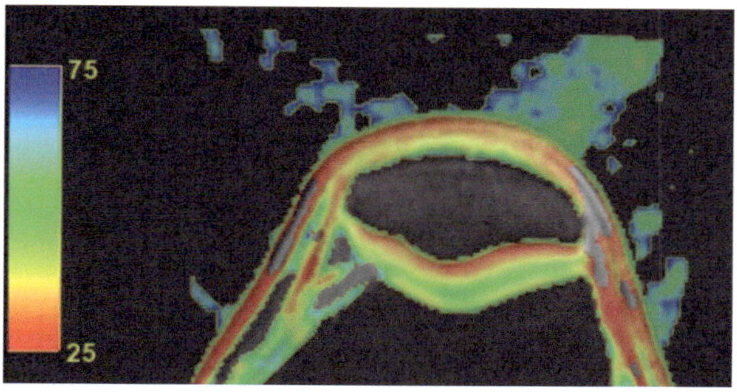

Fig. 5.28 Axial T1 rho color map demonstrating matrix dehydration and collagen degeneration in the patellofemoral joint

lagen and generates higher signal intensity. In abnormal cartilage, this stratification is lost, and the cartilage shows higher T2 values, reflecting greater disorder.

dGEMRIC is a quantitative method for estimating glycosaminoglycan distribution in cartilage. dGEMRIC imaging requires intravenous injection of a contrast agent. These contrast agents commonly contain a negatively charged Gd^2-containing chelate, which diffuses more into areas with low glycosaminoglycan content (diseased cartilage) and diffuses less into areas with high glycosaminoglycan content (healthy cartilage) [33, 60].

Conclusion

Radiographic evaluation of a patient with pain, trauma, or instability of the patellofemoral joint can usually clarify the diagnosis and often narrow treatment options. In most patients, a full set of radiographs are a part of the initial work-up, and in cases involving trauma, persistent symptoms, or instability, a MRI will illustrate the pathology so the appropriate treatment can be followed.

References

1. Antinolfi P, Bartoli M, Placella G, et al. Acute patellofemoral instability in children and adolescents. Joints. 2016;4(1):47–51.
2. Askenberger M, Janarv PM, Finnbogason T, et al. Morphology and anatomic patellar instability risk factors in first-time traumatic lateral patellar dislocations: a prospective magnetic resonance imaging study in skeletally immature children. Am J Sports Med. 2017;45(1):50–8.
3. Black BR, Chong le R, Potter HG. Cartilage imaging in sports medicine. Sports Med Arthrosc. 2009;17(1):68–80.
4. Boutin RD, Januario JA, Newberg AH. MR imaging features of osteochondritis dissecans of the femoral sulcus. AJR Am J Roentgenol. 2003;180(3):641–5.
5. Caton J, Deschamps G, Chambat P. Patella infera. Apropos of 128 cases. Rev Chir Orthop Reparatrice Appar Mot. 1982;68(5):317–25.
6. Chiang H, Liao CJ, Hsieh CH. Clinical feasibility of a novel biphasic osteochondral composite for matrix-associated autologous chondrocyte implantation. Osteoarthr Cartil. 2013;21(4):589–98.

7. Choi YS, Cohen NA, Potter HG. Magnetic resonance imaging in the evaluation of osteochondritis dissecans of the patella. Skelet Radiol. 2007;36(10):929–35.
8. Crema MD, Roemer FW, Marra MD. Articular cartilage in the knee: current MR imaging techniques and applications in clinical practice and research. Radiographics. 2011;31(1):37–61.
9. Davies AP, Vince AS, Shepstone L, et al. The radiologic prevalence of patellofemoral osteoarthritis. Clin Orthop Relat Res. 2002;402:206–12.
10. Dejour H, Walch G, Neyret P, et al. Dysplasia of the femoral trochlea. Rev Chir Orthop Reparatrice Appar Mot. 1990;76:45–54.
11. Dejour H, Walch G, Nove-Josserand L, et al. Factors of patellar instability: an anatomic radiographic study. Knee Surg Sports Traumatol Arthrosc. 1994;2(1):19–26.
12. Dejour D, Reynaud P, Lecoultre B. Douleurs et instabilite rotulienne: Essai de classification. Med Hyg. 1998;56:1466–71.
13. Dejour D, Saggin P. The sulcus deepening trochleoplasty—the Lyon's procedure. Int Orthop. 2010;34(2):311–6.
14. De Smet AA, Fisher DR, Graf BK, et al. Osteochondritis dissecans of the knee: value of MR imaging in determining lesion stability and the presence of articular cartilage defects. AJR Am J Roentgenol. 1990;155:549–53.
15. De Smet AA, Ilahi OA, Graf BK. Reassessment of the MR criteria for stability of osteochondritis dissecans in the knee and ankle. Skelet Radiol. 1996;25:159–63.
16. Dunn TC, Lu Y, Jin H, Ries MD, et al. T2 relaxation time of cartilage at MR imaging: comparison with severity of knee osteoarthritis. Radiology. 2004;232(2):592–8.
17. Eagle S, Potter HG, Koff MF. Morphologic and quantitative magnetic resonance imaging of knee articular cartilage for the assessment of post-traumatic osteoarthritis. J Orthop Res. 2016;35(3):412–23.
18. Endo Y, Shubin Stein BE, Potter HG. Radiologic assessment of patellofemoral pain in the athlete. Sports Health. 2011;3:195–210.
19. Faletti C, De Stefano N, Giudice G, et al. Knee impingement syndromes. Eur J Radiol. 1998;27(Suppl 1):S60–9.
20. Grawe B, Shubin Stein B. Tibial tubercle osteotomy: indication and techniques. J Knee Surg. 2015;28(4):279–84.
21. Grelsamer RP, Proctor CS, Bazos AN. Evaluation of patellar shape in the sagittal plane. A clinical analysis. Am J Sports Med. 1994;22:61.
22. Gustas CN, Blankenbaker DG, Rio AM, et al. Evaluation of the articular cartilage of the knee joint using an isotropic resolution 3D fast spin-echo sequence with conventional and radial reformatted images. AJR Am J Roentgenol. 2015;205:371–9.
23. Heyse TJ, Figiel J, Hähnlein U, Timmesfeld N, Lakemeier S, Schofer MD, Fuchs-Winkelmann S, Efe T. MRI after patellofemoral replacement: the preserved compartments. Eur J Radiol. 2012;81(9):2313–7.
24. Hong E, Kraft MC. Evaluating anterior knee pain. Med Clin N Am. 2014;98:697–717.
25. Hunter DJ, Guermazi A, Lo GH, et al. Evolution of semi-quantitative whole joint assessment of knee OA: MOAKS (MRI osteoarthritis knee score). Osteoarthr Cartil. 2011;19(8):990–1002.
26. Insall J, Salvati E. Patella position in the normal knee joint. Radiology. 1971;101:101–4.
27. Kavanagh EC, Zoga A, Omar I, et al. MRI findings in bipartite patella. Skelet Radiol. 2007;36:209–14.
28. Kijowski R, Blankenbaker DG, Shinki K, et al. Juvenile versus adult osteochondritis dissecans of the knee: appropriate MR imaging criteria for instability. Radiology. 2008;248(2):571–8.
29. Kim T-H, Sobti A, Lee S-H, et al. The effects of weight-bearing conditions on patellofemoral indices in individuals without and with patellofemoral pain syndrome. Skelet Radiol. 2014;43(2):157–64.
30. LaPrade RF, Cram TR, James EW, et al. Trochlear dysplasia and the role of trochleoplasty. Clin Sports Med. 2014;33(3):531–45.
31. Laurin CA, Dussault R, Levesque HP. The tangential x-ray investigation of the patellofemoral joint: x-ray technique, diagnostic criteria and their interpretation. Clin Orthop Relat Res. 1979;144:16–26.

32. Li X, Benjamin Ma C, Link TM. In vivo T(1rho) and T(2) mapping of articular cartilage in osteoarthritis of the knee using 3 T MRI. Osteoarthr Cartil. 2007;15(7):789–97.
33. Matzat SJ, van Tiel J, Gold GE, et al. Quantitative MRI techniques of cartilage composition. Quant Imaging Med Surg. 2013;3(3):162–74.
34. McAlindon TE, Snow S, Cooper C, et al. Radiographic patterns of osteoarthritis of the knee joint in the community: the importance of the patellofemoral joint. Ann Rheum Dis. 1992;51(7):844–9.
35. McIlvain GE, Lavender CD, Boukhemis KW. Bilateral Osteochondritis Dissecans in a 16-year-old female basketball player. Int J Athl Ther Train. 2013;18(4):23–7.
36. Merchant AC, Mercer RL, Jacobsen RH, et al. Roentgenographic analysis of patellofemoral congruence. J Bone Joint Surg Am. 1974;56:1391–6.
37. Obedian RS, Grelsamer RP. Osteochondritis dissecans of the distal femur and patella. Clin Sports Med. 1997;16:157–74.
38. Outerbridge RE. The etiology of chondromalacia patellae. J Bone Joint Surg Br. 1961;43-B:752–7.
39. Pakin SK, Xu J, Schweitzer ME, Regatte RR. Rapid 3D-T1rho mapping of the knee joint at 3.0 T with parallel imaging. Magn Reson Med. 2006;56(3):563–71.
40. Pavlov H. Orthopaedist's guide to plain film imaging. New York: Thieme Publishers; 1999.
41. Peterfy CG, Guermazi A, Zaim S, et al. Whole-organ magnetic resonance imaging score (WORMS) of the knee in osteoarthritis. Osteoarthr Cartil. 2004;12(3):177–90.
42. Peters TA, McLean ID. Osteochondritis dissecans of the patellofemoral joint. Am J Sports Med. 2000;28:63–7.
43. Pfirrmann CW, Zanetti M, Romero J, et al. Femoral trochlear dysplasia: MR findings. Radiology. 2000;216(3):858–64.
44. Potter HG, Linklater JM, Allen AA, et al. Magnetic resonance imaging of articular cartilage in the knee. An evaluation with use of fast-spin-echo imaging. J Bone Joint Surg Am. 1998;80:1276–84.
45. Reider B, Marshall JL, Koslin B, et al. The anterior aspect of the knee joint. J Bone Joint Surg Am. 1981;63:351–6.
46. Saddik D, McNally EG, Richardson M. MRI of Hoffa's fat pad. Skelet Radiol. 2004;33(8):433–44.
47. Samim M, Smitaman E, Lawrence D. MRI of anterior knee pain. Skelet Radiol. 2014;43(7):875–93.
48. Schwaiger BJ, Gersing AS, Mbapte Wamba J, et al. Can signal abnormalities detected with MR imaging in knee articular cartilage be used to predict development of morphologic cartilage defects? 48-month data from the osteoarthritis initiative. Radiology. 2016;281(1):158–67.
49. Sherman SL, Plackis AC, Nuelle CW. Patellofemoral anatomy and biomechanics. Clin Sports Med. 2014;33(3):389–401.
50. Shindle MK, Foo LF, Kelly BT, et al. Magnetic resonance imaging of cartilage in the athlete: current techniques and spectrum of disease. J Bone Joint Surg Am. 2006;88(Suppl 4):27–46.
51. Stefanik JJ, Gross KD, Guermazi A, et al. The relation of MRI-detected structural damage in the medial and lateral patellofemoral joint to knee pain: the multicenter and Framingham osteoarthritis studies. Osteoarthr Cartil. 2015;23(4):565–70.
52. Stefanik JJ, Guermazi A, Roemer FW, et al. Changes in patellofemoral and tibiofemoral joint cartilage damage and bone marrow lesions over 7 years: the multicenter osteoarthritis study. Osteoarthr Cartil. 2016;424(7):1160–6.
53. Stephen JM, Urquhart DW, van Arkel RJ, et al. The use of Sonographically guided botulinum toxin type a (Dysport) injections into the tensor fasciae Latae for the treatment of lateral Patellofemoral overload syndrome. Am J Sports Med. 2016;44(5):1195–202.
54. van de Loo AA, Arntz OJ, Otterness IG, et al. Proteoglycan loss and subsequent replenishment in articular cartilage after a mild arthritic insult by IL-1 in mice: impaired proteoglycan turnover in the recovery phase. Agents Actions. 1994;41:200–8.
55. van der Heijden RA, de Kanter JL, Bierma-Zeinstra SM, et al. Structural abnormalities on magnetic resonance imaging in patients with Patellofemoral pain: a cross-sectional case-control study. Am J Sports Med. 2016;44(9):2339–46.

56. Wang L, Chang G, Xu J, et al. T1rho MRI of menisci and cartilage in patients with osteoarthritis at 3T. Eur J Radiol. 2012;81(9):2329–36.
57. Wheaton AJ, Dodge GR, Borthakur A, et al. Detection of changes in articular cartilage proteoglycan by T(1rho) magnetic resonance imaging. J Orthop Res. 2005;23(1):102–8.
58. White BJ, Sherman OH. Patellofemoral instability. Bull NYU Hosp Jt Dis. 2009;67(1):22–9.
59. Wiberg G. Roentgenographic and anatomic studies on the femoropatellar joint. Acta Orthop Scand. 1941;12:319–410.
60. Williams A, Gillis A, McKenzie C. Glycosaminoglycan distribution in cartilage as determined by delayed gadolinium-enhanced MRI of cartilage (dGEMRIC): potential clinical applications. AJR Am J Roentgenol. 2004;182(1):167–72.

Part II
Patellofemoral Instability

Chapter 6
Instability in the Skeletally Immature Patient

Lauren H. Redler and Christopher S. Ahmad

Natural History

Adolescents represent the highest risk group for acute traumatic patellar dislocation with a peak incidence occurring between 15 and 19 years of age [1, 2]. While several studies have found females to have a higher rate of patellar instability [1], others have found no gender differences [2]. Fithian reported the incidence of patellar instability to be 33/100,000 (95% CI 22–44) in females compared to 25/100,000 (95% CI 16–34) in males in the 10–17 year age group [1].

Young age at the time of primary dislocation is a risk factor for recurrence, with redislocation rates ranging from 16 to 69% despite physical therapy and conservative treatment [3–9]. Lewallen [6] showed that in patients with open physes and trochlear dysplasia, the recurrence rate is 69%. Cartilage injuries may occur in as many as 95% of cases of patellar dislocation [10] and can range from simple fissures to full thickness defects. The incidence of an associated osteochondral fracture in the pediatric and adolescent age group is thought to be higher than adults, and studies have reported rates anywhere from 25% to 75% [11].

The pathoanatomy of patellofemoral instability has many anatomic factors that are challenging to modify in the skeletally immature patient. The tibial tubercle-trochlear groove (TT-TG) distance is the distance between the center of the trochlear groove and the center of the attachment of the patellar tendon to the tibial tubercle. Elevated TT-TG indicates excessive lateralization of the tibial tubercle with a high valgus vector on the patella which contributes to patellar instability. In contrast to older patients, skeletally immature patients with an elevated TT-TG must

L. H. Redler (✉) · C. S. Ahmad
Columbia University Medical Center, Department of Orthopedic Surgery, New York, NY, USA

B. E. Shubin Stein, S. M. Strickland (eds.), *Patellofemoral Pain and Instability*, https://doi.org/10.1007/978-3-319-97640-2_6

be counseled that this feature, which predisposes them to patellar instability, is not something that can be surgically addressed with a medializing tibial tubercle osteotomy until completion of growth. Similarly, patella alta, an independent risk factor for patellar instability [5], cannot be treated with a tibial tubercle distalization procedure due to the open tibial tubercle apophysis and risk of a growth arrest leading to a recurvatum deformity. In addition, trochlear dysplasia is a risk factor for patellar instability [5]. While trochleoplasties are performed more comonly in Europe compared to the USA, most surgeons delay them until skeletal maturity due to the risk of injury to the open distal femoral physis.

Surgical Indications

Standard non-operative treatment includes activity restriction, patellar taping or bracing, and physical therapy focused on stretching the iliotibial band and strengthening the vastus medialis obliquus (VMO), gluteal muscles, and core. Failure to improve after conservative management and repeat dislocations are the most common indications for surgical intervention for patellar instability in the skeletally immature patient. The type of surgery performed should be individualized and take each patient's anatomy into consideration. Anatomic abnormalities including patella alta, tibial tubercle-trochlear groove (TT-TG) distance, and trochlear dysplasia should be noted but rarely affect surgical planning in this age group for the reasons previously discussed [12, 13]. It is still important to recognize these features and counsel patients appropriately with regard to potential failure of surgical intervention.

A primary dislocation with an intra-articular cartilaginous or osteochondral fragment warrants immediate surgical intervention to remove or repair the fragment [3]. In skeletally immature patients, fixation of loose fragments, even those that appear chondral only in nature, should be considered [14–18]. Due to the high risk of recurrence in this patient population, it is vital to also stabilize these patients with either a MPFL repair or reconstruction at the time of treatment for the osteochondral fracture, even after first-time patellar dislocation. This was recently corroborated in a survey of the International Patellofemoral Study Group (IPSG) [19].

Operative Techniques

Surgical Considerations

In the pediatric population, a thorough understanding of the distal femoral and proximal tibial physes as well as the tibial tubercle apophysis is critical when considering the multitude of available operative techniques. The distal femoral physis has a characteristic undulating structure with relatively proximal medial and lateral

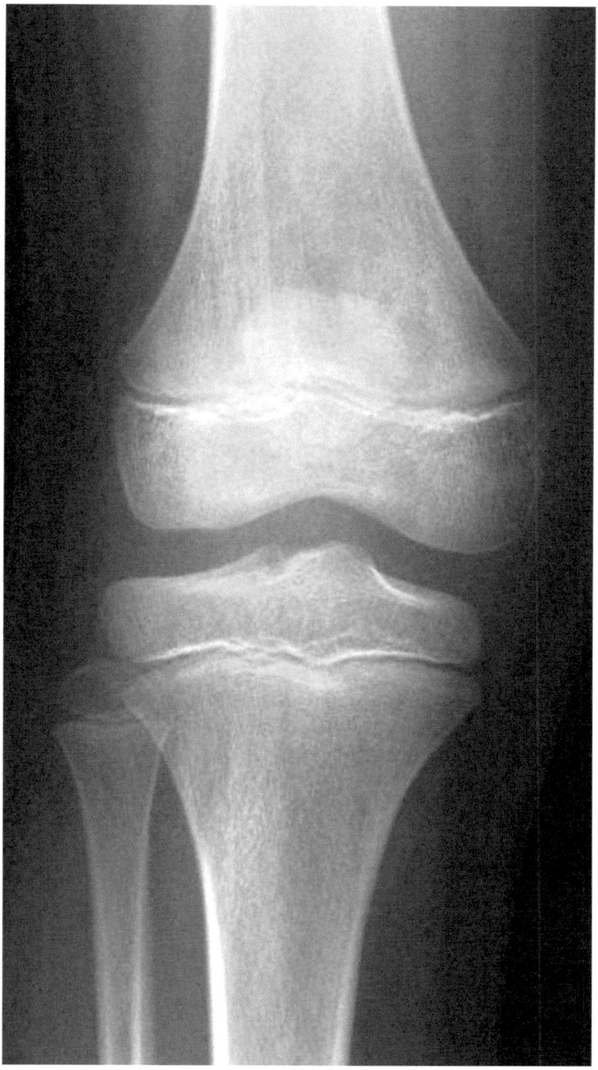

Fig. 6.1 Anteroposterior (AP) view of a skeletally immature knee illustrating the undulating course of the distal femoral physis

borders (Fig. 6.1). It is the largest and fastest growing physis in the body and contributes 70% of the length of the femur and 37% of the overall lower limb growth, which amounts to approximately 1 cm/year during skeletal immaturity. This growth plate fuses between 14 and 16 years in females and 16 and 18 years in males [20]. The proximal tibial physis contributes approximately 55% of the length of the tibia and 25% of the length of the entire limb. On average it contributes 0.65 cm of growth per year. This physis fuses between 13 and 15 years in females and 15 and 19 years in males [20]. The tibial tubercle apophysis fuses between 13 and 15 years in females and 15 and 19 years in males [20].

The MPFL insertion on the medial distal femur is typically described as being distal to the adductor tendon insertion and proximal to the femoral origin of the medial collateral ligament (MCL), which is in very close proximity to the medial aspect of the distal femoral physis. Shea et al. [21] reported in an indirect radiographic study using a lateral x-ray that the insertion of the MPFL was 2–5 mm proximal to the distal femoral physis. Several others [22–25], however, have shown both radiographically and in cadaveric specimens that the MPFL inserts approximately 5 mm distal to the distal femoral physis. Fixation of the reconstructed MPFL proximal to the distal femoral physis has been reported to result in proximal migration in a growing patient, causing excessive graft tension, loss of graft isometry, and loss of knee motion [23]. Thus, it is critically important to fix the graft distal to the distal femoral physis, both to avoid physeal injury, and subsequent growth arrest, and avoid proximal migration.

Isolated proximal (Insall procedure, medial reefing +/− lateral release) and distal realignments (Galeazzi, Nietosvaara, and Roux-Goldthwait) have fallen out of favor due to their non-anatomic nature and high recurrence rates. Currently utilized surgical options for patellofemoral instability in the skeletally immature athlete include MPFL repair, MPFL reconstruction, medial quadriceps tendon femoral ligament (MQTFL) reconstruction, and combinations of the above procedures. As previously discussed, skeletally immature patients are not candidates for a tibial tubercle osteotomy as the proximal tibial physis and the tibial tubercle apophysis will be violated and result in a recurvatum deformity [26]. Instead, soft-tissue procedures must be considered. Implant-mediated guided growth with tension-band plates can be done concomitantly to address pathologic valgus deformity contributing to patellar instability. Additionally, derotational femoral osteotomies can be considered for patients with pathologic femoral anteversion.

Soft-Tissue Surgeries

The emergence of soft-tissue procedures designed to respect physeal and apophyseal integrity has advanced our ability to address this problem in the skeletally immature athlete.

MPFL Repair

Medial patellofemoral ligament repair can be indicated in patients with first-time dislocation in whom concomitant injuries are also being addressed. Early studies showed success with MPFL repair for acute patellar dislocation [27]. However, data exist showing MPFL repair to be less strong than several reconstruction techniques in cadaver models [28]. Christiansen et al. [4] published a prospective randomized controlled trial evaluating the effect of MPFL repair versus conservative treatment in patients with primary patellar dislocations. The authors concluded that delayed MPFL repair (mean, 50 days after injury) did not reduce the risk of redislocation or improve subjective functional outcome scores. Sillanpaa et al. subsequently published a randomized controlled trial also looking at acute MPFL repair versus conservative treatment in an active military recruit population. Surgical stabilization included either medial reefing or a Roux-Goldthwait procedure based on surgeon preference. While they did see fewer redislocations in these skeletally mature patients in the surgical stabilization group, they had no long-term subjective benefits. Similarly, Camp et al. [29] found that the recurrence of dislocation after primary repair of the MPFL in the setting of recurrent instability was 28%, and subjectively 41% of their patients rated their result as either fair or poor.

MPFL Reconstructions

MPFL reconstruction is favored over repair in patients with recurrent patellofemoral instability because the chronically injured medial retinacular tissues are insufficient to establish a checkrein against lateral dislocation. Because of the adjacent physis near the insertion of the MPFL on the distal femur, different techniques for MPFL reconstruction have been described (Fig. 6.2). Various graft choices have been utilized for MPFL reconstruction, including hamstrings [24, 30–32], patellar tendon [33–35], quadriceps tendon [36–41], adductor magnus tendon [42–44], and allograft [45]. Various sling techniques have also been described utilizing either the MCL [46] or the adductor tendon [47–49] as a pulley to reroute a hamstring grafts to the patella.

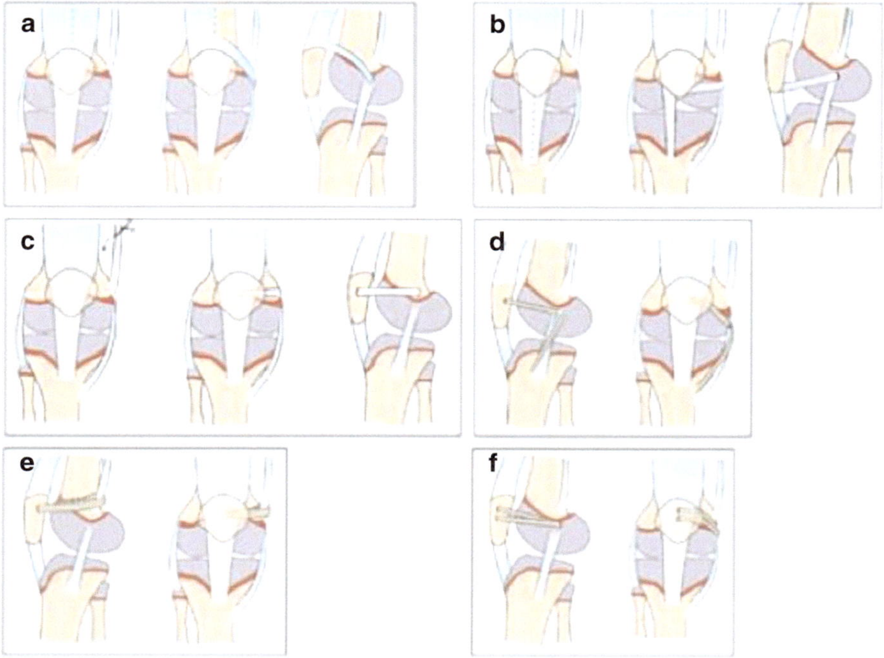

Fig. 6.2 Various physeal-sparing MPFL reconstruction techniques. (**a**) Hemiquadriceps tendon transfer, (**b**) hemipatellar tendon transfer, (**c**) adductor tendon pedicle graft, (**d**) hamstring graft using MCL as pulley, (**e**) hamstring graft using adductor tendon as a pulley, (**f**) double-bundle hamstring allograft using patellar and femoral sockets. (Used with permission from *Pediatric and Adolescent Knee Surgery*, Cordasco/Green (Ed). 2015)

Despite the variety of graft choices listed, many of these techniques require the use of bone tunnels for femoral fixation. If MPFL reconstruction with a femoral bone tunnel is considered, fluoroscopic guidance is mandatory to avoid physeal disturbance in addition to determining appropriate tunnel placement [24, 50].The direction for drilling of the socket should be angulated distally so as to be parallel and below the distal femoral physis (Fig. 6.3).

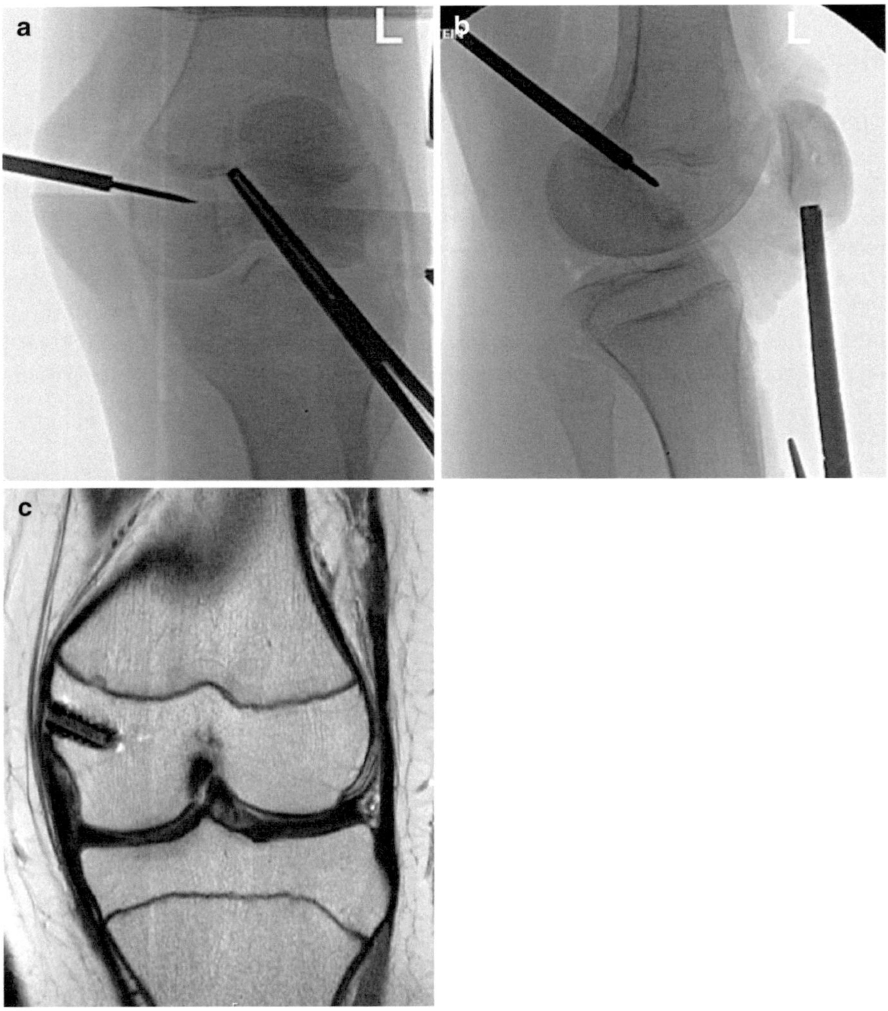

Fig. 6.3 Physeal-sparing drilling of the femoral socket at Schottle's point. (**a**) Anteroposterior intra-operative fluoroscopy showing drilling of the femoral socket away from the physis. (**b**) Lateral intra-operative fluoroscopy showing the drill located at Schottle's point. (**c**) Postoperative coronal MRI showing location of the interference screw on the distal medial femur distal to the physis. (Images courtesy of Beth Shubin Stein, MD)

Free Hamstring Autograft

Several authors have investigated MPFL reconstruction using a free hamstring autograft that is positioned anatomically and anchored to the patella and femur and have shown excellent postoperative improvements in Kujala scores and low postoperative dislocation rates [24, 30–32]. The free hamstring autograft (semitendinosus or gracilis) can be used to form a single bundle reconstruction [32], or the graft can be looped over to form a double bundle graft [24, 30, 31]. The double bundle graft can then be oriented one of two ways – with the center of the graft fixed to the femur and the two free ends fixed to the patella separately (Y-graft) [30] (see Fig. 6.2f above) or with the center of the graft secured to the medial border of the patella at two points and the two free ends fixed at the femur together (C-graft) [31]. Suture anchors are gaining favor over docking in the patella as they avoid the risk of patella fracture. Additionally, if any cartilage restoration procedures are concurrently performed on the patella (osteochondral fracture fixation, OATS, minced chondral allograft), particularly if medial, avoiding bone tunnels in the patella removes the possible complication of these tunnels communicating and compromising the repair.

Hemipatellar Tendon Autograft

Many authors [33–35] have described using a pedicled medial patellar tendon graft to reconstruct the MPFL (see Fig. 6.2b). Camanho et al. [34] was the first to describe this technique and reported initial short-term good results in 25 patients. In a prospective randomized controlled trial, Bitar et al. [33] showed improved Kujala scores and no recurrent instability at a minimum follow-up of 2 years in patients with an average age of 24.5 years. More recently, Witonski et al. [35] similarly reported good clinical outcomes at a minimum follow-up of 2 years in patients with an average age of 27.2 years. Given the older population in these studies, the applicability and viability in the skeletally immature patient population remains unclear.

Quadriceps Turndown

Steensen et al. [40] have described a surgical technique utilizing the quadriceps tendon to reconstruct the MPFL (see Fig. 6.2a). Noyes and Albright [39] described a similar technique which does not require femoral bone tunnels and thus minimizes risk to the distal femoral physis. Both groups harvest an 8x70mm strip of the medial quadriceps tendon, leaving the patellar insertion intact. The free end is shuttled between the capsular and retinacular layers and fixed with an interference screw [40] or sutured to the medial intermuscular septum adjacent to the medial femoral epicondyle [39]. Goyal [37] has advocated for use of a 10–12 mm-wide superficial slip of the quadriceps tendon instead of a full-thickness graft and has shown good results in 38 patients (average age 25 years) with mean follow-up of 38 months. More recently, others have shown similarly good outcomes using only the superficial layer of the quadriceps tendon [36, 41]. Nelitz and Williams [38] describe the advantages of this technique to include avoiding bony patellar complications (from bone tunnels that place the proportionally smaller patellar at higher risk for fracture), an anatomically "truer" reconstruction, and sparing of the hamstring tendons for reconstruction of any future ligamentous injuries.

Hinckel et al. [51] have advocated for a combined MPFL and medial patellotibial ligament (MPTL) reconstruction in patients with patellar subluxation in extension, flexion instability, children with anatomic risk factors, and knee hyperextension associated with generalized ligamentous laxity. They describe a novel technique using the quadriceps tendon for MPFL reconstruction and the patellar tendon for MPTL reconstruction. However, there are no published clinical outcomes on this technique.

Adductor Magnus Autograft

A pedicled adductor magnus tendon graft has also been proposed for pediatric MPFL reconstruction. Steiner et al. [44] described harvesting the medial two-thirds of the adductor tendon, leaving the distal insertion on the femur intact, and reflecting the cut end of the tendon and securing it to the medial side of the patella (see Fig. 6.2c above). In their case series of 34 patients, they found no difference in recurrence rates when compared to hemipatellar tendon autograft or the quadriceps turndown technique. In Sillanpaa's series, 3 of 18 had recurrent subluxation or dislocation [43]. In a cadaveric study, Jacobi et al. [42] explored the potential anatomic dangers of this technique. Damage to the neurovascular bundle of the adductor hiatus, the saphenous nerve, or the saphenous branch of the descending genicular artery, during graft harvest must be considered.

Allograft Hamstring

Use of allograft tissue can preserve autogenous tissues and may be preferable in patients with connective tissue disorders or generalized ligamentous laxity. There is limited published data on the outcomes of allograft MPFL reconstruction in pediatric and adolescent patients.

Soft-Tissue Slings

Deie et al. [46] described a unique way to reconstruct the MPFL using a semitendinosus autograft left attached distally and transferred to the patella using the posterior one-third of the femoral origin of the medial collateral ligament as a pulley (see Fig. 6.2d above). Follow-up results of the first six knees had no recurrent dislocations, and mean Kujala scores were excellent. While potentially a good option, this was a very small sample size and requires violation of a vital medial structure, the MCL, which would otherwise not be at risk during MPFL reconstruction.

Alternatively, to avoid risking injury to the MCL, other authors [47–49] have proposed using the adductor magnus tendon as a sling (see Fig. 6.2e above). A free hamstring autograft is harvested, passed through drill holes in the patella, and looped around the adductor magnus tendon and back to the patella. Monllau et al. [49] reported initial results in 36 patients (average age 25.6 years) with a minimum of 27 months follow-up and reported no recurrent dislocations. Just recently, Lind et al. [48] reported on 24 MPFL reconstructions in 20 children (age 8–16) utilizing the same technique. They compared the outcomes with a cohort of 179 adult patients with recurrent patellar instability treated with MPFL reconstruction using bony femoral fixation. Four patients (20%) in the pediatric group experience redislocation in the first postoperative year compared with 5% in the adult population. The authors concluded that MPFL reconstruction using femoral soft-tissue graft fixation in pediatric patients was inferior to MPFL reconstruction using bony femoral fixation in adult patients.

MQTFL Reconstruction

Tanaka recently published a cadaveric study showing variability in the patellar origin of the MPFL [52]. In 33 cadavers, the author showed that MPFL fibers attach to both the patella and quadriceps tendon, with 57.3% ± 19.5% of the fibers attaching to the patella. This highlights the recent interest in reconstruction both the MPFL and the medial quadriceps tendon femoral ligament (MQTFL). MQTFL reconstruction has been proposed as an alternative or adjunct to MPFL reconstruction to better reestablish the broad origin of the MPFL while avoiding the risk of patella fracture (see Fig. 6.4). Short-term clinical outcomes are promising [53].

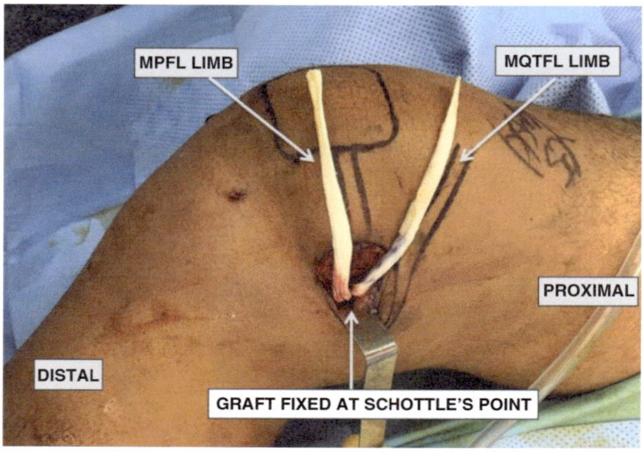

Fig. 6.4 Combined MPFL and MQTFL reconstruction (Image courtesy of Mininder S. Kocher, MD, MPH)

Complications

A recent systematic review by Stupay et al. [54] of MPFL reconstruction for recurrent patellar instability showed that the rate of major complications dropped from 2.01% to 0.46% and the rate of minor complications decreased from 6.53% to 4.00% despite the number of MPFL reconstructions being performed nearly doubling in recent years. Analysis of the literature reveals that a majority of the complications reported can be attributed to patellar fixation of the graft. Patellar fracture was the most devastating complication reported after MPFL reconstruction with a hamstring graft [4, 55–58]. Other reported complications like violation of the chondral surface [55] can result in poor postoperative results and the early onset of patellofemoral arthritis. Parikh et al. [59] specifically looked at complications of MPFL reconstruction in 179 young patients. The authors reported 38 complications in 29 knees (16.2%), with 34 major and 4 minor. Major complications, requiring either hospitalization or further surgery, included recurrence of instability (eight patients), stiffness (eight patients), patella fracture (six patients), and patellofemoral arthrosis/pain (five patients). Eighteen of 38 (47%) complications were secondary to technical factors and were considered preventable. Female sex and bilateral MPFL reconstructions were risk factors associated with postoperative complications. The authors recommended avoiding transverse drill holes in the patella.

Author's Preferred Technique

Our preferred technique is a free hamstring auto or allograft with 2 suture anchors on the patella and a 6.25 × 15 mm PEEK or biocomposite interference screw on the femur. Examination under anesthesia is performed preoperatively to assess the lateral retinacular structures. A lateral release is *only* performed if the patella is unable to be everted to neutral and is especially avoided in ligamentously lax patients. An Esmarch bandage is used to exsanguinate the limb, and a pneumatic thigh tourniquet is inflated. Diagnostic arthroscopy is first performed to address any intra-articular chondral injuries and remove loose bodies if necessary.

With the leg in full extension, a 3-cm longitudinal incision is then made just off the medial border of the patella. The layer between the medial retinaculum and capsule is identified, taking care to remain extracapsular. It is helpful at this point to place 0-vicryl sutures both on the cuff of tissue remaining on the patella and on the medial retinacular structures to aid in retraction. This layer is then developed with scissor dissection toward the MPFL insertion on the medial distal femur. Electrocautery is used to expose the medial border of the patella, and it is prepared with a curette to stimulate bony bleeding and enhance soft-tissue graft healing. A small capsulotomy is then made large enough for your index finger, and the center (superior-inferior) of the patella is identified. Using the hard bone drill, the inferior suture anchor is placed at that central point, and the second suture anchor is placed more proximally. With our technique, the allograft does not require any special preparation other than to make sure that when doubled, it is 6 mm in diameter. The center of the graft is then placed between the two suture anchors, and the graft is secured in place by tying the sutures around the allograft tendon (Fig. 6.5).

With the knee in flexion, the medial epicondyle is palpated, and a small 2-cm longitudinal incision is made. Subcutaneous tissue is dissected until both the medial epicondyle and adductor tubercle can be palpated. If there is difficulty in identifying either of these landmarks, the adductor magnus tendon can be palpated and tracked distally to identify its insertion on the adductor tubercle. The sulcus between these

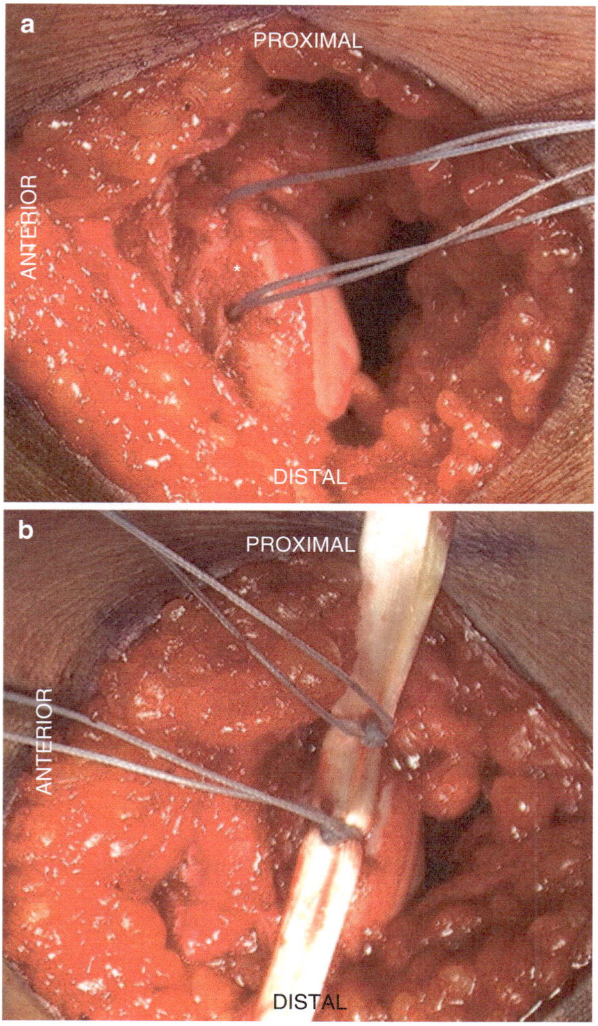

Fig. 6.5 Suture anchor fixation of the hamstring graft to the medial border of the patella. (**a**) Suture anchor placement. (**b**) Graft fixation (* = medial border of patella)

structures is identified, and a guide pin is placed with fluoroscopic guidance, taking care to aim slightly distally, parallel to the physis, to avoid the physis and anteriorly to avoid penetration of the condyle posteriorly (see Fig. 6.3). A curved clamp is then used to pass a passing suture between the medial retinaculum and the capsule, between both incisions. The two limbs of the graft are then shuttled from the patellar incision to the medial epicondyle incision. Next, the patella is seated in the trochlea at 30 degrees of flexion, and both limbs of the graft are passed around the pin with the ends secured with snaps, and the graft is marked with a marker adjacent to the pin. The knee is then taken through a range of motion, ensuring that the mark on the graft does not move excessively (>2 mm), signifying graft isometry. With the isometric point established, fluoroscopy is then used to obtain a lateral image to confirm Schottle's point. Placing any drill bit over the pin with the back end at the pin-bone interface can aid in identifying the point of entry of the guide pin, as the large diameter of the drill is easily differentiated from the small diameter of the pin as it enters bone. Due to the undulating nature of the distal femoral physis, it will appear that the drill is proximal to the physis on the lateral view. We use the AP view to confirm that we are distal to the physis and the lateral view to confirm we are at Schottle's point. We believe isometry to be of paramount importance and thus advocate for it to be used as the primary validation of the appropriate femoral insertion with fluoroscopy used only for secondary verification. A 6 mm reamer is then used to ream a 20 mm socket over the guide pin. A Yankauer suction tip fits perfectly to sound the socket, ensure that there is a good back wall, and remove any debris.

The two limbs of the graft are marked at the entrance of the femoral socket and whipstitched for 2 cm – this is the length of the graft that will be seated in the socket. Excess graft after this point is excised. The graft is then loaded on a 6.25 × 15 mm PEEK tenodesis screw and fixed with the knee in 30 degrees of flexion. The sutures exiting the tenodesis screw are then tied over the screw to the sutures in the graft, thereby creating a combined interference screw and suture anchor construct. With the knee in full extension, we confirm that the graft is not overtensioned by ensuring there are still two quadrants of patellar mobility and that the knee can still attain full range of motion. The medial retinacular split is then closed over the graft, and the two incisions are closed in standard fashion.

Postoperatively we place the knee in a hinged knee brace and allow weight-bearing as tolerated with the brace locked in full extension. Under direction of a physical therapist, active and passive range of motion exercises are initiated 1 week postoperatively, with a goal of achieving 90 degrees flexion by 6 weeks post-operatively. Hamstring and quadriceps strengthening begins at 6 weeks followed by running and agility training at 4–5 months. Patients typically return to full activity between 6–9 months postoperatively. While not as well defined as in the post-ACL reconstruction population, functional movement assessments are critical to determine patients' readiness to return to training for sports after an MPFL reconstruction. We typically perform this as a two-part evaluation. The first occurs around 5 months postoperatively to identify specific areas that need continued work. The second part is done 6–8 weeks later to determine the patient's readiness to return to training for sport.

Guided Growth for Coronal Plane Malalignment

Indications

In young athletes, genu valgum >10° has been associated with patellofemoral instability [60]. Temporary hemiepiphysiodesis through the application of an extra-physeal tension-band plate is a safe, effective, and minimally invasive technique to correct abnormal valgus and can be used in skeletally immature patients with at least 12 months of growth remaining [61, 62]. This technique can be done in isolation or in combination with a soft-tissue procedure detailed above to treat patellofemoral instability in the skeletally immature patient.

Tension-band plates are extra-physeal and result in reproducible improvement in angulation [63]. Hemiepiphysiodesis is most often done at the distal medial femur but can also be applied to the proximal medial tibia in cases in which both the femur and tibia are contributing to the valgus deformity. The concept of the tension band plate with two non-locking screws to bring about temporary hemiepiphysiodesis was introduced by Stevens in 2007 [63] to avoid the complications that had previously been seen with staples [64]. Unlike staples, which bracket the physis, this system of plate and screws does not compress the physis, thus reducing the concern for permanent physeal damage [65]. Instead, this method prevents growth on one side of the physis while allowing unhindered growth on the opposite side until full angular correction is achieved.

Correction of approximately 0.7° per month in the femur and 0.3° per month in the tibia can be expected [61]. Said differently, you can improve valgus alignment on average 8° per year with a femoral hemiepiphysiodesis and an extra 4° per year if you add a tibial hemiepiphysiodesis. Most studies advocate for an overcorrection of 5 degrees to take into consideration the rebound phenomenon.

Guided growth is contraindicated in patients with a physeal bar, patients with closed physes, or patients who are within 6–12 months of physeal closure (14 years bone age for females, 16 years bone age for males) (Goldman, 2010). These principles are summarized in Table 6.1.

Table 6.1 Principles of guided growth

Minimally invasive
Temporary
Extraphyseal
Minimum of 12 months remaining growth
For genu valgum >10°
Femur: correct 0.7°/month, 8°/year
Tibia: correct 0.3°/month, 4°/year
Overcorrect 5° to avoid rebound

Surgical Technique

The technical steps are fairly standard but differ slightly depending on the implant choice due to a variety of plate designs. Guided growth constructs and available sizes are listed in Table 6.2. The periosteal surface of the distal medial femur and/or the proximal medial tibia is carefully exposed with blunt dissection to avoid injury to this layer. A small localizing pin is placed in the physis, and its position is verified with fluoroscopy. The guided growth plate is then placed over the K-wire. Using a drill guide, epiphyseal and metaphyseal guide wires are placed, aiming away from the physis. The central guide wire is removed, and plate position is then checked with fluoroscopy. A cannulated drill is then used to drill to the predetermined screw length, and cannulated screws are then sequentially placed and tightened. The guide wires are removed, and the final construct is checked using fluoroscopy, ensuring the screws are fully seated, and there is no gap between the screw-plate-bone interface (Fig. 6.6).

Technical Considerations

When performing guided growth with an MPFL reconstruction, the guide growth plate should be placed prior to femoral fixation of the ligament, as it will lie deep to the ligament after MPFL reconstruction. At the time of planned hardware removal, it is vitally important to maintain the integrity of the MPFL reconstruction.

Derotational Femoral Osteotomies

Indications

In young patients, increased femoral anteversion, or internal torsion, has been associated with recurrent patellar instability [67]. A derotational femoral osteotomy can be used to correct pathologic anteversion and can safely be used in skeletally immature patients [67]. Similar to growth modulation, this technique can be done in isolation or in combination with a soft-tissue procedure detailed above to treat patellofemoral instability in the skeletally immature patient. Derotational femoral osteotomy is indicated with internal femoral torsion of more than 15–25° [67].

Measurement Technique

The Waidelich technique [68] is the most commonly cited method for measuring femoral torsion, and normative values are reported in the literature. The center of the femoral head on an axial image (CT or MRI) is connected to the center of an

Table 6.2 Guided growth constructs

Plate name	Manufacturer	Available sizes	Image
Eight-Plate and quad-Plate	Orthofix (McKinney, TX)	Eight-plate: 12 mm, 16 mm Quad-plate: 16 mm, 22 mm	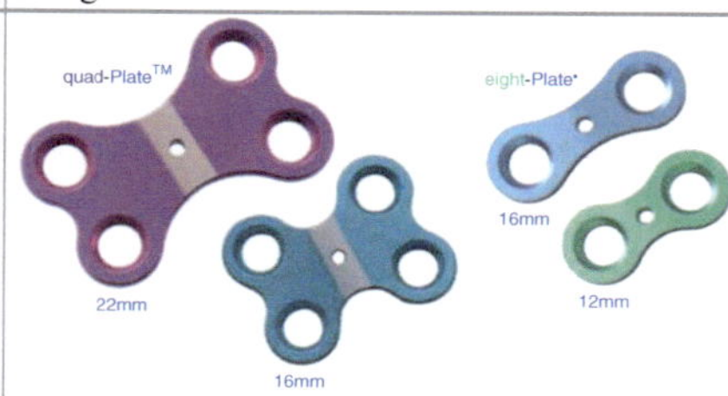
Hinge Plate	Pega Medical (Quebec, Canada)	12 mm, 16 mm, 20 mm	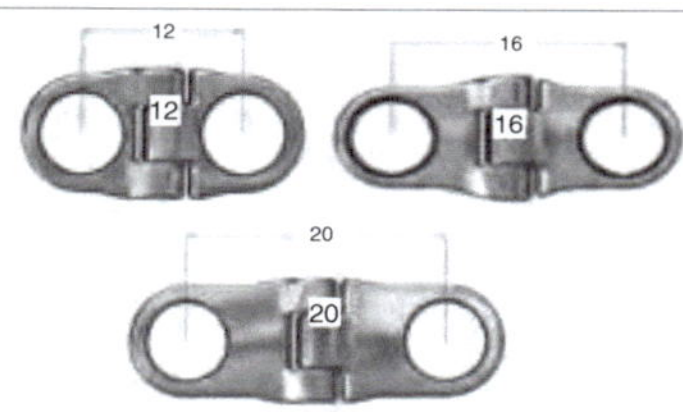
Peanut Plate	Biomet (Warsaw, IN)	Arched (purple): 12 mm, 16 mm Stepped (blue): 12 mm, 16 mm	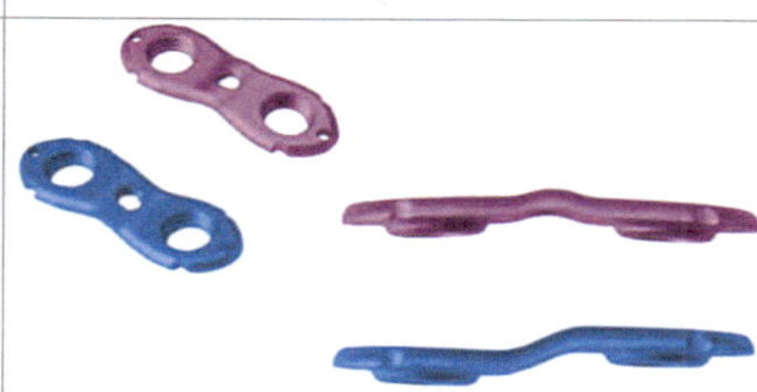
PediPlates	OrthoPediatrics (Warsaw, IN)	O-Plate: 12 mm, 16 mm I-Plate: 16 mm, 22 mm	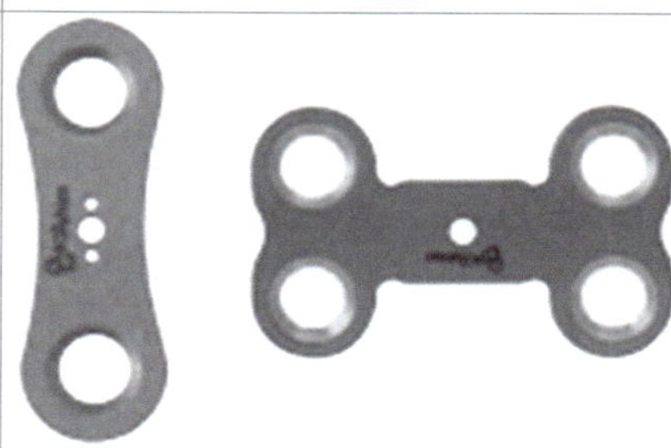

Adapted from Haskel et al. [66]

[a]From http://web.orthofix.com/Products/Products/Guided%20Growth%20System/EP-1004-PL-E0.pdf

[b]From http://www.pegamedical.com/medias/iw/hinge-plate_surgical_techniques_en.pdf

[c]From http://www.biomet.com/wps/wcm/connect/internet/dba65ca5-cb26-4718-83e0-55b11e78e368/Peanut%C2%AE+Growth+Control+Plating+System+Surgical+Technique.pdf?MOD=AJPERES&CACHEID=dba65ca5-cb26-4718-83e0-55b11e78e368

[d]From https://258413772373414384.s3.amazonaws.com/pdf/2015/5/ST-1010-01-01_Rev_C_PediPlates_Surgical_Technique.pdf

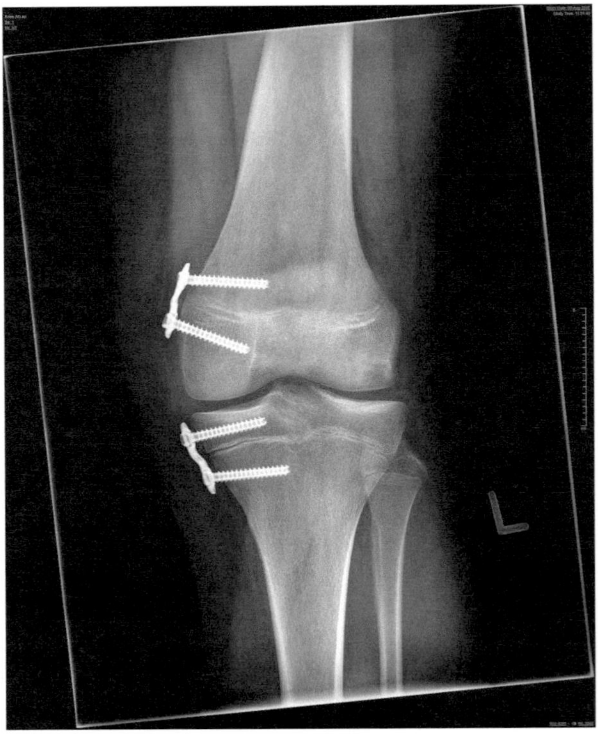

Fig. 6.6 Postoperative AP x-ray showing distal medial femoral and proximal medial tibial hemiepiphysiodesis for correction of a valgus deformity

ellipse around the greater trochanter on another axial slice (taken between the greater and lesser trochanter). The angle between this line and a line tangential to the posterior femoral condyles gives the femoral torsion. Kaiser et al. [69] showed a high level of intraobserver and interobserver agreement with this measurement method. Clinically, this can also be measured with the trochanteric prominence angle test [70]. With the patient in the prone position, the examiner internally rotates the hip until the greater trochanter is most prominent laterally. This degree of hip internal rotation correlates with three-dimensional imaging measurements of femoral torsion.

Special Considerations

Normal femoral anteversion at birth is between 30° and 40°, and this decreases to the normal adult average of 15° by skeletal maturity [67]. This factor needs to be taken into account when deciding to use a derotational femoral osteotomy in the skeletally immature patient.

Surgical Technique

Derotation can be achieved with a diaphyseal osteotomy and derotation over a nail [71, 72] or distally on the medial femur with a locking compression plate [73]. Small vertical marks should be made with a sagittal saw crossing the level of the planned osteotomy to accurately measure the amount of derotation.

Conclusion

Patellar dislocation is the most common acute knee disorder in children and adolescents [1]. Predisposing factors for patellofemoral instability are multifactorial. Nonsurgical treatment is typically used to treat a first-time acute patellar dislocation in a skeletally immature athlete. However, there is growing literature that may eventually support more aggressive treatment in this high-risk population. A recent systematic review showed that surgical treatment of first-time patella dislocation in children and adolescents is associated with a lower risk of recurrent dislocation and higher health-related quality of life and sporting function [74]. In the setting of recurrent instability, surgical reconstruction of the MPFL is recommended and should be tailored to the physeal growth status. Surgical treatment in skeletally immature athletes has evolved from non-anatomic extensor mechanism realignment procedures to anatomic procedures to recreate the MPFL and more recently the MQTFL. Lower limb alignment continues to be an important factor, and adjunct surgical treatment options, including implant-mediated guided growth, should be considered on a case-by-case basis.

References

1. Fithian DC, Paxton EW, Stone ML, et al. Epidemiology and natural history of acute patellar dislocation. Am J Sports Med. 2004;32(5):1114–21. PMID:15262631
2. Waterman BR, Belmont PJ Jr, Owens BD. Patellar dislocation in the United States: role of sex, age, race, and athletic participation. J Knee Surg. 2012;25(1):51–7. PMID:22624248
3. Apostolovic M, Vukomanovic B, Slavkovic N, et al. Acute patellar dislocation in adolescents: operative versus nonoperative treatment. Int Orthop. 2011;35(10):1483–7. PMID:21574051
4. Christiansen SE, Jakobsen BW, Lund B, Lind M. Isolated repair of the medial patellofemoral ligament in primary dislocation of the patella: a prospective randomized study. Arthroscopy. 2008;24(8):881–7. PMID:18657736
5. Colvin AC, West RV. Patellar instability. J Bone Joint Surg Am. 2008;90(12):2751–62. PMID:19047722
6. Lewallen LW, McIntosh AL, Dahm DL. Predictors of recurrent instability after acute patellofemoral dislocation in pediatric and adolescent patients. Am J Sports Med. 2013;41(3):575–81. PMID:23339838

7. McManus F, Rang M, Heslin DJ. Acute dislocation of the patella in children. The natural history. *Clin Orthop Relat Res*. 1979;139:88–91. PMID:378498
8. Palmu S, Kallio PE, Donell ST, Helenius I, Nietosvaara Y. Acute patellar dislocation in children and adolescents: a randomized clinical trial. J Bone Joint Surg Am. 2008;90(3):463–70. PMID:18310694
9. Sillanpaa PJ, Mattila VM, Maenpaa H, Kiuru M, Visuri T, Pihlajamaki H. Treatment with and without initial stabilizing surgery for primary traumatic patellar dislocation. A prospective randomized study. J Bone Joint Surg Am. 2009;91(2):263–73. PMID:19181969
10. Nomura E, Inoue M, Kurimura M. Chondral and osteochondral injuries associated with acute patellar dislocation. Arthroscopy. 2003;19(7):717–21. PMID:12966379
11. Kramer DE, Pace JL. Acute traumatic and sports-related osteochondral injury of the pediatric knee. Orthop Clin North Am. 2012;43(2):227–36. vi. PMID:22480471
12. Balcarek P, Jung K, Frosch KH, Sturmer KM. Value of the tibial tuberosity-trochlear groove distance in patellar instability in the young athlete. Am J Sports Med. 2011;39(8):1756–61. PMID:21566067
13. Bollier M, Fulkerson JP. The role of trochlear dysplasia in patellofemoral instability. J Am Acad Orthop Surg. 2011;19(1):8–16. PMID:21205763
14. Chotel F, Knorr G, Simian E, Dubrana F, Versier G, French AS. Knee osteochondral fractures in skeletally immature patients: French multicenter study. Orthop Traumatol Surg Res. 2011;97(8 Suppl):S154–9. PMID:22041573
15. Khormaee S, Kramer DE, Yen YM, Heyworth BE. Evaluation and management of patellar instability in pediatric and adolescent athletes. Sports Health. 2015;7(2):115–23. PMID:25984256
16. Nakamura N, Horibe S, Iwahashi T, Kawano K, Shino K, Yoshikawa H. Healing of a chondral fragment of the knee in an adolescent after internal fixation. A case report. J Bone Joint Surg Am. 2004;86-A(12):2741–6. PMID:15590863
17. Rorabeck CH, Bobechko WP. Acute dislocation of the patella with osteochondral fracture: a review of eighteen cases. J Bone Joint Surg Br. 1976;58(2):237–40. PMID:932087
18. Uchida R, Toritsuka Y, Yoneda K, Hamada M, Ohzono K, Horibe S. Chondral fragment of the lateral femoral trochlea of the knee in adolescents. Knee. 2012;19(5):719–23. PMID:22321389
19. Liu JN, Steinhaus ME, Kalbian IL, Post WR, Green DW, Strickland SM, Shubin Stein BE. Patellar instability management: a survey of the International Patellofemoral Study Group. Am J Sports Med. 2018;46(13):3299–306. https://doi.org/10.1177/0363546517732045. Epub 2017 Oct 6.
20. Pritchett JW. Longitudinal growth and growth-plate activity in the lower extremity. Clin Orthop Relat Res. 1992;275:274–9. PMID:1735225
21. Shea KG, Grimm NL, Belzer J, Burks RT, Pfeiffer R. The relation of the femoral physis and the medial patellofemoral ligament. Arthroscopy. 2010;26(8):1083–7. PMID:20678706
22. Kepler CK, Bogner EA, Hammoud S, Malcolmson G, Potter HG, Green DW. Zone of injury of the medial patellofemoral ligament after acute patellar dislocation in children and adolescents. Am J Sports Med. 2011;39(7):1444–9. PMID:21372313
23. Nelitz M, Dornacher D, Dreyhaupt J, Reichel H, Lippacher S. The relation of the distal femoral physis and the medial patellofemoral ligament. Knee Surg Sports Traumatol Arthrosc. 2011;19(12):2067–71. PMID:21594662
24. Nelitz M, Dreyhaupt J, Reichel H, Woelfle J, Lippacher S. Anatomic reconstruction of the medial patellofemoral ligament in children and adolescents with open growth plates: surgical technique and clinical outcome. Am J Sports Med. 2013;41(1):58–63. PMID:23111806
25. Nelitz M, Reichel H, Dornacher D, Lippacher S. Anatomical reconstruction of the medial patellofemoral ligament in children with open growth-plates. Arch Orthop Trauma Surg. 2012;132(11):1647–51. PMID:22878896
26. Harrison MH. The results of a realignment operation for recurrent dislocation of the patella. J Bone Joint Surg Br. 1955;37-B(4):559–67. PMID:13271482
27. Ahmad CS, Stein BE, Matuz D, Henry JH. Immediate surgical repair of the medial patellar stabilizers for acute patellar dislocation. A review of eight cases. Am J Sports Med. 2000;28(6):804–10. PMID:11101102

28. Mountney J, Senavongse W, Amis AA, Thomas NP. Tensile strength of the medial patellofemoral ligament before and after repair or reconstruction. J Bone Joint Surg Br. 2005;87(1):36–40. PMID:15686235
29. Camp CL, Krych AJ, Dahm DL, Levy BA, Stuart MJ. Medial patellofemoral ligament repair for recurrent patellar dislocation. Am J Sports Med. 2010;38(11):2248–54. PMID:20716682
30. Ahmad CS, Brown GD, Stein BS. The docking technique for medial patellofemoral ligament reconstruction: surgical technique and clinical outcome. Am J Sports Med. 2009;37(10):2021–7. PMID:19546481
31. Song SY, Kim IS, Chang HG, Shin JH, Kim HJ, Seo YJ. Anatomic medial patellofemoral ligament reconstruction using patellar suture anchor fixation for recurrent patellar instability. Knee Surg Sports Traumatol Arthrosc. 2014;22(10):2431–7. PMID:24154711
32. Wylie JD, Burks RT. Medial patellofemoral ligament reconstruction with semitendinosus autograft. Arthrosc Tech. 2013;2(4):e417–21. PMID:24400192
33. Bitar AC, D'Elia CO, Demange MK, Viegas AC, Camanho GL. Randomized prospective study on traumatic patellar dislocation: conservative treatment versus reconstruction of the medial patellofemoral ligament using the patellar tendon, with a minimum of two years of follow-up. Rev Bras Ortop. 2011;46(6):675–83. PMID:27027072
34. Camanho GL, Bitar AC, Hernandez AJ, Olivi R. Medial patellofemoral ligament reconstruction: a novel technique using the patellar ligament. *Arthroscopy*. 2007;23(1):108 e101–4. PMID:17210439
35. Witonski D, Keska R, Synder M, Sibinski M. An isolated medial patellofemoral ligament reconstruction with patellar tendon autograft. Biomed Res Int. 2013;2013:637678. PMID:24224173
36. Fink C, Veselko M, Herbort M, Hoser C. MPFL reconstruction using a quadriceps tendon graft: part 2: operative technique and short term clinical results. Knee. 2014;21(6):1175–9. PMID:24927675
37. Goyal D. Medial patellofemoral ligament reconstruction: the superficial quad technique. Am J Sports Med. 2013;41(5):1022–9. PMID:23460327
38. Nelitz M, Williams SR. Anatomic reconstruction of the medial patellofemoral ligament in children and adolescents using a pedicled quadriceps tendon graft. Arthrosc Tech. 2014;3(2):e303–8. PMID:24904782
39. Noyes FR, Albright JC. Reconstruction of the medial patellofemoral ligament with autologous quadriceps tendon. *Arthroscopy*. 2006;22(8):904 e901–7. PMID:16904594
40. Steensen RN, Dopirak RM, Maurus PB. A simple technique for reconstruction of the medial patellofemoral ligament using a quadriceps tendon graft. Arthroscopy. 2005;21(3):365–70. PMID:15756193
41. Vavalle G, Capozzi M. Isolated reconstruction of the medial patellofemoral ligament with autologous quadriceps tendon. J Orthop Traumatol. 2016;17(2):155–62. PMID:26387113
42. Jacobi M, Reischl N, Bergmann M, Bouaicha S, Djonov V, Magnussen RA. Reconstruction of the medial patellofemoral ligament using the adductor magnus tendon: an anatomic study. Arthroscopy. 2012;28(1):105–9. PMID:22001735
43. Sillanpaa PJ, Maenpaa HM, Mattila VM, Visuri T, Pihlajamaki H. A mini-invasive adductor magnus tendon transfer technique for medial patellofemoral ligament reconstruction: a technical note. Knee Surg Sports Traumatol Arthrosc. 2009;17(5):508–12. PMID:19165466
44. Steiner TM, Torga-Spak R, Teitge RA. Medial patellofemoral ligament reconstruction in patients with lateral patellar instability and trochlear dysplasia. Am J Sports Med. 2006;34(8):1254–61. PMID:16567459
45. Hohn E, Pandya NK. Does the utilization of allograft tissue in medial patellofemoral ligament reconstruction in pediatric and adolescent patients restore patellar stability? Clin Orthop Relat Res. 2017;475(6):1563–9.
46. Deie M, Ochi M, Sumen Y, Yasumoto M, Kobayashi K, Kimura H. Reconstruction of the medial patellofemoral ligament for the treatment of habitual or recurrent dislocation of the patella in children. J Bone Joint Surg Br. 2003;85(6):887–90. PMID:12931813

47. Gomes JE. Comparison between a static and a dynamic technique for medial patellofemoral ligament reconstruction. Arthroscopy. 2008;24(4):430–5. PMID:18375275
48. Lind M, Enderlein D, Nielsen T, Christiansen SE, Fauno P. Clinical outcome after reconstruction of the medial patellofemoral ligament in paediatric patients with recurrent patella instability. Knee Surg Sports Traumatol Arthrosc. 2016;24(3):666–71. PMID:25416673
49. Monllau JC, Masferrer-Pino A, Ginovart G, Perez-Prieto D, Gelber PE, Sanchis-Alfonso V. Clinical and radiological outcomes after a quasianatomical reconstruction of medial patellofemoral ligament with gracilis tendon autograft. Knee Surg Sports Traumatol Arthrosc. 2017;25(8):2453–9.
50. Schottle PB, Schmeling A, Rosenstiel N, Weiler A. Radiographic landmarks for femoral tunnel placement in medial patellofemoral ligament reconstruction. Am J Sports Med. 2007;35(5):801–4. PMID:17267773
51. Hinckel BB, Gobbi RG, Demange MK, Bonadio MB, Pecora JR, Camanho GL. Combined reconstruction of the medial patellofemoral ligament with Quadricipital tendon and the medial Patellotibial ligament with patellar tendon. Arthrosc Tech. 2016;5(1):e79–84. PMID:27073782
52. Tanaka MJ. Variability in the patellar attachment of the medial patellofemoral ligament. Arthroscopy. 2016;32(8):1667–70. PMID:27132768
53. Fulkerson JP, Edgar C. Medial quadriceps tendon-femoral ligament: surgical anatomy and reconstruction technique to prevent patella instability. Arthrosc Tech. 2013;2(2):e125–8. PMID:23875137
54. Stupay KL, Swart E, Shubin Stein BE. Widespread implementation of medial patellofemoral ligament reconstruction for recurrent patellar instability maintains functional outcomes at midterm to long-term follow-up while decreasing complication rates: a systematic review. Arthroscopy. 2015;31(7):1372–80. PMID:25703288
55. Ellera Gomes JL, Stigler Marczyk LR, Cesar de Cesar P, Jungblut CF. Medial patellofemoral ligament reconstruction with semitendinosus autograft for chronic patellar instability: a follow-up study. Arthroscopy. 2004;20(2):147–51. PMID:14760346
56. Mikashima Y, Kimura M, Kobayashi Y, Miyawaki M, Tomatsu T. Clinical results of isolated reconstruction of the medial patellofemoral ligament for recurrent dislocation and subluxation of the patella. Acta Orthop Belg. 2006;72(1):65–71. PMID:16570897
57. Siebold R, Chikale S, Sartory N, Hariri N, Feil S, Passler HH. Hamstring graft fixation in MPFL reconstruction at the patella using a transosseous suture technique. Knee Surg Sports Traumatol Arthrosc. 2010;18(11):1542–4. PMID:20411374
58. Thaunat M, Erasmus PJ. Recurrent patellar dislocation after medial patellofemoral ligament reconstruction. Knee Surg Sports Traumatol Arthrosc. 2008;16(1):40–3. PMID:17973099
59. Parikh SN, Nathan ST, Wall EJ, Eismann EA. Complications of medial patellofemoral ligament reconstruction in young patients. Am J Sports Med. 2013;41(5):1030–8. PMID:23539043
60. Guzman H, Yaszay B, Scott VP, Bastrom TP, Mubarak SJ. Early experience with medial femoral tension band plating in idiopathic genu valgum. J Child Orthop. 2011;5(1):11–7. PMID:21415941
61. Ballal MS, Bruce CE, Nayagam S. Correcting genu varum and genu valgum in children by guided growth: temporary hemiepiphysiodesis using tension band plates. J Bone Joint Surg Br. 2010;92(2):273–6. PMID:20130322
62. Stevens PM, Klatt JB. Guided growth for pathological physes: radiographic improvement during realignment. J Pediatr Orthop. 2008;28(6):632–9. PMID:18724199
63. Stevens PM. Guided growth for angular correction: a preliminary series using a tension band plate. J Pediatr Orthop. 2007;27(3):253–9. PMID:17414005
64. Kulkarni RM, Ilyas Rushnaiwala FM, Kulkarni GS, Negandhi R, Kulkarni MG, Kulkarni SG. Correction of coronal plane deformities around the knee using a tension band plate in children younger than 10 years. Indian J Orthop. 2015;49(2):208–18. PMID:26015611
65. Wiemann JM, Tryon C, Szalay EA. Physeal stapling versus 8-plate hemiepiphysiodesis for guided correction of angular deformity about the knee. J Pediatr Orthop. 2009;29(5):481–5. PMID:19568021

66. Haskel JD, Shin YW, Green DW. Applications of implant-mediated guided growth in pediatric knee surgery. In: Cordasco FA, Green DW, editors. Pediatric and adolescent knee surgery. New York: Wolters Kluwer; 2015.
67. Dejour D, Le Coultre B. Osteotomies in patello-femoral instabilities. Sports Med Arthrosc. 2007;15(1):39–46. PMID:17301701
68. Waidelich HA, Strecker W, Schneider E. Computed tomographic torsion-angle and length measurement of the lower extremity. The methods, normal values and radiation load. Rofo. 1992;157(3):245–51. PMID:1391819
69. Kaiser P, Attal R, Kammerer M, et al. Significant differences in femoral torsion values depending on the CT measurement technique. Arch Orthop Trauma Surg. 2016;136(9):1259–64. PMID:27501703
70. Delialioglu MO, Tasbas BA, Bayrakci K, et al. Alternative reliable techniques in femoral torsion measurement. J Pediatr Orthop B. 2006;15(1):28–33. PMID:16280716..
71. Pailhe R, Bedes L, Sales de Gauzy J, Tran R, Cavaignac E, Accadbled F. Derotational femoral osteotomy technique with locking nail fixation for adolescent femoral antetorsion: surgical technique and preliminary study. J Pediatr Orthop B. 2014;23(6):523–8. PMID:25153645
72. Stambough JB, Davis L, Szymanski DA, Smith JC, Schoenecker PL, Gordon JE. Knee Pain and Activity Outcomes After Femoral Derotation Osteotomy for Excessive Femoral Anteversion. J Pediatr Orthop. 2016. PMID:27636916.
73. Nelitz M, Dreyhaupt J, Williams SR, Dornacher D. Combined supracondylar femoral derotation osteotomy and patellofemoral ligament reconstruction for recurrent patellar dislocation and severe femoral anteversion syndrome: surgical technique and clinical outcome. Int Orthop. 2015;39(12):2355–62. PMID:26156717
74. Nwachukwu BU, So C, Schairer WW, Green DW, Dodwell ER. Surgical versus conservative management of acute patellar dislocation in children and adolescents: a systematic review. Knee Surg Sports Traumatol Arthrosc. 2016;24(3):760–7. PMID:26704809

Chapter 7
Acute Patellar Dislocation (First-Time Dislocator)

Jacqueline Munch Brady

Natural History

The incidence of patellar dislocation is 29 per 100,000 in the adolescent age group, and recurrence rates with nonoperative treatment after a first-time dislocation have been reported from 15% to 70% [1–5]. Most authors describe the patient population suffering from patellofemoral instability as predominantly female [2], although Atkin et al. described an equal male and female patient population in the primary or first-time patella dislocator [3]. The incidence of chondral or osteochondral injury after first-time dislocation is approximately 70% [4], ranging from cracking or fissure formation to full-thickness chondral and osteochondral injury [6]. This chondral injury predisposes patients to an increased risk of posttraumatic arthritis, particularly if the instability becomes recurrent.

The anatomy or pathoanatomy of the patellofemoral joint itself contributes to patellar instability. Trochlear dysplasia, indicating an abnormally shallow or convex femoral trochlear groove, has been demonstrated to be the number one more predictive risk factor for recurrence after first-time dislocation, particularly in young patients [1, 5]. According to a study by Askenberger et al., trochlear dysplasia is the most common anatomic factor found in skeletally immature first-time patellar dislocators [7]. Li et al. demonstrated secondary trochlear dysplasia following iatrogenic patellar dislocation in a rabbit model, suggesting that skeletally immature patients may be particularly at risk of recurrence after their first instability episode in part due to an alteration of the normal joint contact forces and secondary changes in trochlear architecture [8]. Likewise, patella alta, or an abnormally high-riding patella in the sagittal plane, can increase the instability of the patellofemoral joint by requiring more knee flexion before patellar engagement. Coronal malalignment can be demon-

J. M. Brady (✉)
Department of Orthopaedics and Rehabilitation, Oregon Health and Science University, Portland, OR, USA
e-mail: munch@ohsu.edu

B. E. Shubin Stein, S. M. Strickland (eds.), *Patellofemoral Pain and Instability*,
https://doi.org/10.1007/978-3-319-97640-2_7

strated clinically by testing a patient for a "J-sign" during knee range of motion: the centralized patella in a flexed knee shifts laterally with knee extension, when it becomes disengaged from the underlying trochlea. Coronal malalignment can also be measured statically using the quadriceps or "Q" angle on physical examination or the tibial tubercle-to-trochlear groove (TT-TG) distance on cross-sectional imaging.

Patellofemoral stability is highly dependent on the integrity of the soft tissues surrounding the joint. The medial patellofemoral ligament (MPFL) has been shown to provide 60% of the restraint to lateral patellar translation [9]. As the force required to rupture the MPFL in biomechanical testing is lower than the force required to dislocate the patella [10, 11], the MPFL is considered to be injured in all cases of patellofemoral dislocation. The retinacular expansion of the extensor mechanism of the knee is known to be an important stabilizing force as well. While the lateral retinacular release gained popularity as a treatment intervention for patellofemoral instability when arthroscopy became more widely used, biomechanical evidence has demonstrated that the procedure actually reduces the stability of the patellofemoral joint [9] and thus isolated lateral release is not an appropriate procedure to treat patellar instability.

Patient factors also contribute to patellar instability. Patients with collagen abnormalities such as Ehlers-Danlos Syndrome are known to have higher rates of joint instability, likely due to laxity of the retinaculum and medial patellofemoral ligament in particular [12]. The mechanical factors—such as upright landing and positioning in valgus and internal rotation—that have been shown to contribute to risk of ACL rupture are also thought to have a role in patellofemoral instability, though studies are forthcoming on the utility of intervention. Finally, age has recently become better recognized as a risk factor for recurrence after first-time dislocation: patients under the age of 25 have been demonstrated to have a four times higher rate of recurrence than their older counterparts, and this risk increases if the patients exhibit any degree of trochlear dysplasia [1, 5].

The mechanism of injury of patellofemoral instability often involves positioning in valgus and internal rotation and predominantly non-contact [13]. While a transient subluxation episode may be a comparatively subtle diagnosis, patellar dislocation is often dramatic, requiring manipulation to achieve anatomic reduction. Patients experience significant swelling, which may cause quadriceps inhibition and buckling of the knee. On examination, patients exhibit increased patellar translation and apprehension to lateral translation in particular. X-rays may be unremarkable but may show a loose body caused by an osteochondral injury, or an avulsion injury to the medial patellar bone (Fig. 7.1) may be identified. MRI demonstrates injury to

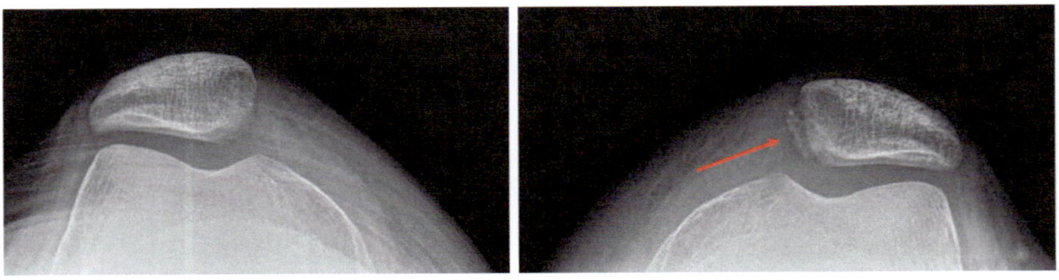

Fig. 7.1 Bilateral knee Merchant view demonstrating an avulsion injury to the medial patella (red arrow)

the medial patellofemoral ligament and retinacular complex, along with the typical bony contusions to the medial patella and lateral trochlea or lateral femoral condyle (Fig. 7.2a, b). MRI can also demonstrate a bony patellar avulsion injury or a chondral/osteochondral defect (Fig. 7.3).

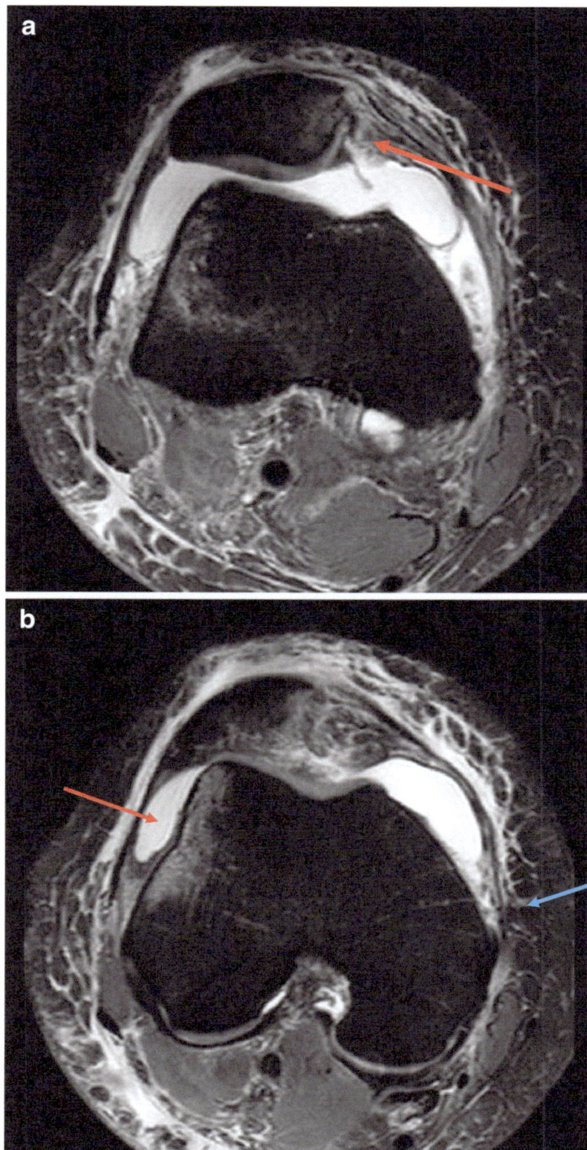

Fig. 7.2 Axial MRI images depicting (**a**) a medial patellar bony contusion (red arrow) and (**b**) a lateral trochlear contusion (red arrow) with a femoral-sided injury to the medial patellofemoral complex (blue arrow)

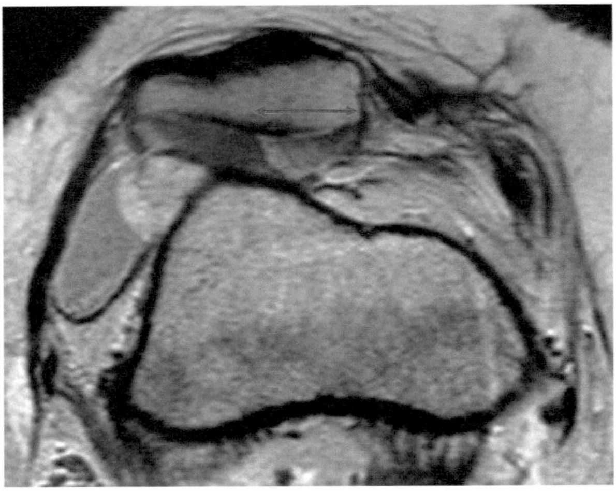

Fig. 7.3 Axial MRI image depicting a full-thickness central and medial patellar chondral injury (red arrow) in a patient with recurrent patellofemoral instability

Treatment Options

Closed reduction of a fixed dislocation can be performed in the field or in an emergency room/urgent care setting. The knee is gently and progressively extended, and lateral pressure is applied to the patella. Patients may elect to undergo anesthesia for the closed reduction procedure if they are in significant pain. The patella generally reduces into its anatomic position without incident. Immobilization in full extension can help prevent the patient from suffering a buckling episode in the setting of significant swelling and quadriceps inhibition but should not be prolonged, as it can lead to stiffness and atrophy and thus delay the return to function [14]. Patients are instructed on crutch use to prevent falls and encourage pain-free ambulation with as much protected quadriceps activation as possible.

First-time dislocators are generally treated conservatively, unless an additional injury such as a loose body or osteochondral fracture warrants surgical intervention. Physical therapy is a mainstay of patellofemoral rehabilitation. Initial interventions include the normalization of gait and restoration of motion. Core and hip strengthening are begun early, to prepare the patient for more coordinated activities. Once the patient is exhibiting normal muscle activation and near-normal motion, strengthening efforts around the knee begin. When strength is approaching baseline, more complex exercises and return-to-sport efforts begin.

Surgical Indications

If a patellofemoral instability episode results in a loose chondral or osteochondral fragment, surgery is indicated to prevent further chondral injury from impingement of the loose fragment. If the osteochondral fragment is large (Fig. 7.4a–c), repair is

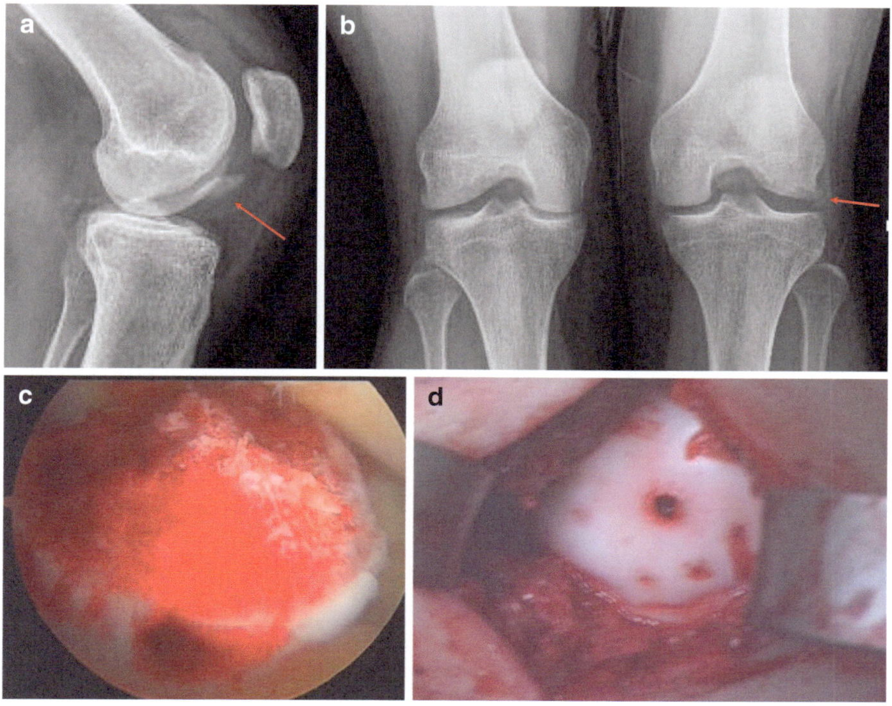

Fig. 7.4 (**a**) and (**b**): Radiographs demonstrating a lateral femoral condyle osteochondral injury in the setting of patellar dislocation. (**c**): Intraoperative view of the bony bed at the base of the injury. (**d**): Repair of the osteochondral fragment, which was performed concomitantly with patellar stabilization surgery

undertaken. The surgical repair generally requires a small arthrotomy (Fig. 7.4d) and is completed in the early post-injury period for the best result. The base of the lesion is debrided of any fibrous tissue; the fragment is reduced into its anatomical position, and the construct is secured with small absorbable tacks, headless compression screws, or a combination thereof, depending on size and depth. This early surgical intervention in an inflamed and acutely injured knee may increase the risk of postoperative stiffness, so an appropriate balance must be struck between protection of the repair and restoration of motion. Improvements in implants for repair of even small osteochondral lesions have allowed surgeons to allow early postoperative range of motion in most cases.

Some controversy still exists regarding whether a patient who is undergoing a simple loose body removal or a more involved osteochondral repair should also undergo stabilization of the patellofemoral joint. The risks of the additional procedure must be considered, but the case for prevention of posttraumatic arthritis in the setting of potential recurrent instability is compelling. Generally, the surgical intervention, when stabilizing a patellofemoral joint after the first intervention episode, is targeted at restoring the function of the medial patellofemoral ligament (MPFL) via either repair or reconstruction. Based on a recently published survey of the Internation Patellofemoral Study Group, the consensus opinion was to also stabilize patients when treating the loose body or osteochondral fracture [15].

MPFL Repair

MRI studies have demonstrated variability in the location of the MPFL injury following patellofemoral dislocation, with a majority of patellar-sided injuries in skeletally immature patients [16, 17]. MPFL disruption has been demonstrated at the patellar insertion, at the femoral origin, within the midsubstance of the ligament, or in more than one of the aforementioned locations. Careful scrutiny of the patient's imaging to locate the site of injury is therefore crucial if repair is to be undertaken [18, 19].

MPFL Reconstruction

One study has shown that MPFL repair after first-time dislocation does not affect the rate of recurrent instability [20], but Arendt et al. demonstrated in 2011 that the rate of failure of MPFL repair is high in the setting of recurrent patellofemoral instability [21]. Thus, if the location of the injury to the MPFL is combined or unclear on imaging or if the patient has any history of possible pre-existing patellar instability, MPFL reconstruction should be considered. Please see Chapter 6 for more detail on the technique of MPFL reconstruction.

Recommendations for Treatment of First-Time Patellofemoral Dislocators

After successful reduction of a dislocated patella, x-rays are obtained of the affected knee, including an axial patellofemoral view in early flexion (Merchant view) to evaluate for residual patellofemoral malalignment and any osteochondral injury. The knee is placed into an extension brace, which is worn for ambulation until the return of quadriceps function (at our institution, the ability to perform a straight leg raise is used as the criterion for allowing ambulation with normal knee flexion). The patient is instructed on crutch use, which should continue until any alteration in normal gait resolves. The patient may then be discharged from the acute setting and allowed to follow up on a more elective basis.

Given the high rate of chondral and osteochondral injury associated with patellar dislocation, patients generally undergo MRI to investigate the chondral surfaces and evaluate any additional soft tissue injury. If a small chondral or osteochondral fragment is discovered, the patient undergoes arthroscopy with loose body removal to prevent mechanical symptoms and further injury. Because of the high rate of recurrent instability and potential for resultant cumulative chondral injury in the absence of stabilization, concurrent MPFL reconstruction is generally undertaken if patients proceed to surgery for loose body removal. Likewise, if a larger osteochondral fragment is discovered on imaging, patients proceed to surgery for arthroscopic evaluation followed by fracture fixation via a small arthrotomy, along with MPFL reconstruction.

In cases of first-time dislocation without a displaced chondral or osteochondral injury, the patient is carefully evaluated via physical examination and imaging for risk factors associated with recurrent instability: generalized laxity as measured by the Beighton criteria, patella alta, coronal malalignment (J-sign or TT-TG), and trochlear dysplasia. Operative intervention for these patients is uncommon and remains controversial, but some surgeons elect to proceed with MPFL reconstruction in patients with significant risk factors and/or a history of contralateral instability. In the case of skeletally mature patients with dramatic malalignment (patella alta or coronal malalignment), distal realignment in the form of tibial tubercle osteotomy may be combined with MPFL reconstruction to improve patellar tracking and stability.

For the majority of first-time patellofemoral dislocators, who are treated without surgery, a dedicated rehabilitation protocol is prescribed. Gentle range of motion and control of knee pain and swelling are prescribed first, along with strengthening of the core and hip musculature. Gait training is an early focus as well: patients walk with one or two crutches and place as much weight on the walking aid as is necessary to contract the quadriceps muscles with each step. Once the swelling and pain have subsided, quadriceps function has returned, and normal gait is restored, the physical therapist proceeds with more focused strengthening of the quadriceps and hamstrings, proprioception exercises, and training for return to sports and activities for work. Experienced therapists may recommend taping, supportive bracing, and modalities for accelerated quadriceps activation and improved comfort during the recovery process.

Bibliography

1. Lewallen LW, McIntosh AL, Dahm DL. Predictors of recurrent instability after acute patellofemoral dislocation in pediatric and adolescent patients. Am J Sports Med. 2013;41(3):575–81. https://doi.org/10.1177/0363546512472873.
2. Fithian DC, Paxton EW, Stone ML, et al. Epidemiology and natural history of acute patellar dislocation. Am J Sport Med. 2004;32:1114–21.
3. Atkin DM, Fithian DC, Marangi KS, Stone ML, Dobson BE, Mendelsohn C. Characteristics of patients with primary acute lateral patellar dislocation and their recovery within the first 6 months of injury. Am J Sports Med. 2000;28(4):472–9. http://www.ncbi.nlm.nih.gov/pubmed/10921637.

4. Elias DA, White LM. Acute lateral patellar dislocation at MR imaging: injury patterns of medial patellar soft-tissue restraints and osteochondral injuries of the inferomedial patella. Radiology. 2002;225(3):736–43.
5. Lewallen L, Mcintosh A, Dahm D. First-time patellofemoral dislocation: risk factors for recurrent instability. J Knee Surg. 2015;28(4):303–9. https://doi.org/10.1055/s-0034-1398373.
6. Nomura E, Inoue M. Second-look arthroscopy of cartilage changes of the patellofemoral joint, especially the patella, following acute and recurrent patellar dislocation. Osteoarthr Cartil. 2005;13(11):1029–36. https://doi.org/10.1016/j.joca.2005.07.004.
7. Askenberger M, Janarv P-M, Finnbogason T, Arendt EA. Morphology and anatomic patellar instability risk factors in first-time traumatic lateral patellar dislocations: a prospective magnetic resonance imaging study in skeletally immature children. Am J Sports Med. 2016;45:50–8. https://doi.org/10.1177/0363546516663498.
8. Li W, Wang Q, Wang F, Zhang Y, Ma L, Dong J. Femoral trochlear dysplasia after patellar dislocation in rabbits. Knee. 2013;20(6):485–9. https://doi.org/10.1016/j.knee.2013.05.016.
9. Desio SM, Burks RT, Bachus KN. Soft tissue restraints to lateral patellar translation in the human knee. Am J Sport Med. 1998;26(1):59–65.
10. Arendt EA. MPFL reconstruction for PF instability: the soft (tissue) approach. Orthop Traumatol Surg Res. 2009;95(8):97–100.
11. Amis AA, Firer P, Mountney J, Senavongse W, Thomas NP. Anatomy and biomechanics of the medial patellofemoral ligament. Knee. 2003;10:215–20. https://doi.org/10.1016/S0968-0160(03)00006-1.
12. Cattalini M, Khubchandani R, Cimas R. When flexibility is not necessarily a virtue: a review of hypermobility syndromes and chronic or recurrent musculoskeletal pain in children. Pediatr Rheumatol Online J. 2015;13(1):40.
13. Mitchell J, Magnussen RA, Collins CL, et al. Epidemiology of overuse injuries among high school athletes in the United States. Am J Sports Med. 2015;43(7):1676–82. https://doi.org/10.1177/0363546515577786.
14. Rood A, Boons H, Ploegmakers J, van der Stappen W, Koeter S. Tape versus cast for non-operative treatment of primary patellar dislocation: a randomized controlled trial. Arch Orthop Trauma Surg. 2012;132(8):1199–203.
15. Liu JN, Steinhaus ME, Kalbian IL, Post WR, Green DW, Strickland SM, Shubin Stein BE. Patellar instability management: a survey of the International Patellofemoral Study Group. Am J Sports Med. 2018;46(13):3299–306. https://doi.org/10.1177/0363546517732045. Epub 2017 Oct 6.
16. Kepler CK, Bogner EA, Hammoud S, Malcolmson G, Potter HG, Green DW. Zone of injury of the medial patellofemoral ligament after acute patellar dislocation in children and adolescents. Am J Sports Med. 2011;39(7):1444–9. https://doi.org/10.1177/0363546510397174.
17. Askenberger M, Arendt EA, Ekstro MW, Voss U, Finnbogason T, Janarv P-M. Medial patellofemoral ligament injuries in children with first-time lateral patellar dislocations: a magnetic resonance imaging and arthroscopic study. Am J Sports Med. 2016;44(1):152–8. https://doi.org/10.1177/0363546515611661.
18. Camanho GL, Viegas ADC, Bitar AC, Demange MK, Hernandez AJ. Conservative versus surgical treatment for repair of the medial patellofemoral ligament in acute dislocations of the Patella. Arthroscopy. 2009;25(6):620–5. https://doi.org/10.1016/j.arthro.2008.12.005.
19. Christiansen SE, Jakobsen BW, Lund B, Lind M. Isolated repair of the medial patellofemoral ligament in primary dislocation of the Patella: a prospective randomized study. Arthroscopy. 2008;24(8):881–7. https://doi.org/10.1016/j.arthro.2008.03.012.
20. Palmu S, Kallio PE, Donell ST, et al. Treatment with and without initial stabilizing surgery for primary traumatic patellar dislocation. A prospective randomized study. J Bone Joint Surg Am. 2008;24(12):620–5. https://doi.org/10.1016/j.arthro.2008.03.012.
21. Arendt EA, Moeller A, Agel J. Clinical outcomes of medial patellofemoral ligament repair in recurrent (chronic) lateral patella dislocations. Knee Surg Sports Tramatol Arthrosc. 2011;19:1909–14.

Chapter 8
Recurrent Patellar Instability

Robin West, Ryan S. Murray, and Daniel M. Dean

Introduction

Recurrent patellar instability has an incidence of 5.8 per 100,000; in individuals age 10–17 years, the incidence increases to 29 per 100,000 [1, 2]. The rate of recurrence after a single episode of patellar dislocation ranges from 15% to 69% if the initial injury is treated nonoperatively [2]. If a second patellar dislocation occurs, there is a 50% incidence of further recurrent patellar dislocations [1]. Although the rate of recurrence following primary patellar dislocation is low in some patients, many patients may continue to have pain and mechanical symptoms of instability following the initial dislocation episode [3]. Patellar dislocation can result in articular cartilage injuries, osteochondral fractures, and patellofemoral arthritis in addition to the risk of recurrent instability [1, 2, 4]. Atkin et al. found that 58% of patients had limitations in strenuous activity at 6 months following a single episode of patellar dislocation [5]. In addition, up to 55% of patients fail to return to sporting activity after a primary patellar dislocation event [5].

The etiology of patellar instability is multifactorial and is related to limb alignment, the osseous structure of the patella and trochlea, and the integrity of the static and dynamic soft tissue constraints [4, 6]. The management of recurrent patellar instability is challenging due to the complex relationship of the predisposing factors as well as a dearth of long-term, robust, clinical outcome studies. This chapter will provide an understanding of the factors affecting recurrent patellar instability and an algorithmic approach to managing these injuries.

R. West (✉)
Inova Sports Medicine, Georgetown University Medical Center, Washington, DC, USA

Virginia Commonwealth University School of Medicine, Richmond, VA, USA
e-mail: robin.west@inova.org

R. S. Murray · D. M. Dean
Department of Orthopedic Surgery, Georgetown University Hospital, Washington, DC, USA

B. E. Shubin Stein, S. M. Strickland (eds.), *Patellofemoral Pain and Instability*,
https://doi.org/10.1007/978-3-319-97640-2_8

Treatment

Nonoperative Management

When considering the management of patellar dislocations in general, there is strong evidence to support nonoperative management for first-time patellar dislocators [7]. There is a shortage of evidence indicating whether physical therapy or bracing is effective in the management of acute, first-time, patellar dislocations. However, the aim of nonoperative treatment of a patellar dislocation is to decrease swelling, promote vastus medialis and gluteus activity, and increase knee range of motion [6]. Swelling negatively affects quadriceps function, so the faster the swelling is controlled and reduced, the more expedient the expected recovery.

Before making recommendations regarding treatment, plain radiographs should be performed to include a 45° flexion weight bearing, a flexion lateral, and bilateral Merchant views to assess joint space narrowing, patellar height, patellar tilt, and trochlear dysplasia (Figs. 8.1, 8.2 and 8.3). An MRI is usually performed in addition to the radiographs to better assess articular cartilage, medial patellofemoral ligament, and other associated findings.

Few studies have directly addressed the efficacy of various nonoperative treatment modalities [6]. Treatment regimens range from immediate mobilization without a brace to cast immobilization in extension for a period of 6 weeks, with countless variations in between. Immobilization in extension may help the medial soft tissue structures heal but can result in stiffness. Maenpaa and Lehto treated 100 patients with three modalities, cast immobilization, posterior splint, or a patella brace. The casts and splints were worn for 6 weeks, and the patients were followed an average of 13 years post injury. There was a three times higher rate of redislocation in patients treated with a brace. However, cast immobilization resulted in an expected higher rate of stiffness [8].

There is also a role for nonoperative modalities, including physical therapy in patients with recurrent patellar instability. This is especially true when evaluating in-season athletes who desire to continue to participate. However, they need to be

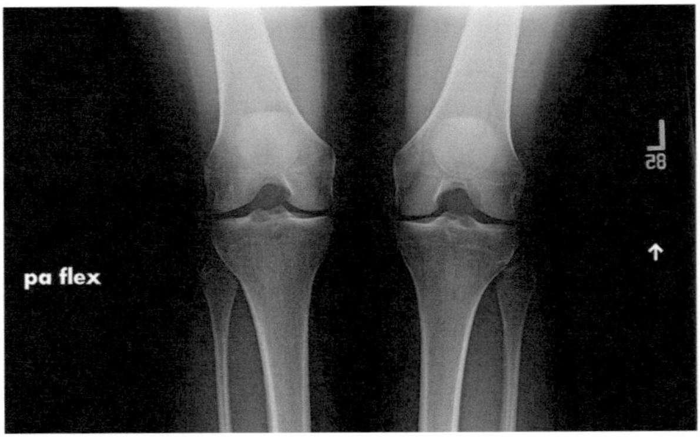

Fig. 8.1 PA flexion weight-bearing radiograph to assess joint space narrowing, patellar height

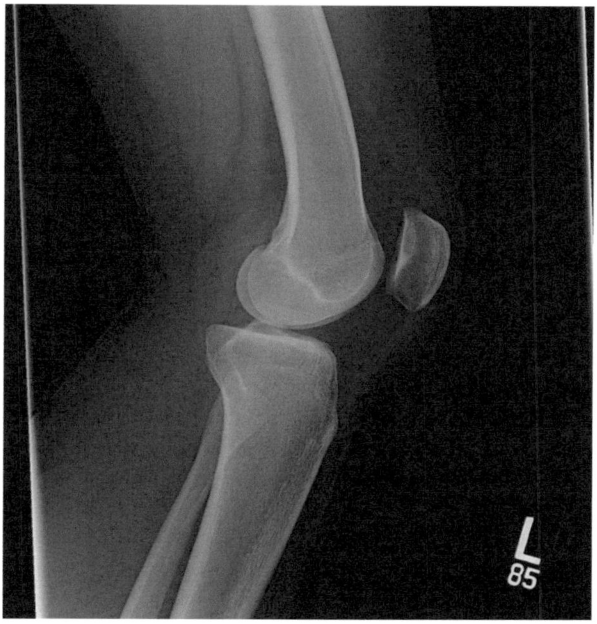

Fig. 8.2 Lateral flexion weight-bearing radiograph to assess patellar height/tilt, trochlear dysplasia, joint space narrowing/spurring

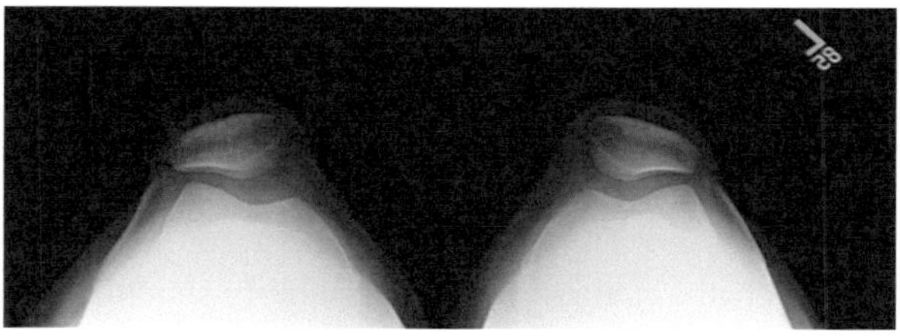

Fig. 8.3 Bilateral Merchant view radiograph to assess patellar tilt, patellar subluxation, trochlear dysplasia, joint space narrowing

informed as to the risks, including recurrent dislocation as well as the potential for cartilage and soft tissue damage [4]. Patients with chronic patellar instability may benefit from physical therapy which can help to regain strength, motion, and proprioception. Therapy should consist of a gradual progression to full range of motion and strength followed by a graduated return to play. Patellar taping such as McConnell taping may help to control excessive patellar motion during therapy and has been shown to increase quadriceps muscle torque while activating the vastus medialis earlier than the vastus lateralis with repetitive resisted flexion and extension [9–11]. Hinged knee braces or lateral stabilization braces may also enhance the patient's sense of stability and should be employed especially in the case of an in-season athlete hoping to progress through rehabilitation more aggressively [4, 6]. Muscle specific physical therapy should focus not only on the medial quadriceps but also on the gluteal muscles, which are often weak in recurrent patellar dislocators. This weakness results in adduction and internal rotation of the femur, which may exacerbate patellar instability with weight-bearing activities. Strengthening the gluteal muscles, and in some cases taping the hip, helps to promote external rotation of the femur to help address this problem [10].

There is a growing body of evidence to support weight-bearing or closed chain exercises for rehabilitation rather than open chain exercises. It has been shown that closed chain knee extension promotes simultaneous electromyographic activity in the four different muscles of the quadriceps in asymptomatic subjects. The rectus femoris has the earliest response, while the vastus medialis obliquus has the latest and weakest response with open chain exercises, which is not optimal in rehabilitation of a recurrently unstable patella [12]. Closed chain exercises, however, produce more vastus activity which promotes patellar stability and allows for training of the vastus muscles as well as the gluteal muscles and core trunk muscles simultaneously to better control limb position [13].

Despite the potential for a reasonably good response to nonoperative methods in first-time patellar dislocators, there is a significant rate of failure. Atkin et al. reviewed their results of nonoperative management at 6 months following patellar dislocation and found that 58% of patients continued to have limitations with strenuous activity and that 55% had not returned to sports [5]. Therefore it is generally thought that operative intervention is indicated in patients who continue to experience recurrent patellar instability with or without progressive worsening osteochondral injury [4]. Thus, the benefit of avoiding surgery should be weighed against the risks of recurrent dislocation and further secondary injury.

Operative Management

Patients with recurrent patellar instability should be thoroughly evaluated to determine the optimal surgical approach to address their pathology. More than 100 different operations have been described for the treatment of patellar instability, and typically, a combination of procedures is necessary to achieve a satisfactory outcome. Given the multifactorial and dynamic problems associated with recurrent patellar instability, the approach to a surgical evaluation should be algorithmic in nature. A thorough algorithm to approach these patients will be discussed briefly, and the specific techniques will be covered in detail subsequently.

There are several clinical and radiographic metrics that must be incorporated into the initial evaluation of surgical treatment options for recurrent patellar instability. First a determination of skeletal maturity should be made. For skeletally immature patients, the coronal and rotational alignment should be determined as well as any isolated or concomitant soft tissue injury to the medial patellofemoral ligament

(MPFL). In skeletally immature patients with a coronal malalignment greater than 10°, with more than a year of growth remaining, a guided growth hemiepiphysiodesis should be done and will be covered more thoroughly in the pediatrics section. If excessive femoral anteversion (absolute value of greater than 20–25°) is present, a femoral derotational osteotomy may be considered as a component of the management of the recurrent patellar instability. Finally, in the setting of medial patellofemoral ligament disruption in the skeletally immature patient, an anatomic medial patellofemoral ligament reconstruction should be undertaken. In cases where there is a concern for potential physeal injury, a non-anatomic procedure can be pursued.

In the skeletally mature patient, important anatomic metrics including trochlear dysplasia, patella alta, patella tilt, and tibial tubercle-trochlear groove distance should be compiled to determine the best procedure(s) to address their recurrent patellar instability. A general brief overview of the indications will be outlined and again reviewed in detail in later sections. The tibial tubercle-trochlear groove distance should be considered as a part of the equation, and if it is close to, or above, 20 millimeters and/or if there is a lateral patellar or trochlear chondral lesion, a tibial tubercle transfer should be considered. If there is significant patella alta, the tubercle may also be distalized in isolation or in combination with medialization. If Dejour Types B or D trochlear dysplasia is present, a groove deepening trochleoplasty can be considered; however, it is important to realize that this procedure has significant potential complications including early arthritis and chondral damage and should be considered only if other well done stabilization procedures have failed. Patients with a medial patellofemoral ligament injury should undergo a medial patellofemoral ligament reconstruction in conjunction with any necessary osseous procedures. In cases of patellar tilt greater than 20° that is not flexible, but fixed, a lateral release or lengthening can be done in combination with other definitive procedures. Finally, in cases of rotational alignment abnormalities, such as excessive tibial external rotation or femoral anteversion, derotational osteotomies should be considered.

The subsequent sections will provide a detailed review of the various procedures to address each facet of the pathology inherent to recurrent patellar instability. It should be noted that these procedures do not always occur in isolation so a thorough review of the underlying pathology should be undertaken prior to selecting the corrective surgical procedure(s). Prior to performing any surgical treatment, a diagnostic knee arthroscopy should be performed to assess for associated meniscal, ligamentous, or articular cartilage injuries. The 70° scope placed into the superolateral portal gives a view of the entire patellofemoral joint and allows for excellent visualization to assess the articular cartilage of the trochlea and patella and the patellar tracking through a range of motion (Figs. 8.4 and 8.5).

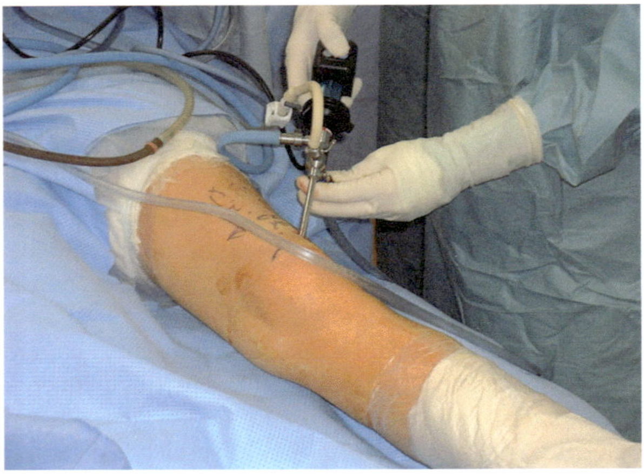

Fig. 8.4 Diagnostic arthroscopy from the superolateral portal with the 70° arthroscope to assess patellar tracking throughout range of motion, status of articular cartilage

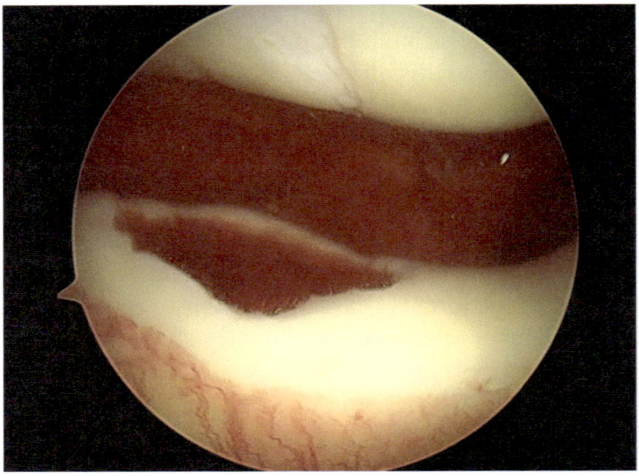

Fig. 8.5 Diagnostic arthroscopy from the superolateral portal with the 70° arthroscope shows large cartilage shear injury that occurred during patellar subluxation event

Lateral Release

Lateral release is commonly mistaken as a surgical treatment option for recurrent patellar instability. In fact, an isolated lateral release is the only surgical procedure that has been proven ineffective in the treatment of patellar instability. Despite the utility of a lateral release in treating lateral patellar compression syndrome, there is no utility of an isolated lateral release in the setting of patellar instability [14]. In a series of 28 patients by Kolowich et al., 100% of patients who underwent lateral release for patellar instability had persistent instability [14]. In a review of 14 studies evaluating lateral release as a surgical treatment for patellar instability, there was 80% satisfaction in the short term; however, this dropped to 63.5% at 4 years postoperatively [15].

These poor results can be attributed to several factors, with the principal one being that the lateral release fails to align the patella more medially. In addition, lateral release can be complicated by medial instability if the release extends proximally into the attachment of the vastus lateralis obliquus [15]. Despite these poor results, lateral release or lateral lengthening can be used in conjunction with other medial sided procedures such as medial patellofemoral ligament reconstruction. Furthermore, if there is osseous malalignment, a bony procedure and a lateral release can be combined successfully.

Medial Repair

Repair of the medial sided structures following patellar dislocations is less commonly performed today compared with reconstructive procedures. However, there is value in exploring and considering the body of literature surrounding these procedures. Advocates of a medial sided repair or imbrication as an alternative to reconstruction cite the potential to overload the patella with graft reconstruction [16]. The native medial patellofemoral ligament has a load to failure of 208 Newtons, while a hamstring graft used in medial patellofemoral ligament reconstruction can withstand up to 1600 Newtons [16]. Medial imbrication is non-anatomic and can result in over medialization of the patella and lead to abnormal tracking and pressures. Ostermeier et al. showed biomechanically that the combination of a medial imbrication and lateral release resulted in a significantly medialized and internally tilted patella compared with the native knee [17]. In addition, medial imbrication fails to address the most common etiology of medial sided instability which is disruption of the medial patellofemoral ligament [18].

There are two randomized controlled trials comparing medial repair with nonoperative treatment of acute patellar dislocations. In these studies, 127 first-time patellar dislocators were evaluated at 2 and 7 years [19, 20]. At both intervals, there was no difference in the rate of recurrent instability. There were also no significant differences in objective outcome scores. In a study by Palmu et al., the rates of recurrent dislocation (70%) were similar between patients who had undergone medial sided repair and those who were managed nonoperatively [7]. At 14-year follow-up, both groups had similar good to excellent subjective outcome scores. These studies illustrate that there is no significant advantage to primary medial sided repair in comparison with nonoperative treatment for first-time dislocators.

Despite these results, there are proponents of medial sided repair for acute first-time dislocators. In a small series by Ahmad et al., patients who underwent an acute medial sided repair with repair of any torn vastus medialis obliquus muscle had no episodes of recurrent instability [21]. In a survey of the National Football League Physician's Society, 6% or 1 out of 32 surgeons suggested that they would perform a medial sided repair for an acute patellar dislocation on a competitive athlete without a loose body [6, 22]. Furthermore, early operative intervention for an acute patellar dislocation was not indicated for athletes at any level by 58 percent of surgeons surveyed.

Thus medial sided repair or imbrication has a fairly robust degree of evidence to suggest that it fails to provide adequate restoration of patellofemoral stability in the setting of patellar dislocation. There is seldom an instance given modern techniques of reconstruction where such a procedure would be indicated given the non-anatomic nature of the procedure and the failed randomized trials suggesting no improvement over nonoperative management.

In addition, repair has been looked at for recurrent patella instability. A study by Arendt et al. retrospectively reported on MPFL repair in 55 knees in 48 patients in the setting of chronic (recurrent) patella instability. They demonstrated a 46% failure rate as defined by recurrent instability at or before 2 years. In another similar study, Camp et al. looked at isolated MPFL repair in the setting of recurrent patella instability. The study comprised 27 patients and 29 knees with an average follow-up of 4 years (minimum, 2 years). They found a 28% rate of recurrence in this relatively young (average age, 19 years old) population. Both studies concluded that repair in the chronic or recurrent setting yielded unsatisfactory high rates of recurrence.

Medial Patellofemoral Ligament Reconstruction

The medial patellofemoral ligament is the most important restraint to lateral patellar displacement with knee range of motion between 0° and 30° of flexion [4, 23, 24]. Therefore when addressing soft tissue pathology related to recurrent patellar instability, it is important to address the integrity of this stabilizing structure. One advantage of MPFL reconstruction over medial sided repair is that the disrupted native ligament is being replaced with a collagen-containing graft with more structural integrity. The fact that reconstruction depends on more reliable tissue rather than injured native structures is likely responsible for the increased adoption of reconstructive techniques to address medial sided soft tissue injury. Despite the advantages of reconstruction, there is a paucity of literature surrounding the optimal graft choice, graft positioning, tension, or static versus dynamic techniques for MPFL reconstruction.

Selecting the appropriate patient for medial patellofemoral ligament reconstruction is seemingly simple, though can be complicated if a thorough evaluation of the pattern of instability is not performed. In the workup of recurrent patellar instability, most patients will obtain a magnetic resonance imaging study to evaluate the intraarticular and extraarticular soft tissue structures including the medial patellofemoral ligament. Magnetic resonance imaging is a reliable study to detect an injury to the medial patellofemoral ligament, approximately 80% sensitive and 75% specific [25]. However, the presence of a disrupted medial patellofemoral ligament should not be viewed in isolation. Those patients with limb alignment and rotational abnormalities, as well as those with an increased tibial tubercle-trochlear groove distance or patella alta, should be evaluated for concomitant osseous procedures to normalize the bony anatomy. Furthermore, an isolated soft tissue procedure in the presence of significant bony abnormalities can result in a lower success rate as recurrent stress on the graft can lead to early failure and recurrent instability.

Techniques to reconstruct the MPFL are numerous but follow a standard series of principles. The native ligament originates at Schottle's point between the adductor tubercle and medial femoral epicondyle and inserts on the proximal medial half of the patella. Reconstructive approaches for the medial patellofemoral ligament consist of placing a graft between these two points to provide medial sided soft tissue stability. The choice of graft will be discussed in detail in the following section as will the methods of determining appropriate graft tension. Furthermore, the placement of the graft tunnels, particularly the femoral graft placement, is arguably the most important factor when reconstructing the MPFL, and the consequences of malposition will also be discussed. Finally choices for graft fixation will be considered, though this factor is less significant in predicting a successful outcome when compared with the other aforementioned factors.

There are many graft choices, yet there is no validated consensus regarding the efficacy of the various options. Adductor magnus and semitendinosus or gracilis autografts as well as semitendinosus and tibialis anterior allografts have been proposed as potential graft choices [26–31]. Others have advocated for the doubled semitendinosus allograft to replicate the broad patellar attachment of the medial patellofemoral ligament [27]. However the use of this doubled semitendinosus can be problematic if malpositioned as it is significantly stronger and stiffer than the native MPFL [32].

The interplay of the graft choice and the functional role with dynamic motion of the knee is important. Studies suggest that femoral tunnel malposition can result in graft anisometry, resulting in graft laxity, leading to early failure, or early arthrosis as a result of increased patellofemoral compressive forces [31–35]. The radiographic guidelines for femoral tunnel placement have been outlined by Schottle et al. [36] as well as Stephen et al. [35] and provide a reliable guide to femoral tunnel placement. The determination of the femoral origin radiographically is based on the Schottle point which is 1 millimeter anterior to the tangent of the posterior femoral cortex and 2.5 millimeters distal to a line drawn perpendicular to the superior border of the femoral condyle. It is also immediately proximal to a perpendicular line drawn from the superoposterior aspect of Blumensaat line [36]. Stephen et al. based their radiographic reference for the femoral origin on normalized dimensions. They considered the anterior-posterior diameter of the medial femoral condyle to be 100% horizontally and the superior-inferior distance from the superior articular border of the patella to the distal border of the femoral condyle to also be considered 100%. With these dimensions the medial patellofemoral ligament attachment is 40% from the posterior margin and 50% from the distal margin with a reproducible location similar to that described by Schottle [35].

A femoral tunnel placed too far proximally may lead to graft laxity in extension and excessive tension in flexion, which can limit flexion and result in anterior knee pain [37]. This can ultimately result in early attenuation of the graft with repetitive loading and potentially early failure. In contrast, a femoral tunnel placed too distal can have excessive tension in extension and laxity in early flexion which can clinically manifest as an early failure with similarly impaired kinematics and recurrent instabilty [37]. Therefore, it has been recommended that the femoral attachment of the graft be placed 1 cm distal to the adductor tubercle to prevent excessive loading of the medial facet of the patella [31]. This same study by Elias and Cosgarea found that femoral tunnels placed too far distally resulted in a medial patellar tilt from full extension to 90° of flexion which could increase the load on the medial patellofemoral joint and predispose to early joint degeneration [31].

Though femoral tunnel position is undoubtedly an important factor in performing a successful reconstruction of the MPFL, other factors, such as graft length and tension, are also important to understand and consider. There is still a significant question as to what amount of knee flexion is appropriate to tension the graft. While some believe that the medial patellofemoral ligament is isometric, there is also a concept of "favorable" graft anisometry. Therefore, there are varying recommendations for graft tensioning with some authors suggesting tensioning the graft at 30–45°, while others prefer to tension at higher degrees of flexion such as 60–90° [18, 29, 30]. The concept of tensioning the graft at higher degrees of flexion relies on the idea that doing so avoids over tightening and ensures that the patella is engaged in the trochlea. Others, such as LeGrand et al., have advocated tensioning the graft at 45–60° and then checking for symmetric medial and lateral patellar motion at 20° of flexion which provides reassurance that the graft has enough tension [38]. Furthermore, Farr and Schepsis have described the "anatometric" graft tension which is tensioned in 30° of flexion such that it becomes more lax with knee flexion but tensions in terminal extension or the position of highest instability [27]. This was further supported by Thaunat and Erasmus, who introduced the aforementioned favorable anisometry, which conceptually relies on the idea that the graft should be isometric between 0° and 30° of knee flexion, which is the isometric range of the native medial patellofemoral ligament [37]. Measuring graft tension intraoperatively has a subjective element, though the contralateral knee can be used as a control in patients with unilateral pathology. Furthermore, Koh and Stewart suggested that following graft tensioning, the reconstructed MPFL should allow for 1 cm of lateral translation in full extension or two quadrants of lateral deviation with a firm endpoint [39].

Given the ambiguity regarding static tensioning of a medial patellofemoral ligament graft, there have been dynamic techniques of reconstruction described. These techniques are used less commonly but are worth reviewing and understanding. Ostermeier et al. performed a dynamic reconstruction by transferring the distal end of the semitendinosus behind the proximal medial collateral ligament to the medial margin of the patella [17]. They found that this dynamic type reconstruction resulted in significantly less medialization of the patella, which could theoretically protect the medial patellofemoral joint from the deleterious effects of over tensioning. The results of this technique were reported by Deie et al. who found that such a dynamic reconstruction provided significant improvement in knee scores without recurrent dislocation in 46 knees with a mean follow-up of 9.5 years [26].

Despite the apparent success of this approach, Panagopoulos et al. suggested that the medial collateral ligament is not an adequate pulley for the graft since its fibers are in line with the direction of patellar motion. They showed that using the medial collateral ligament as a pulley resulted in splitting of the fibers and subsequent loosening of the graft. They instead used the medial intramuscular septum as a pulley for the semitendinosus autograft with the tendon inserted through a bone tunnel on the patella. In a series of 25 patients, they reported improved knee scores with no cases of redislocation at 13-month follow-up [18]. Despite these encouraging results in small samples, the dynamic medial patellofemoral techniques have yet to be proven superior to static reconstructions.

Static reconstruction of the MPFL has shown great success and is still the most commonly performed surgical technique. In a biomechanical study, Mountney et al. compared several femoral graft fixation techniques including suture repair, suture anchor repair, and reconstruction with either a blind-ended tunnel in the medial femoral condyle or a through tunnel fixation in the lateral femoral condyle [40]. They found that the strength of through tunnel fixation on the lateral femoral condyle was the same as the native intact medial patellofemoral ligament.

Fixation of the graft to the patella is also varied between surgeons. Fixation options include suture fixation and suture anchor fixation, through tunnel fixation and blind-ended tunnel fixation. There are no studies comparing through tunnel fixation with suture anchor fixation and blind-ended tunnels. However, there is a risk of patellar fracture with the through tunnel technique. Mikashima et al. reported two patellar fractures in 24 knees reconstructed with through bone patellar tunnels [28]. Therefore, the ideal fixation method for the reconstructed MPFL is unproven, though through tunnel lateral femoral fixation coupled on the patella with either blind tunnels or suture anchor fixation appears to be the strongest and safest.

Medial patellofemoral ligament reconstruction in skeletally immature patients will be covered in more depth in a different chapter. Nevertheless, it has been shown that anatomic reconstruction is safe in the skeletally immature patient, so long as care is taken to avoid injuring the physis with femoral tunnel placement [41]. Furthermore, suture anchors rather than through bone tunnels can be used if there is a concern for physeal injury or a more distal non-anatomic procedure can be performed. Despite the reported success of non-anatomic distal realignment procedures in the skeletally immature patient, there is a significant risk of graft stretching which might necessitate subsequent revision procedures [42, 43].

In considering all of these factors related to MPFL reconstruction, the overall results of this procedure have been good [18, 29]. In retrospective clinical studies, 80–90% of patients have a good to excellent outcomes following medial patellofemoral ligament reconstruction [44–47].

Biomechanically, medial patellofemoral ligament reconstruction provides more stability than a medial tibial tubercle transfer. In a cadaveric study of knees following a medial tibial tubercle transfer or reconstruction of the medial patellofemoral ligament, the knee motion and strain on the MPFL was tested with and without a 100 Newtown subluxation force in both scenarios. This study found that reconstruction of the medial patellofemoral ligament reduced the ligament load and lateral patellar displacement compared with a medial tibial tubercle transfer at all degrees of flexion. This study concluded that MPFL reconstruction was better at stabilizing patellar movement under laterally directed force [48]. However, this should be taken only as a biomechanical study, as it does not reflect the in vivo condition. Reconstruction of the MPFL in isolation cannot address significant underlying osseous pathology predisposing to recurrent lateral patella dislocation.

Though the results of medial patellofemoral reconstruction are largely positive, the procedure is not without complications. In a recent systematic review, there was a 26.1% complication rate in patients averaging 24 years of age. The most common complications include recurrent apprehension or dislocation, arthrofibrosis, pain, and patellar fracture [49]. The complication rate can be minimized with appropriate patient selection, good surgical technique, in addition to appropriate postoperative rehabilitation that focuses on early mobilization and progressive strengthening to prevent arthrofibrosis and recurrent instability [4]. Patient selection is very important, as patients with preexisting chondromalacia of the patella have predictably poorer results following MPFL reconstruction [29]. Patients with degeneration of the patellar cartilage should be considered for additional or concurrent procedures.

Understanding the biomechanics of the medial patellofemoral ligament and the important points in the reconstructive technique will help lessen potential complications of this procedure. Ultimately, graft selection is surgeon's preference, with most using a semitendinosus auto- or allograft and a static approach to the procedure. Anatomic femoral tunnel placement is paramount, and the biomechanically strongest fixation is through a tunnel in the femur with graft fixation on the lateral femoral cortex. The literature suggests that suture anchors in the patella provide adequate fixation without the risk of patellar fracture associated with through tunnels. Patient selection is the most important factor. Patients with arthrosis or combined osseous and soft tissue abnormalities are less likely to benefit from an isolated MPFL reconstruction.

Trochleoplasty

Trochleoplasty is a technically demanding procedure with significant risks of serious and irreversible articular cartilage or subchondral bone injury and should not be performed without appropriate training and technical expertise. However, despite use with equivocal results in Europe, there has been a renewed interest in trochleoplasty procedures given that more than 85% of patients with recurrent patellar instability have trochlear dysplasia [50]. Indications for trochleoplasty are evolving and include aberrant patellar tracking identified by a clinical J sign and a tibial tubercle-trochlear groove distance of 10–20 millimeters and abnormal trochlear morphology identified on a true lateral radiograph of the knee or cross-sectional imaging [51, 52]. The patient must also have normal or nearly normal trochlear articular cartilage and normal or corrected rotational alignment.

If these criteria are met, a sulcus deepening trochleoplasty can be considered but is technically demanding. During this procedure, cancellous bone is exposed in the trochlea by elevating a strip of cortical bone around the edge of the trochlear. A new sulcus is then created more proximally and 3–6° lateral to the previous sulcus by removing cancellous bone. The trochlear shell with its overlying cartilage is then impacted into the newly formed sulcus and fixed with small staples or with resorbable sutures [53, 54].

Schottle et al. examined the cellular effect of raising an articular cartilage flap in a series of patients evaluated microscopically and histologically at 3, 6, and 9 months. They found that in a well-performed trochleoplasty, the articular cartilage remained viable at short-term follow-up [55]. Despite these positive short-term clinical results, there were subtle variations in the calcified cartilage layer, which warrant further follow-up to determine the long-term significance.

Several clinical studies have reported outcomes following trochleoplasty for recurrent patellar instability. These studies are small and provide results of short-term follow-up, which is equivocal or marginally positive in the early postoperative time frame [52–54]. Verdonk et al. reported equivocal results at an average of 18 months following trochleoplasty in 13 knees in 12 patients. They indicated the operation for patients with patellar pain with or without instability. Their results are not generalizable to other trochleoplasty studies on recurrent patellar instability, because not all of their patients had instability [56].

The subjective outcomes following trochleoplasty have been positive in several short-term study groups [53, 54, 57, 58]. In addition, radiographic parameters such as trochlear depth were improved postoperatively as one might expect [52, 54]. Not surprisingly, preoperative degenerative changes have been associated with poor results following trochleoplasty [53, 58].

Von Knoch et al. have reported the largest series, 45 knees in 38 patients with a mean follow-up of 8.3 years, who underwent trochleoplasty and medial reefing with or without medial patellofemoral ligament reconstruction [54]. They used the scoring system by Kujala et al. [59]. to determine outcome success and reported a mean score of 94.9 points but had no preoperative comparison scores for this cohort. A single patient had subluxation and a positive apprehension test, but there were no instances of recurrent patellar dislocation. Though there were no recurrences of instability, trochleoplasty was ineffective in preventing the progression of patellofemoral arthritis in this study group. At latest follow-up, 10 knees had osteoarthritic changes that were grade two or more, and 43% of the 45 knees had worsening patellofemoral pain compared with their preoperative state. Furthermore, in other studies by Verdonk et al. and Donnell et al., their small cohorts each reported several cases of postoperative arthrofibrosis [52, 56].

The lackluster results of trochleoplasty in conjunction with the significant technical demands of the procedure and high complication rates suggest that trochleoplasty be performed only in patients with complex recurrent patellofemoral instability that has failed previous attempts at stabiization and by surgeons with significant experience with these procedures. Furthermore, patients with trochlear dysplasia can be successfully treated with other procedures that do not jeopardize the articular cartilage of the trochlea. Steiner et al. reported the results of MPFL reconstruction in patients with trochlear dysplasia and showed significant improvement in validated scoring systems without recurrent dislocation at final follow-up

[31]. Furthermore, they showed no difference in the quality of the outcome scores for increasing severity of trochlear dysplasia. Thus, the large percentage of patients with trochlear dysplasia and recurrent patellar instability do not necessarily warrant a trochleoplasty.

Tibial Tubercle Osteotomy

Tibial tubercle osteotomy (TTO) is a powerful bony procedure that can be used in isolation or in conjunction with soft tissue procedures to address patellofemoral instability and abnormal contact pressures in the patellofemoral joint by redirecting the distal force vector acting on the patella. Traditionally, indications for TTO have included a tibial tubercle-trochlear groove (TT-TG) distance greater than 20 millimeters, an excessively high Q-angle, focal patellar or trochlear chondral lesions, patella alta, and patellofemoral arthritis in conjunction with instability or maltracking [60]. The decision to include TTO in surgical correction of recurrent patellar instability is based on patient-specific factors, chondral lesion characteristics, and biomechanical abnormalities requiring offloading of an area of the patellofemoral joint surface [60]. When used in conjunction with MPFL to address instability, Ebied et al. reported 96% good or excellent results 2 years postoperatively [61].

The biomechanics of the patellofemoral joint and patient-specific factors play an important role in determining the type and direction of TTO that can most effectively be used to prevent further instability and pain. The tibial tubercle can be moved in the anterior to posterior plane, the medial to lateral plane, and the proximal to distal plane. As our understanding of the biomechanics of the patellofemoral articulation has evolved, the preferred TTO technique has also changed.

Hauser first described his procedure, a distal and medial transfer of the tibial tubercle to address instability, in 1938. While the Hauser procedure resulted in good short-term resolution of instability, it led to high rates of patellofemoral joint arthritis secondary to posterior translation of the tubercle [60].

The Elmslie-Trillat procedure was a modification of the initial Hauser procedure that relied on an isolated tibial tubercle medialization (TTM). The Elmslie-Trillat procedure is a single plane or flat osteotomy. Flat osteotomies have a significantly higher load to failure when compared to oblique osteotomies of the tibial tubercle [62]. Medialization of the tibial tubercle leads to shifting of contact pressures from medial to lateral and results in a decreased TT-TG distance, which in turn results in decreased lateral instability. Isolated medialization of the tibial tubercle has been used successfully in patients with instability without any cartilaginous defects. Studies of isolated medialization show a 62.5% good to excellent results at long-term follow-up [63].

The Maquet technique, described in 1976, is a straight anteriorization of the tibial tuberosity utilizing iliac bone graft [64]. Anteriorization decreases joint reaction forces by increasing the angle between the patellar and quadriceps tendon, increasing the lever arm for the patellar tendon. Anteriorization also leads to rotation of the patella on its horizontal axis which transfers contact pressures from the distal to the proximal patella. The Maquet technique is complicated by high rates of skin necrosis and should be reserved for large distal patellar chondral defects, kissing bipolar chondral lesions, and patellofemoral arthritis with a TT-TG less than 15 mm [60].

Fulkerson modified the TTO in 1983 by combining the positives of the Maquet and Elmslie-Trillat procedure by describing an anteromedialization (AMZ) TTO [65]. The Fulkerson osteotomy is an oblique plane osteotomy that results in decreased lateral facet pressures, shifting of contact pressures proximally on the patella, and improved tracking of the patella in the trochlea [65]. The Fulkerson osteotomy is now the preferred method of TTO to address patellofemoral instability in conjunction with cartilage defects. In addition to changes in the anterior to posterior and medial to lateral plane, tibial tubercle osteotomies can also alter the proximal to distal positioning of the tibial tubercle. Distalization of the tibial tubercle causes the patella to engage the trochlea earlier in flexion and can be used to increase the osseous restraint, preventing lateral instability.

Contraindications to the Fulkerson osteotomy include any conditions in which increased stress on the medial compartment and proximal patella would be undesirable [60]. Some of these conditions include patients with varus knees, degenerative changes to medial or proximal patella, a prior medial meniscectomy, and patella baja. AMZ osteotomies should also be avoided in patients with an open physis and patients with localized or systemic inflammatory conditions. Fulkerson describes the procedure as using a lateral incision from the level of the distal pole of the patella halfway between Gerdy's tubercle and the tibial tubercle [65]. The incision is extended 10–12 cm distally to a point on the anterior ridge of the tibia. However, a smaller, medially based incision can also be used. An oblique osteotomy of the tibial tubercle is performed and moved anteromedially. The amount of anteriorization and medialization can be altered by the obliquity of the cut with a more oblique osteotomy leading to relatively more anteriorization [65]. The osteotomy is secured with 2–3 partially or fully threaded 3.5–4.5 mm cortical or cancellous screws, with cadaveric studies showing no difference in load to failure between the constructs [66].

Outcome studies in patients who have undergone a TTO have shown generally favorable outcomes. There are no well-designed randomized control trials comparing outcomes in patients who have undergone a TTO, but several well-designed retrospective and prospective studies do exist. Ding et al. retrospectively reviewed young, active patients with recurrent patellar instability who underwent a Fulkerson osteotomy [67]. Patients had good to excellent outcomes in 83.8% of cases based on Kujala scores for anterior knee pain [67]. The authors concluded that Fulkerson osteotomies are effective in reducing pain and improving function in a young, active population.

Other studies have addressed TTO in general. One such study was a systematic review of 38 studies on distal realignment procedures for patellar instability [68]. The authors found an overall recurrence rate of 7% and a short- to medium-term recurrence rate of 5.3%, indicating overall good results [68]. Positive outcomes following TTO are associated with male gender, the absence of chondral defects, longer follow-up, and instability rather than pain as the primary preoperative symptom [69]. While outcomes tend to get worse with time, with some long-term studies reporting good to excellent outcomes in 62.5% of patients, recurrence of instability does not seem to increase when comparing intermediate to long-term follow-up [63, 70].

Although good to excellent outcomes can be expected when utilizing TTO for patellar instability, there are several complications associated with the procedure. Payne et al. published a systematic review in 2015 and identified an overall complication rate of 4.6% with a major complication rate of 3.0% [71]. Hardware was removed in 36.7% of cases, with the Elmslie-Trillat procedure being the only TTO that was significantly associated with less hardware removal [71]. Complications of the procedure include delayed wound healing, infection, tuberosity fractures, proximal tibial fractures, arthrofibrosis, and delayed union of the osteotomy site [60]. Soft tissue complications are of special concern when using the Maquet technique. Fracture of the proximal tibia ranges from 2.6% to 8%, and the importance of a progressive weight-bearing regimen following TTO cannot be overstated in preventing this complication [72, 73]. Also, the osteotomy technique is important in preventing a fracture. Flat osteotomies are more likely to fail through a shingle fracture of the tubercle shingle, while oblique osteotomies are more likely to fail through fracture of the proximal tibia [62].

Overall, tibial tubercle osteotomies result in excellent outcomes when used in isolation or conjunction with soft tissue procedures for patellar instability. When taking into account patient-specific factors, chondral lesion characteristics, and biomechanics of the knee, the tibial tubercle osteotomy can be utilized to offload areas of concern and provide stability to the patellofemoral joint, resulting in improved pain and function.

Femoral Derotational Osteotomy

In addition to tibial tubercle osteotomies for tibial based deformity, femoral anteversion alters the forces across the patellofemoral joint by causing a greater laterally displaced force vector. Excessive femoral anteversion greater than 20° is a well-described cause of recurrent patellar instability [4]. If excessive femoral anteversion is suspected, a CT or MRI should be performed [4]. Derotational osteotomies of the femur can be performed in conjunction with soft tissue reconstruction and other bony procedures. The derotational osteotomy should be performed in the area closest to the source of excessive anteversion and are generally performed in the intertrochanteric or supracondylar region of the femur [4]. Results specific to patellar instability are limited with only one study demonstrating improvements in knee function and high patient satisfaction for patients who underwent femoral derotational osteotomy with MPFL reconstruction for patellar instability [74]. However, overall results for femoral derotational osteotomies indicate good to excellent results [4].

Conclusion

The preceding sections have outlined in detail the surgical options for managing recurrent patellar instability. They are not intended to be viewed in isolation but rather as components of an armamentarium of methods to surgically address recurrent patellar instability. In evaluating the potential surgical options, it is always important to understand the etiology of recurrent patellar instability. These include both the osseous characteristics of the limb and patellofemoral joint and the static and dynamic soft tissue components affecting patellar stability. In the case of recurrent patellar instability, there is almost always some element of medial sided soft tissue injury to the medial patellofemoral ligament or vastus medialis obliquus. The extent to which this soft tissue injury can resolve following a patellar dislocation likely diminishes in cases of multiple, recurrent, episodes of instability as the supporting structures become damaged, stretched, and attenuated. Therefore, in planning a surgical intervention for recurrent patellar instability, one must thoroughly evaluate the MPFL and be prepared to reconstruct, rather than repair, the deficient medial sided soft tissues when indicated.

Furthermore, a common mistake is to plan a medial patellofemoral ligament reconstruction without first considering the potentially abnormal osseous morphologies predisposing patients to this pathology. A thorough assessment of the relationship between the tibial tubercle and trochlear groove, as well as the patellar height, limb alignment, and rotation, is imperative in the surgical workup of this chronic problem. This requires the correlation of clinical and radiographic data points including limb alignment, full-length radiographs, and appropriately selected cross-sectional imaging.

The unique characteristics of the patient including their age, activity level, expectations, and concomitant pathology must also be considered in preoperative planning. The high-level athlete often presents a unique and ultimately rare circumstance where the surgical approach may be influenced significantly by their sport, season, and time frame for rehabilitation and recovery. Each procedure outlined in this chapter has a different time frame for rest, immobilization, rehabilitation, and healing, and this can dictate the timeline for return to play. These instances can often bring about real discussions regarding nonoperative management, at least in the short term, even in the case of recurrent patellar instability. Maximizing and exhausting nonoperative measures such as appropriate physical therapy, bracing, and taping is important in these athletes and all patients with recurrent patellar instability. In conclusion, the management of recurrent patellar instability is rarely, if ever, clear cut and is not to be taken lightly as the complex etiology of this condition, and the surgical management thereof can have profound impact on the life, activity, and livelihood of affected patients.

References

1. Fithian DC, Paxton EW, Stone ML, Silva P, Davis DK, Elias DA, White LM. Epidemiology and natural history of acute patellar dislocation. Am J Sports Med. 2004;32(5):1114–21. Epub 2004 May 18
2. Hawkins RJ, Bell RH, Anisette G. Acute patellar dislocations. The natural history. Am J Sports Med. 1986;14(2):117–20.
3. Cofield RH, Bryan RS. Acute dislocation of the patella: results of conservative treatment. J Trauma. 1977;17:526–31.
4. Weber AE, Nathani A, Dines JS, Allen AA, Shubin-Stein BE, Arendt EA, Bedi A. Current concepts review: an algorithmic approach to the management of recurrent lateral patellar dislocation. J Bone Joint Surg Am. 2016;98:417–27.
5. Atkin DM, Fithian DC, Marangi KS, Stone ML, Dobson BE, Mendelsohn C. Characteristics of patients with primary acute lateral patellar dislocation and their recovery within the first 6 months of injury. Am J Sports Med. 2000;28:472–9.
6. Colvin AC, West RV. Current concepts review: patellar instability. J Bone Joint Surg Am. 2008;90:2751–62.
7. Palmu S, Kallio PE, Donell ST, Helenius I, Nietosvaara Y. Acute patellar dislocation in children and adolescents: a randomized clinical trial. J Bone Joint Surg Am. 2008;90:463–70.
8. Maenpaa H, Lehto MU. Patellar dislocation. The long-term results of nonoperative management in 100 patients. Am J Sports Med. 1997;25:213–7.
9. Lee SE, Cho SH. The effect of McConnell taping on vastus medialis and lateralis activity during squatting in adults with patellofemoral pain syndrome. J Exerc Rehabil. 2013;9(2):326–30. Epub 2013 Apr 25.
10. McConnell J. Rehabilitation and nonoperative treatment of patellar instability. Sports Med Arthrosc. 2007;15(2):95–104.
11. Cowan SM, Bennell KL, Hodges PW. Therapeutic patellar taping changes the timing of vasti muscle activation in people with patellofemoral pain syndrome. Clin J Sport Med. 2002;12:339–47.
12. Stensdotter AK, Hodges PW, Mellor R, Sundelin G. Häger-Ross C. Quadriceps activation in closed and in open kinetic chain exercise. Med Sci Sports Exerc. 2003;35:2043–7.
13. Escamilla RF, Fleisig GS, Zheng N, Barrentine SW, Wilk KE, Andrews JR. Biomechanics of the knee during closed kinetic chain and open kinetic chain exercises. Med Sci Sports Exerc. 1998;30:556–69.
14. Kolowich PA, Paulos LE, Rosenberg TD, Farnsworth S. Lateral release of the patella: indications and contraindications. Am J Sports Med. 1990;18:359–65.
15. Lattermann C, Toth J, Bach BR Jr. The role of lateral retinacular release in the treatment of patellar instability. Sports Med Arthrosc. 2007;15:57–60.
16. Tom A, Fulkerson JP. Restoration of native medial patellofemoral ligament support after patella dislocation. Sports Med Arthrosc. 2007;15:68–71.
17. Ostermeier S, Holst M, Bohnsack M, Hurschler C, Stukenborg-Colsman C, Wirth CJ. In vitro measurement of patellar kinematics following reconstruction of the medial patellofemoral ligament. Knee Surg Sports Traumatol Arthrosc. 2007;15:276–85.

18. Panagopoulos A, van Niekerk L, Triantafillopoulos IK. MPFL reconstruction for recurrent patella dislocation: a new surgical technique and review of the literature. Int J Sports Med. 2008;29:359–65.
19. Nikku R, Nietosvaara Y, Kallio PE, Aalto K, Michelsson JE. Operative versus closed treatment of primary dislocation of the patella. Similar 2-year results in 125 randomized patients. Acta Orthop Scand. 1997;68:419–23.
20. Nikku R, Nietosvaara Y, Aalto K, Kallio PE. Operative treatment of primarily patellar dislocation does not improve medium-term outcome: a 7-year follow-up report and risk analysis of 127 randomized patients. Acta Orthop. 2005;76:699–704.
21. Ahmad CS, Stein BE, Matuz D, Henry JH. Immediate surgical repair of the medial patellar stabilizers for acute patellar dislocation. A review of eight cases. Am J Sports Med. 2000;28:804–10.
22. Colvin AC, West RV. Current concepts review patellar instability. J Bone Joint Surg Am. 2008;90:2751–62. https://doi.org/10.2106/JBJS.H.00211.
23. Desio SM, Burks RT, Bachus KN. Soft tissue restraints to lateral patellar translation in the human knee. Am J Sports Med. 1998;26:59–65.
24. Conlan T, Garth WP Jr, Lemons JE. Evaluation of the medial soft-tissue restraints of the extensor mechanism of the knee. J Bone Joint Surg Am. 1993;75(5):682–93.
25. Sanders TG, Morrison WB, Singleton BA, Miller MD, Cornum KG. Medial patellofemoral ligament injury following acute transient dislocation of the patella: MR findings with surgical correlation in 14 patients. J Comput Assist Tomogr. 2001;25:957–62.
26. Deie M, Ochi M, Sumen Y, Adachi N, Kobayashi K, Yasumoto M. A long-term follow-up study after medial patellofemoral ligament reconstruction using the transferred semitendinosus tendon for patellar dislocation. Knee Surg Sports Traumatol Arthrosc. 2005;13:522–8.
27. Farr J, Schepsis AA. Reconstruction of the medial patellofemoral ligament for recurrent patellar instability. J Knee Surg. 2006;19:307–16.
28. Mikashima Y, Kimura M, Kobayashi Y, Miyawaki M, Tomatsu T. Clinical results of isolated reconstruction of the medial patellofemoral ligament for recurrent dislocation and subluxation of the patella. Acta Orthop Belg. 2006;72:65–71.
29. Nomura E, Inoue M. Hybrid medial patellofemoral ligament reconstruction using the semitendinosus tendon for recurrent patellar dislocation: minimum 3 years' follow-up. Arthroscopy. 2006;22:787–93.
30. Steiner TM, Torga-Spak R, Teitge RA. Medial patellofemoral ligament reconstruction in patients with lateral patellar instability and trochlear dysplasia. Am J Sports Med. 2006;34:1254–61.
31. Elias JJ, Cosgarea AJ. Technical errors during medial patellofemoral ligament reconstruction could overload medial patellofemoral cartilage: a computational analysis. Am J Sports Med. 2006;34:1478–85.
32. Beck P, Brown NA, Greis PE, Burks RT. Patellofemoral contact pressures and lateral patellar translation after medial patellofemoral ligament reconstruction. Am J Sports Med. 2007;35:1557–63.
33. Steensen RN, Dopirak RM, McDonald WG 3rd. The anatomy and isometry of the medial patellofemoral ligament: implications for reconstruction. Am J Sports Med. 2004;32(6):1509–13. Epub 2004 Jul 20
34. Bollier M, Fulkerson J, Cosgarea A, Tanaka M. Technical failure of medial patellofemoral ligament reconstruction. Arthroscopy. 2011;27(8):1153–9. Epub 2011 Jun 12.
35. Stephen JM, Lumpaopong P, Deehan DJ, Kader D, Amis AA. The medial patellofemoral ligament: location of femoral attachment and length change patterns resulting from anatomic and nonanatomic attachments. Am J Sports Med. 2012;40(8):1871–9. Epub 2012 Jun 22.
36. Schottle PB, Schmeling A, Rosenstiel N, Weiler A. Radiographic landmarks for femoral tunnel placement in medial patellofemoral ligament reconstruction. Am J Sports Med. 2007;35(5):801–4. Epub 2007 Jan 31.

37. Thaunat M, Erasmus PJ. Management of overtight medial patellofemoral ligament reconstruction. Knee Surg Sports Traumatol Arthrosc. 2009;17(5):480–3. Epub 2009 Jan 9.
38. LeGrand AB, Greis PE, Dobbs RE, Burks RT. MPFL reconstruction. Sports Med Arthrosc. 2007;15:72–7.
39. Koh JL, Stewart C. Patellar instability. Clin Sports Med. 2014;33(3):461–76. Epub 2014 May 29.
40. Mountney J, Senavongse W, Amis AA, Thomas NP. Tensile strength of the medial patellofemoral ligament before and after repair or reconstruction. J Bone Joint Surg Br. 2005;87:36–40.
41. Weeks KD 3rd, Fabricant PD, Ladenhauf HN, Green DW. Surgical options for patellar stabilization in the skeletally immature patient. Sports Med Arthrosc. 2012;20(3):194–202.
42. Fondren FB, Goldner JL, Bassett FH 3rd. Recurrent dislocation of the patella treated by the modified roux-Goldthwait procedure. A prospective study of forty seven knees. J Bone Joint Surg Am. 1985;67(7):993–1005.
43. Hinton RY, Sharma KM. Acute and recurrent patellar instability in the young athlete. Orthop Clin North Am. 2003;34(3):385–96.
44. Drez D Jr, Edwards TB, Williams CS. Results of medial patellofemoral ligament reconstruction in the treatment of patellar dislocation. Arthroscopy. 2001;17(3):298–306.
45. Fernandez E, Sala D, Castejon M. Reconstruction of the medial patellofemoral ligament for patellar instability using a semitendinosus autograft. Acta Orthop Belg. 2005;71(3):303–8.
46. Schöttle PB, Fucentese SF, Romero J. Clinical and radiological outcome of medial patellofemoral ligament reconstruction with a semitendinosus autograft for patella instability. Knee Surg Sports Traumatol Arthrosc. 2005;13(7):516–21. Epub 2005 Jun 15.
47. Slenker NR, Tucker BS, Pepe MD, Marchetto PA, Cohen SB. Short−/intermediate-term outcomes after medial patellofemoral ligament reconstruction in the treatment of chronic lateral patellofemoral instability. Phys Sportsmed. 2013;41(2):26–33.
48. Ostermeier S, Stukenborg-Colsman C, Hurschler C, Wirth CJ. In vitro investigation of the effect of medial patellofemoral ligament reconstruction and medial tibial tuberosity transfer on lateral patellar stability. Arthroscopy. 2006;22:308–19.
49. Shah JN, Howard JS, Flanigan DC, Brophy RH, Carey JL, Lattermann C. A systematic review of complications and failures associated with medial patellofemoral ligament reconstruction for recurrent patellar dislocation. Am J Sports Med. 2012;40(8):1916–23. Epub 2012 Jun 7.
50. Dejour H, Walch G, Nove-Josserand L, Guier C. Factors of patellar instability: an anatomic radiographic study. Knee Surg Sports Traumatol Arthrosc. 1994;2:19–26.
51. Dejour D, Le Coultre B. Osteotomies in patello-femoral instabilities. Sports Med Arthrosc. 2007;15(1):39–46.
52. Donell ST, Joseph G, Hing CB, Marshall TJ. Modified Dejour trochleoplasty for severe dysplasia: operative technique and early clinical results. Knee. 2006;13(4):266–73. Epub 2006 Apr 24.
53. Schottle PB, Fucentese SF, Pfirrmann C, Bereiter H, Romero J. Trochleoplasty for patellar instability due to trochlear dysplasia: a minimum 2-year clinical and radiological follow-up of 19 knees. Acta Orthop. 2005;75:693–8.
54. von Knoch F, Bohm T, Burgi ML, von Knoch M, Bereiter H. Trochleoplasty for recurrent patellar dislocation in association with trochlear dysplasia. A 4- to 14-year follow-up study. J Bone Joint Surg Br. 2006;88:1331–5.
55. Schöttle PB, Schell H, Duda G, Weiler A. Cartilage viability after trochleoplasty. Knee Surg Sports Traumatol Arthrosc. 2007;15(2):161–7. Epub 2006 Sep 2.
56. Verdonk R, Jansegers E, Stuyts B. Trochleoplasty in dysplastic knee trochlea. Knee Surg Sports Traumatol Arthrosc. 2005;13:529–33.
57. Koeter S, Pakvis D, van Loon CJ, van Kampen A. Trochlear osteotomy for patellar instability: satisfactory minimum 2-year results in patients with dysplasia of the trochlea. Knee Surg Sports Traumatol Arthrosc. 2007;15:228–32.
58. Utting MR, Mulford JS, Eldridge JD. A prospective evaluation of trochleoplasty for the treatment of patellofemoral dislocation and instability. J Bone Joint Surg Br. 2008;90:180–5.

59. Kujala UM, Jaakkola LH, Koskinen SK, Taimela S, Hurme M, Nelimarkka O. Scoring of patellofemoral disorders. Arthroscopy. 1993;9:159–63.
60. Sherman SL, Erickson BJ, Cvetanovich GL, Chalmers PN, Farr J, Bach BR, Cole BJ. Tibial tuberosity osteotomy: indications, techniques, and outcomes. Am J Sports Med. 2014;42:2006–17.
61. Ebied AM, El-Kholy W. Reconstruction of the medial patello-femoral and patello-tibial ligaments for treatment of patellar instability. Knee Surg Sports Traumatol Arthrosc. 2011;20:926–32.
62. Cosgarea J, Schatzke MD, Seth K, Litsky S. Biomechanical analysis of flat and oblique tibial tubercle osteotomy for recurrent patellar instability. Am J Sports Med. 1999;27(4):507–12.
63. Naveed MA, Ackroyd CE, Porteous AJ. Long-term (ten- to 15-year) outcome of arthroscopically assisted Elmslie-Trillat tibial tubercle osteotomy. Bone Joint J. 2013;95(4):478–85.
64. Maquet P. Advancement of the tibial tuberosity. Clin Orthop Relat Res. 1976;115:225–30.
65. Fulkerson JP. Anteromedialization of the tibial tuberosity for patellofemoral malalignment. Clin Orthop Relat Res. 1983;177:176–81.
66. Warner BT, Kamath GV, Spang JT, Weinhold PS, Creighton RA. Comparison of fixation methods after anteromedialization osteotomy of the tibial tubercle for patellar instability. Arthroscopy. 2013;29(10):1628–34.
67. Ding DY, Kanevsky R, Strauss EJ, Jazrawi LM. Anteromedialisation tibial tubercle osteotomy for recurrent patellar instability in young active patients: a retrospective case series. Injury. 2016;47(3):737–41.
68. Longo UG, et al. Medial patellofemoral ligament reconstruction combined with bony procedures for patellar instability: current indications, outcomes, and complications. Arthroscopy. 2016;32:1421–7.
69. Pritsch T, Haim A, Arbel R, Snir N, Shasha N, Dekel S. Tailored tibial tubercle transfer for patellofemoral malalignment: analysis of clinical outcomes. Knee Surg Sports Traumatol Arthrosc. 2007;15:994–1002.
70. Carney JR, Mologne TS, Muldoon M, Cox JS. Long-term evaluation of the roux-Elmslie-Trillat procedure for patellar instability: a 26-year follow-up. Am J Sports Med. 2005;33:1220–3.
71. Payne J, Rimmke N, Schmitt LC, Flanigan DC, Magnussen RA. The incidence of complications of tibial tubercle osteotomy: a systematic review. Arthroscopy. 2015;31:1819–25.
72. Stetson WB, Friedman MJ, Fulkerson JP, Cheng M, Buuck D. Fracture of the proximal tibia with immediate weight bearing after a Fulkerson osteotomy. Am J Sports Med. 1997;25:570–4.
73. Bellemans J, Cauwenberghs F, Brys P, Victor J, Fabry G. Fracture of the proximal tibia after Fulkerson anteromedial tibial tubercle transfer: a report of four cases. Am J Sports Med. 1998;26(2):300–2.
74. Nelitz M, Dreyhaupt J, Williams SRM, Dornacher D. Combined supracondylar femoral derotation osteotomy and patellofemoral ligament reconstruction for recurrent patellar dislocation and severe femoral anteversion syndrome: surgical technique and clinical outcome. Int Orthop. 2015;39:2355–62.

Chapter 9
Patellofemoral Instability Surgery Complications: How to Avoid Them

Michael S. Laidlaw, David R. Diduch, and Brian C. Werner

Introduction

Both soft tissue and bone anatomy confer stability to the patella during the knee arc of motion. While high-energy trauma can result in damage to these constraints, low-energy forces can also result in recurrent patellar instability if there is underlying pathology to the basic architecture. Maltracking, or malalignment, of the patellofemoral articulation can not only contribute to potential instability but can also predispose to excessive cartilage wear, resulting in the progression of chondromalacia related disease and pain. While there are a myriad of soft tissue, bone stabilization, and realignment procedures that can confer stability to the patellofemoral joint, these procedures also have inherent risks and potential complications. This chapter details the most commonly observed complications reported in the literature associated with patellofemoral surgery as it pertains to soft tissue and bony stabilization and realignment procedures. It will also review the technical causes of these complications and provide guidance on how to avoid and troubleshoot their occurrence in the operating room.

Complications of Soft Tissue Surgery

Previous chapters have detailed the non-operative and operative measures available to treat patellofemoral pain and instability. Given the unpredictable results of MPFL repair or imbrication in the setting of recurrent patellar instability, MPFL reconstruction with graft augmentation has become more widely used [1–3]. Proximal

M. S. Laidlaw · D. R. Diduch (✉) · B. C. Werner (✉)
Department of Orthopedic Surgery, Universtiy of Virginia, Charlottesville, VA, USA
e-mail: DRD5C@hscmail.mcc.virginia.edu; BCW4X@hscmail.mcc.virginia.edu

B. E. Shubin Stein, S. M. Strickland (eds.), *Patellofemoral Pain and Instability*,
https://doi.org/10.1007/978-3-319-97640-2_9

soft tissue patellar stabilization procedures achieve graft fixation to the patella by utilizing either tunnel techniques or suture techniques. Tunnel techniques can include a graft alone within tunnels, or, alternatively, the graft may be fixed with an interference screw within tunnels. Suture techniques can include suture anchor fixation to the medial patellar border or quadriceps turndown maintaining its proximal patellar soft tissue attachment. Most surgical techniques gain femoral-sided fixation by interference screws; however, some techniques obviate the need for this by looping the graft around the adductor magnus at its attachment on the adductor tubercle, although this is in a nonanatomic location [4]. It should be noted that there are inherent risks associated when utilizing procedures that use patellar tunnels to secure the MPFL reconstruction to the patella. In a systematic review of 25 studies primarily evaluating MPFL reconstructions for patellar instability, which also included tibial tubercle osteotomies, VMO advancement, lateral retinacular release, retinacular plication, and chondroplasty, a total of 164 complications occurred in 629 knees (26.1%) [5]. These major complications included patellar fracture, postoperative instability, flexion loss, and pain.

Patella Fracture

The Complication

Patella fracture is one of the most frequently reported complications to date with MPFL reconstructions that utilize patellar tunnel techniques [6–8]. In general, transpatellar tunnels have a higher risk of fracture given the potential stress riser placed by drilling transversely across the patella. Direct trauma to the patella or even maximal eccentric quadriceps contractures in poorly placed tunnels or in poor quality bone can result in a patella fracture postoperatively (Fig. 9.1). Shah reported 4 patella fractures in 629 knees (0.6%), with each patella fracture occurring in association with patellar tunnel use [5]. These fractures occurred with techniques using 3.2 mm transverse patellar tunnels, 4.5 mm diameter tunnels that exited anteriorly, and also two 4.5 mm transverse tunnels separated by a 10–15 mm bone bridge [5]. However, studies that recorded tunnels size drilled at 2.4 mm did not report any patellar fractures. No patellar fractures were reported in association with a docking technique, suture anchor, or soft tissue attachment on the patella. Fractures can and do exist with these techniques, especially if the anchor or tunnel is placed too anteriorly, though it is much less common compared to the tunnel techniques described above.

Schiphouwer et al. has provided the single largest retrospective case series to date examining 192 knees and reporting on the complications associated with isolated MPFL reconstruction using two 4.5 mm patellar tunnels drilled from the medial patellar border and exited on the anterior patellar cortex. Overall, there was a 20.3% complication rate, 14.1% of which were considered major [4]. Seven patella fractures were reported with this technique (3.6%) [4]. All patients who sustained a patellar fracture were male, and the mean time from surgery to fracture was

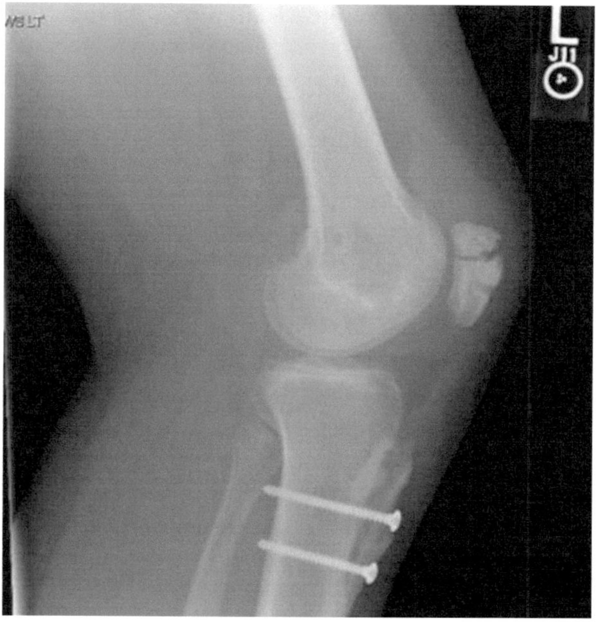

Fig. 9.1 Patella fracture seen with anterior oblique drill holes

5.8 months. With the limited number of complications reported in the literature and the vast heterogeneity of studies and surgical techniques employed, a true prevalence of this complication is difficult to determine. However, the research we currently have can be used to guide our techniques and help limit this major complication [5].

How to Avoid It

Biomechanical cadaveric studies have demonstrated the native MPFL maximum load to failure at the patellar insertion to be 144–210 N. Studies have shown suture anchors, interference screws, and bone tunnels all provide satisfactory graft fixation strength above that of the native MPFL [2, 9–11].

Blind-ended docking tunnel fixation can be achieved by small interference screws and negates the need to drill across the patella reducing the potential for patellar fracture compared to through tunnels. Usual modes of fixation failure upon biomechanical testing are graft slippage at the interference screw interface or graft-suture construct failure at the suture anchor [10, 11]. While drilling tunnels that converge intraosseously or that exit the patellar cortex have shown higher loads to failure, when they do fail, it is usually with bone bridge fracture or fracture in general. Although the cost of implants is a consideration, if this complication is to be avoided, then patellar tunnels should be small and short if used at all. Drilling patellar tunnels smaller than 4.5 mm in diameter reduces this risk and is advised. Other options are to only suture the graft to the medial patellar retinaculum/periosteum or to perform a quadriceps turndown, which obviates the need for any patellar tunnels or fixation devices on the patellar side of the soft tissue reconstruction [12, 13].

The available literature suggests that fully transverse patellar tunnels have an increased risk of associated patellar fracture, and therefore the authors do not recommend this surgical technique. If tunnels are used, then short oblique tunnels 4.5 mm or less in size could potentially decrease fracture risk. Conversely, existing literature suggests that either suture anchors or docking techniques with interference screws can help further mitigate this risk.

Take-Home Points

1. Patella fracture is the most common and severe complication associated with MPFL reconstruction
2. Avoid large or transverse patellar tunnels
3. Use short blind-ended patellar tunnels with interference screws or suture anchors *or* consider short, oblique tunnels less than 4.5 mm with looped graft placement

Malpositioned Tunnels, Anisometry, and Recurrent Instability

The Complication

Anisometry and malpositioned tunnels can present clinically as a loss of flexion or tightness *or* as recurrent instability. While direct palpation of anatomic structures is beneficial and worthwhile in understanding the native anatomy in reconstructing the MPFL at its origin, sometimes body habitus or revision surgery with scar makes this challenging and difficult to do. Schottle's point, Fig. 9.2, helps to alleviate some of this variability by providing a radiographic reference of the anatomic origin of the native MPFL using intraoperative C-arm imaging [14].

Malposition of the femoral attachment can have devastating consequences to the postoperative range of motion. A systematic review has shown that 3.4% of patients developed postoperative loss of knee flexion, which ultimately resulted in an overall 1.4% procedural complication rate of manipulation under anesthesia (MUA) for loss of flexion [5]. Meaning, for those patients who developed postoperative arthrofibrosis or stiffness, 40% ultimately required a MUA. Mulliez et al. also reported postoperative stiffness rates of 1.5% resulting from MPFL reconstructive with concomitant TTO [6].

Shah et al. reported that 32% of all reported complications were associated with recurrent apprehension [5]. There were 3.7% clinical failures with frank repeat subluxation/dislocation events reported across 11 studies [5]. 8.3% of their study population continued to report subjective apprehension on postoperative examination

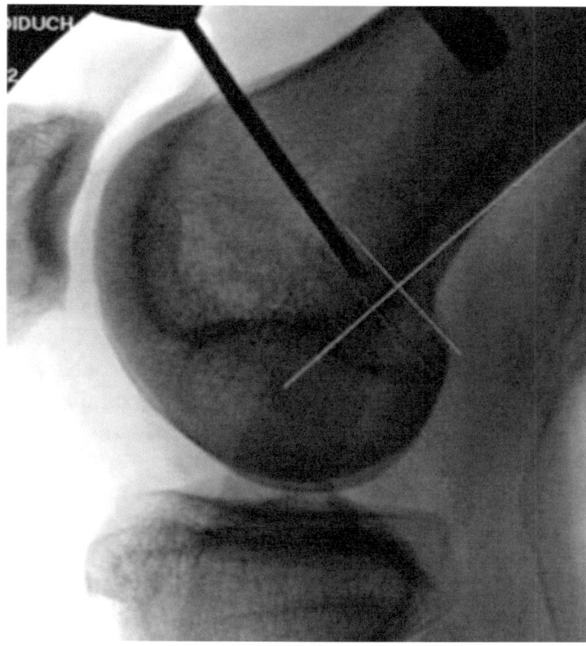

Fig. 9.2 Appropriate lateral radiograph with tunnel placed at Schottle's point

without documented re-dislocation [5]. Ultimately, reoperation rates for recurrent instability by subluxation or dislocation were 0.9% [5]. Schiphouwer et al. stated across a series of patients 5.2% had objective recurrence of instability and a significantly higher recurrence rate of patellar instability in skeletally immature vs mature patients, 33.3% vs 3.8%, respectively, but there was no difference between the isolated MPFL reconstruction vs combined procedure results [4]. Lower re-dislocation rates have also been reported at 0.8%, with similar surgical techniques reported as a soft tissue proximal stabilization procedure by MPFL reconstruction combined with a TTO distally [6]. The heterogeneity across the literature once again makes comparisons difficult; yet, these values are within reasonably reported data for MPFL reconstruction failure rates for recurrent instability.

This systematic study also reported that suture techniques compared to tunnel technique demonstrated an increased rate of recurrent subluxation/dislocation at 4.8% and hypermobility/apprehension at 24%, versus 3.3% and 8.6%, respectively [5]. While clear comparisons cannot be gleamed from this information given the differences of techniques, concomitant procedures recorded, and lack of overall sample sizes reported, it does raise the question as to bone tunnels providing better inherent stability with or without fixation. This could be attributed to the soft tissue graft-suture fixation construct failing or stretching out. Biomechanical studies have shown lower implant load to failure rates, which could contribute to these higher rates of symptomatic apprehension and dislocation seen clinically [10, 11].

How to Avoid It

Limiting the complication of tunnel malposition (with resultant anisometry/loss of flexion or recurrent instability) is vital. Patellar graft placement has been shown to be less critical in determining graft isometry as long as the graft is fixed in the upper medial one-third to one-half of the patella. The crucial part of the procedure is the correct placement of the femoral tunnel for the insertion of the MPFL reconstruction. A key part of this is obtaining a perfect lateral intraoperative C-arm image of the knee. Significant deviation from Schottle's point, as described in the previous chapter's surgical techniques, can result in either recurrent instability from early graft loosening or may have untoward effects of increasing patellar contract pressures and resultant loss of range of motion secondary to graft malposition and tightness. Correctly placed, there will not be any significant graft lengthening throughout range of motion (Fig. 9.3). Intraoperatively this can be assessed after the guide pin is drilled in the femur and the graft wrapped around the beath pin and the knee taken through its arc of motion. Assessing for graft length displacement will help determine its isometry and the relative positioning of the femoral tunnel.

Troubleshooting graft position intraoperatively can be aided by remembering two catchphrases that describe graft behavior as the knee is flexed: "high and tight" or "low and loose." If the graft is placed 1 cm too proximal, it will be loose in extension and the patella will be unstable. The converse will be true as the knee is flexed, where it will be tight, resulting in loss of terminal flexion, graft rupture, or patella chondrosis (Fig. 9.4). This proximal femoral placement would result in a graft that tightens with flexion and result in a "high and tight" pattern. If instead the graft is secured 1 cm distal to the anatomic origin, it will be too tight in extension and will be loose in flexion, unable to control the patella, which may result in recurrent instability (Fig. 9.5). Hence a "low and loose" picture would be seen intraoperatively as the knee is flexed through a range of motion [15]. Having correctly placed the femoral bone tunnel will help to ensure that the graft length and isometry are appropriate and limit the risk of continued patellar instability or excessive compressive forces. The position of the knee when the graft is fixed and the "tension" placed also play a role, and these will be discussed in the next section.

Take-Home Points

1. The true anatomic insertion of the graft on the femur needs to be determined and confirmed as the knee is fully ranged (check graft length change throughout arc of knee motion to ensure proper positioning of the femoral tunnel). Fluoroscopy should be used to help confirm or localize the femoral insertion point.
2. Perfect lateral every time.
3. Schottle's point is key.

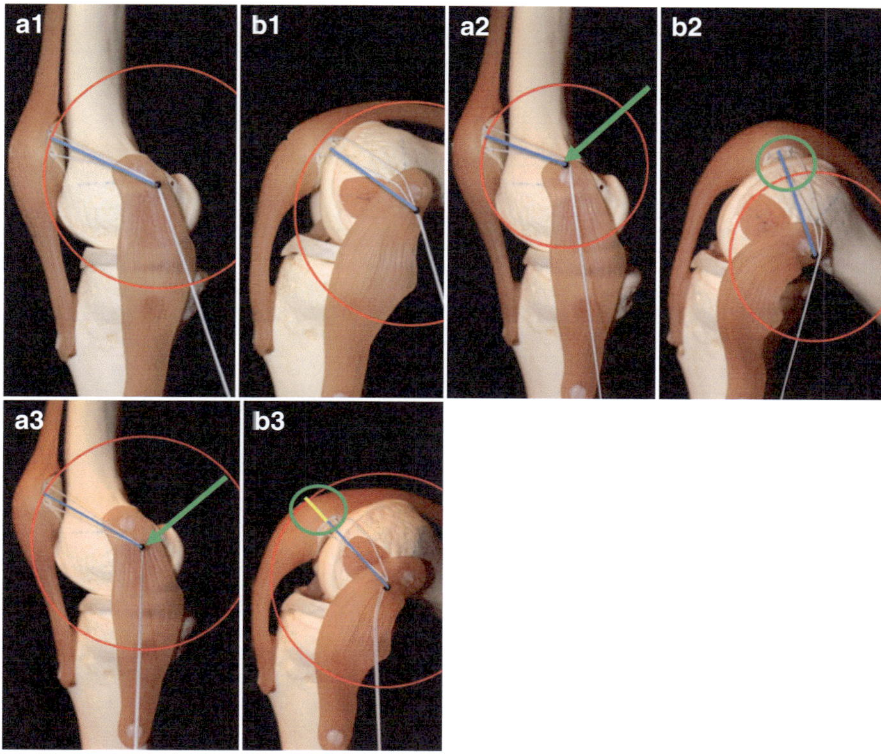

Figs. 9.3, 9.4, and 9.5 Notice graft isometry placed. In these models, the red circle represents the length of the graft at the time it is fixed, whereas the line indicates the length of graft actually needed to reach from femur to patella. Graft tunnel at Schottle's point with the closest isometry present fixed at 30° of flexion (Fig. 9.3**a1**, **b1**); graft tunnel too proximal and anisometric; tight in flexion, loose in extension (Fig. 9.4**a2**, **b2**); graft tunnel too distal and anisometric; tight in extension and loose in flexion (Fig. 9.5**a3**, **b3**)

Medial Overload OA

The Complication

Medial patellar overload and resultant osteoarthritis is an avoidable iatrogenic injury to the cartilage that occurs more often than not when over tensioning of the graft is performed. This can also be influenced by the knee flexion angle at the time of femoral graft fixation. It has been shown that only 2 N, or 0.5lbs, of force is all that is required to effectively restore the normal tension and patellar contact pressures and that short and malpositioned grafts can adversely increase medial patellar contact

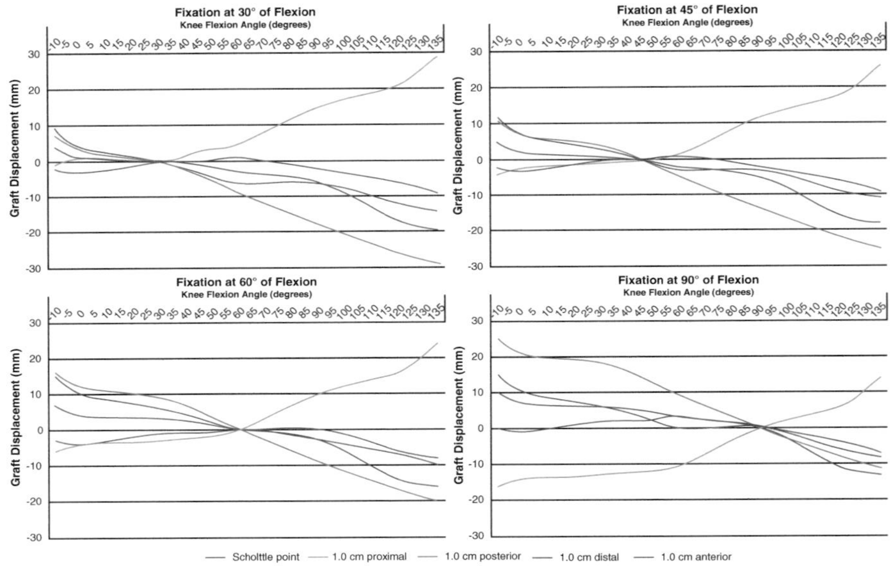

Fig. 9.6 Graphic depictions of various femoral attachments with the model medial patellofemoral ligament (MPFL) fixed at different knee flexion angles. For grafts fixed at >45° of knee flexion, substantial variation in graft lengths occurs during the 0–30° range if the femoral attachment is not exactly at the Schottle's point. As the MPFL is most important during the first 30° of flexion, deviations from proper kinematics will have significant clinical implications. (Permission request submitted to OJSM Ref. [15])

pressures by more than 50% [16, 17]. There are no long-term studies to date that report on long-term outcomes of resultant medial patellar arthritis as it relates to MFPL reconstruction. The MPFL functions predominantly and exerts its force as a "check rein" at 0–30° of knee flexion. During further knee flexion, trochlear morphology provides the necessary constraint and control to provide stability to the patella [18]. In a recent study, Burrus et al. provided guidance as to the knee flexion angle at the time when femoral graft fixation is placed (Fig. 9.6). This study took into consideration the relationship of femoral tunnel placement and showed that at the time of femoral graft fixation, higher angles of knee flexion resulted in substantial graft length variability between 0° and 30° of knee flexion and magnified the errors in the femoral tunnel placement if malpositioned [19]. As the MPFL is most important during the first 30° of knee flexion, these significant variations in graft length would not only result in changes in normal kinematics but would also impact clinical results.

How to Avoid It

Given the findings of graft length displacement with fixation at higher degrees of knee flexion, the recommendation was to flex the knee to 30–45° prior to graft fixation. This is also in line with where the MPFL exerts its most active role in patellar stability during early flexion. Only 2 N or 0.5 lb of force is required to tension the graft. This is not like tensioning an ACL reconstruction.

Another subtle point to help avoid complication when placing the interference screw, the graft can inadvertently be pulled into the tunnel during the final turns so that it over-tightens the construct and can medialize the patella. It is important to watch for this and if necessary, slightly back out the screw to ensure the graft is at the correct length and tension. Finally, it is crucial to assess the lateral retinaculum after the MPFL fixation is completed. It is important not to release the lateral retinaculum prior to MPFL fixation to help limit iatrogenic over-medialization and iatrogenic medial instability as the graft is tensioned without a lateral restraint. Furthermore, a lateral retinacular "Z" lengthening rather than a simple release allows the benefit of releasing the lateral excessive tightness but still provides satisfactory soft tissue restraint without completely destabilizing the lateral structures as a complete lateral release does. While there are no studies directly comparing the two methods with MPFL reconstructions, a lengthening would be the safer of the two options to limit destabilizing the patella further.

Take-Home Points

1. 0.5lbs of force is all it takes to tension the MPFL graft.
2. Knee angle flexion at 30–45° during femoral graft fixation. Any mistakes in femoral tunnel position are magnified if the graft is fixed in higher degrees of flexion.
3. Consider lateral lengthening over lateral release if indicated

Medial Instability/Lateral Retinacular Reconstruction

The Complication

While rare, medial instability is iatrogenic and can be caused by excessively releasing the lateral retinaculum. Hughston et al. reported on the destabilizing effect of lateral retinacular releases in isolation as treatment for patellar instability, noting up to 50% medial patellar subluxation [20]. MRI studies have also confirmed the medial subluxation of the patella when treated with isolated lateral retinacular release for patellar instability [21]. Medial instability can also be seen from over-tensioning the graft with associated lateral release at the time of MPFL reconstruction. This is a rarely reported complication in the literature, with brief mentioning in case series and reports. Schiphouwer et al. reported one case of medial dislocation after a failed repair of a lateral retinaculum at the time of MPFL reconstruction [4]. In treating this complication, there are several reports of surgical techniques, using local IT band or even quadriceps tendon, aimed at stabilizing the patella as salvage operations in treating this debilitating condition, known as iatrogenic medial patellar instability (IMPI) [22, 23]. Current long-term follow-up is lacking but short-term results show improvements in pain and psychological symptoms associated with the surgical treatment of IMPI [22].

How to Avoid It

To avoid this complication, it is advised to limit the tension placed on the graft during fixation to only 2 N as previously discussed. Do not perform lateral release prior to MPFL fixation, and if a lateral release has been performed previously, ensure that the patella is centered in the trochlea and not medialized at the time of femoral fixation. A quick guide is to palpate the lateral border of the patella, which should be in line and nearly flush with the lateral border of the trochlea; however, in trochlea dysplasia cases, this can be difficult to ascertain. As always, after completing the reconstruction, assess patellar glide both medial and lateral to assess for gross asymmetry, and observe the patella behavior through a full ROM. Lastly, a lateral "Z" lengthening rather than release is preferred to maintain restraint.

Take-Home Points

1. Assess for lateral sided soft tissue lengthening/releases after femoral fixation to limit over-medialization with resultant instability.
2. "Z" lengthening is preferred over lateral release.
3. Know your patients prior surgical history – it will impact your case.

General Complications (MPFL Reconstructions)

Shah et al. detailed generalized wound complications in roughly 2% of patients undergoing MPFL reconstructions including wound infection, wound dehiscence, subcutaneous hematoma, and graft harvest-related neuroma [5]. Significant postop pain was also seen in 5.4% of patients, where symptomatic hardware was present in 3.0% of patients and 1.1% required an additional procedure of hardware removal for persistent pain [5]. Given the soft tissue envelope and hamstring tendons, adductor tendons, and MCL present medially, the medial femoral fixation is often the location of symptomatic hardware for isolated reconstructions and tibial tubercle osteotomy screw fixation when combined procedures are performed. Other studies have reported on wound infections and wound healing complications in association with soft tissue reconstruction stabilization procedures listed between 1.5% and 5.7% [4, 6].

Complications of Tibial Tubercle Osteotomies

Tibial tubercle osteotomies are powerful and versatile surgical techniques that can both address patellar instability as well as other pathologies associated with maltracking such as overload and cartilage wear. As previously discussed, there are differing obliquities of osteotomies, each allowing a different type of planar correction to be performed, specified to the particular offending pathology at hand. Tibial tubercle osteotomies (TTO), unfortunately, can also result in serious complications, many of which can prolong the recovery course. Payne et al. provided a systematic review of the literature as it pertains to early complications associated with TTO and reported on 19 studies, totaling 787 TTOs. The majority of the patients treated were for patellar instability, and the remaining were for patellar pain and malalignment. The overall complication rate reported was 4.6% or 36/787 procedures [24]. Direct surgical techniques were reported as 472 Elmslie-Trillat, 193 Fulkerson, and 102 complete detachments as a medialization, distalization, or a combination of such. Of note, the risk of major complications trended higher when the tibial tubercle shingle was completely detached (5.7%) than with an Elmslie-Trillat (2.3%) or Fulkerson (3.1%), but this was not statistically significant [24]. In addition to potential complications with the osteotomy itself, potential sequelae of the TTO such as overcorrection have been reported, where forces were transferred to the medial and proximal patellar facets in patients where there was pre-existing medial chondral disease [25, 26]. Resultant anterior knee pain and disability with painful hardware have also been reported.

Nonunions/Delayed Unions

The Complication

There are many baseline risk factors for nonunion development that have been established in the acute trauma fracture literature [27]. As a controlled fracture, an osteotomy relies on relative bone apposition and a healing bed of bone to unite. TTOs have a large cancellous bone bed for healing to occur, and with adequate fixation, this usually occurs without event. Patient risk factors such as smoking, obesity, malnutrition, and weight-bearing status are modifiable to an extent; however, the surgical technique of shingle length, obliquity, "step cut" versus "feather," soft tissue attachment preservation, shingle depth, and screw placement can all influence healing as well. In a systematic review of the literature, the nonunion rate was reported as 0.8% [24]. Subdividing the techniques into distinct risks, the complete shingle detachment had the highest risk of nonunion at 2.4% compared to the Fulkerson technique at 1.0% and the Elmslie-Trillat slide at 0.2%. Delayed unions can also occur as evidenced by prolonged healing, most notably at the distal aspect of the osteotomy shingle. This can be seen in patella alta correction with distalization procedures [28]. A horizontal step cut as performed for distalization to allow docking of the tubercle fragment results in lengthy healing across this mainly cortical bone interface. Fisher et al., in their 2016 retrospective review of military servicemembers undergoing TTO for patellar chondral pathology, found a 2.3% delayed union rate of their osteotomy sites [29]. An example of a delayed union can be seen in Fig. 9.7a, b. These transverse cuts in cortical bone routinely take 6 months or longer to fully heal.

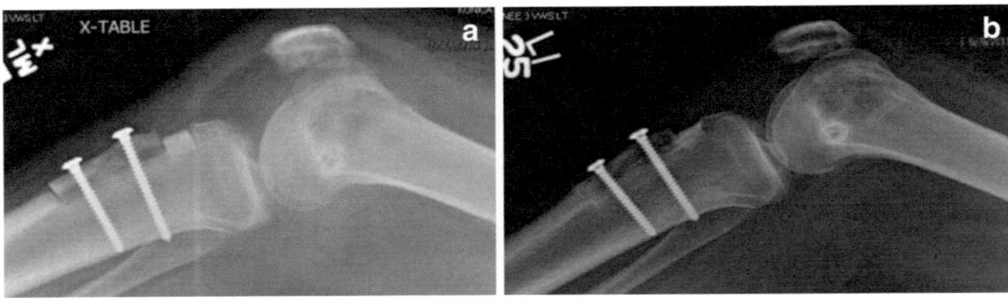

Fig. 9.7 (**a**, **b**) Note the sclerotic distal osteotomy "step cut" without full consolidation at 3 months or at 6 months

How to Avoid It

In order to help limit the risk of nonunion, particular attention is needed to ensure that satisfactory fixation is placed orthogonal to the osteotomy site's obliquity and that adequate compression is maintained with fixation for relative bone apposition. Additional allograft bone grafting can be placed to fill any voids left at the osteotomy site or autograft from the local exposed lateral cavity to help ensure bony incorporation. An additional technique can be used with distalizing the osteotomy for patella alta, where the distal shingle edge is "feathered" instead of an abrupt "step cut." See Figs. 9.8 and 9.9. This allows a 4–5 mm shingle to slide distally which keeps a good bone surface area for healing instead of a step cut which might be a risk factor for delayed healing given it is a transverse cortical cut. Any further distalization generally requires a step cut, however.

Take-Home Points

1. Rigid osteotomy fixation and compression.
2. Bone graft as needed.
3. Can feather and slide the shingle to overlap bone.

Tibial Fractures

The Complication

When performing TTOs, tibial fractures can occur at the time of surgery or postoperatively and involve the osteotomy shingle or the tibial shaft. Tibial shingle fractures can occur at the time of surgery from propagation of the osteotomy site distally with osteotome use. When placing fixation, if the shingle is too thin or aggressive compression is placed with hardware, this can cause a fracture of the shingle, requiring additional fixation at times. Limiting the shingle length to no more than 6–8 cm helps to limit violating the anterior tibial cortical bow as it starts to transition into the higher tension-sided meta-diaphyseal region of the bone. Postoperatively, disuse osteopenia, premature full weight-bearing, and eccentric quad contractures can cause shingle fracture or displacement. Still, the most likely fracture is due to a stress riser at the inferior site of the osteotomy cut or through one of the screw holes (Fig. 9.9). This could be influenced by too long of

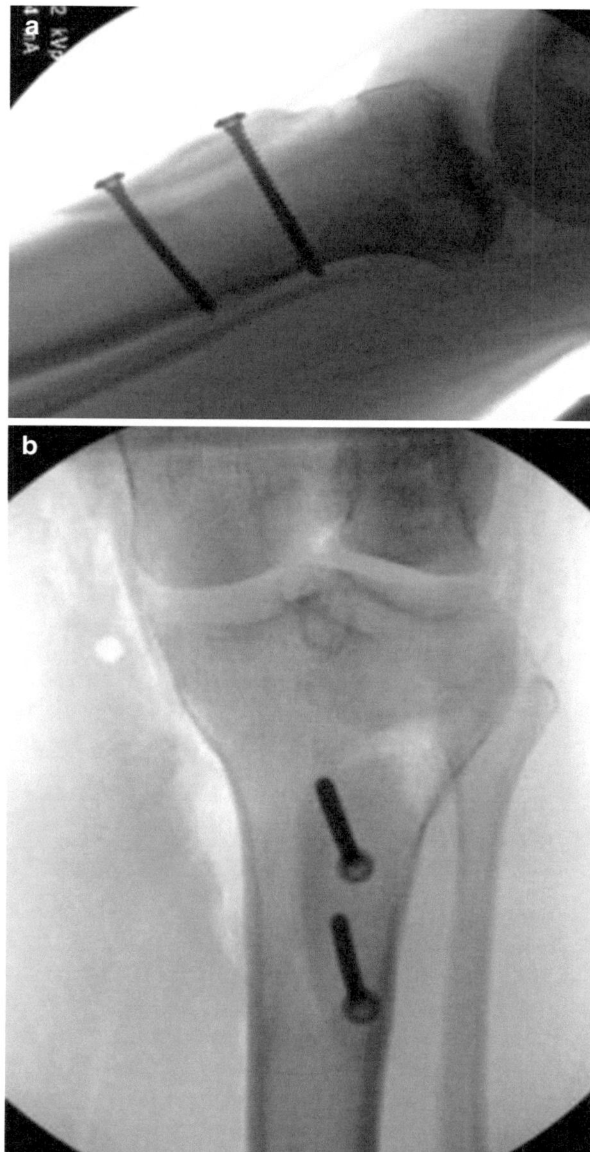

Fig. 9.8 (**a**, **b**) Note the feathered distal edge of the shingle, distalized without "step cut"

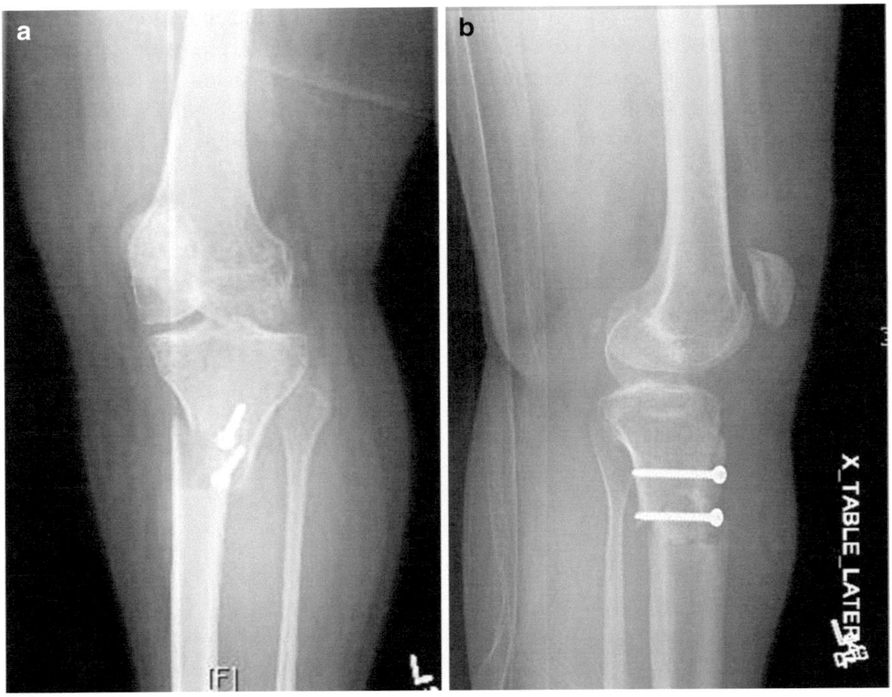

Fig. 9.9 (**a**, **b**) Tibial shaft fracture at the distal most screw/osteotomy site. (courtesy of Beth E. Shubin Stein, MD)

an osteotomy shingle, which violates the distal cortical bow, or premature weight-bearing. In a systematic review of the literature, the ibial fracture rate in the setting of TTO was reported as 8 out of 787 patients, 1.0% [24]. In a recent retrospective review of military servicemembers undergoing TTO, there was a 2.3% reported osteotomy shingle fracture rate, which underscores its very real occurrence [29].

How to Avoid It

To help limit the risks of tibial shaft fracture, use an oscillating saw after adequately defining the patellar ligament insertion on the tibial tubercle. The osteotomy's distal extent can be tapered or "feathered" with use of the saw and lateral side completed with osteotomes. Alternatively, small "stress relaxation" drill holes can be made in the anterior cortex to limit fracture propagation distally as the osteotomy is completed with an osteotome. Appropriate width shingle creation is key to limit the risk of shingle fracture, with a thick enough cut being taken even for an Elmslie-Trillat osteotomy to limit fracture during screw use and osteotomy compression. Feathering and tapering the distal edge of the shingle and to limit its length will help to not violate the transition into the anterior cortical bow of the tibia, which could be a stress riser and result in a tibia fracture during the recovery phase. Most importantly, patients need to restrict weight-bearing until the osteotomy has adequately healed, which is typically 6 weeks.

Take-Home Points

1. Use oscillating saw and taper distally – complete with osteotome.
2. Create satisfactory shingle thickness but limit its distal extent.
3. Restrict full weight-bearing for 6 weeks or radiographic bony union.

Generalized Complications (Tibial Tubercle Osteotomies)

Wound complication rates have been reported in the literature at 0.8%, which includes dehiscence. Wound infection rates have been reported at 1.0% [24]. Additional, more rare complications were also reported as saphenous neuromas and temporary peroneal nerve palsies, and DVT/PE seen in other lower extremity surgeries performed [24]. Payne et al. reported an overall risk of 36.7% hardware removal secondary to symptomatic painful hardware [24]. The Elmslie-Trillat and detached shingle technique had the least amount of painful hardware (26.8% and 48.3%, respectively) compared to the Fulkerson osteotomy technique, which had the most at 49% [24].

Complications of Trochleoplasty and Femoral Osteotomies

While the MPFL has a vital role in guiding the patella during the first 30° of knee flexion, the trochlea also has an important role in the remaining arc of flexion in providing patellar stability. Trochleoplasty is a novel approach as a proximal bone realignment procedure that can also lateralize the mechanical axis as a way to reduce the TT-TG. Previous chapters have focused on indications and trochleoplasty surgical techniques. Given its inherent ability to change the underlying trochlear morphology, it also comes with risk of complications as an intra-articular procedure as well.

Arthrofibrosis

The Complication

Each surgical technique is a variation upon the same basic concept of reshaping the trochlea to provide a better congruent trough for the patella to glide in. Subtle variations allow for changes in the center of the trochlear trough and axis; however, each must be fixated to allow for satisfactory healing to occur. As such, the potential for postoperative adhesions, loss of range of motion, and resultant pain can occur [30, 31]. This can require an arthroscopic lysis of adhesions (LOA) and manipulation under anesthesia (MUA), which also carries with it its own inherent risks of peri-genu fracture but also could damage other concomitant procedures such as TTO fixation or even stretch out a scarred in MPFL reconstruction. The literature has reported a wide range of postoperative arthrofibrosis rates from 0% to 46% [31–34]. This wide range of reported levels very well could be attributable to varying surgical techniques and evolving physical therapy regimens. More recent studies trend that number to closer to 0–20%, which also correlates to unpublished data by the senior author of this chapter at a LOA/MUA rate of 19% in a series of over 50 procedures to date.

How to Avoid It

Some newer surgical techniques negate the need for potential hardware removal by utilizing suture anchor fixation and absorbable suture (Fig. 9.10). Studies have shown that intra-articular absorption of vicryl occurs upon repeat arthroscopy and that satisfactory healing of the subchondral trochlear flap occurs [34–36]. Also, presuming stable fixation of the trochlea has been achieved, the importance of a regimented and progressive physical therapy program starting immediately with regaining range of motion cannot be underscored enough. Working closely with a physical therapist will maximize patient outcomes, especially when multiple

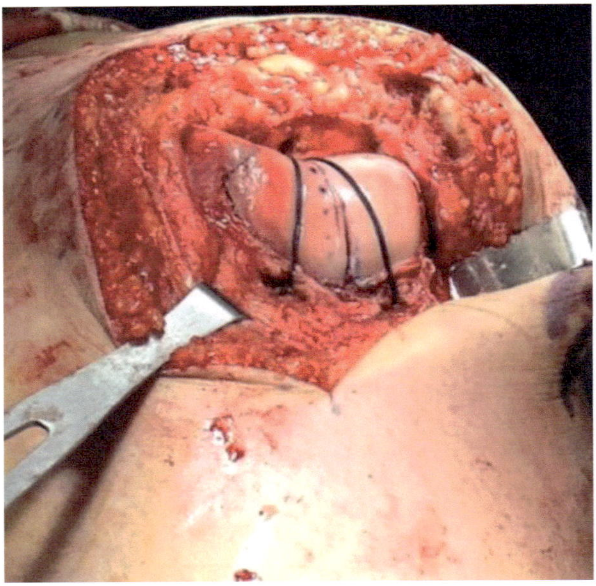

Fig. 9.10 Note the placement of #1 vicryl preloaded into knotless suture anchors, specifically placed to gain maximum sulcus reduction/recreation with bone apposition while healing

procedures have been performed on a single knee to address a multiple pathologic process for their patellar instability and pain.

Take-Home Points
1. Choose a reproducible surgical technique in your hands that recreates the trochlear morphology that the patient requires.
2. Review absorbable fixation devices that might negate the need for revision surgery for hardware removal.
3. Even in the best of hands, arthrofibrosis occurs, manage it appropriately.

Cartilage Perforation/Subchondral Fracture Propagation/ Loss of Sulcus Morphology/Arthritis

The Complication

When performing trochleoplasty procedures, it is imperative to choose your patients appropriately, as it is for all surgical procedures. While indications have been discussed previously, it has been noted that pre-existing arthritis is a contraindication, namely, because of the brittle subchondral bone that is sometimes present. Sometimes, when using a 20 blade for incising the cartilage and the subchondral plate, there will be subchondral cysts which can split anywhere along the path of least resistance and can cause an unintended osteochondral fracture line propagation. The bone can also be so sclerotic that a 20 blade cannot perforate it. Additional complications that occur during the postoperative recovery period can be seen and assessed on postoperative routine radiographs, such as a change and increase in the sulcus angle caused by settling of the trochleoplasty margins. This effectively reverses the procedure from the morphology the trochlea had been placed in intraoperatively as it settles and returns to a more flat and dysplastic shape, potentially placing any soft tissue medial reconstruction at risk and recurrent instability at redeveloping.

Also, with the use of a high-speed burr to create the sulcus deepening osteotomy, there is the potential for heat transference, which could cause thermal necrosis to the chondral surface if too close to the subchondral bone (Fig. 9.11a, b). This could result in the possible development of an osteochondral loose fragment or chondromalacia, progressing to symptomatic arthritis.

The most concerning complication from performing a trochleoplasty is the development of osteoarthritis. At baseline, patellar dislocations and trochlear dysplasia are risk factors for the development of patellofemoral arthrosis and arthritis. However, the act of intervening to correct the underlying bony and articular morphology also could result in a negative cartilage outcome, despite its primary purpose of providing better patellofemoral congruency to limit maltracking and

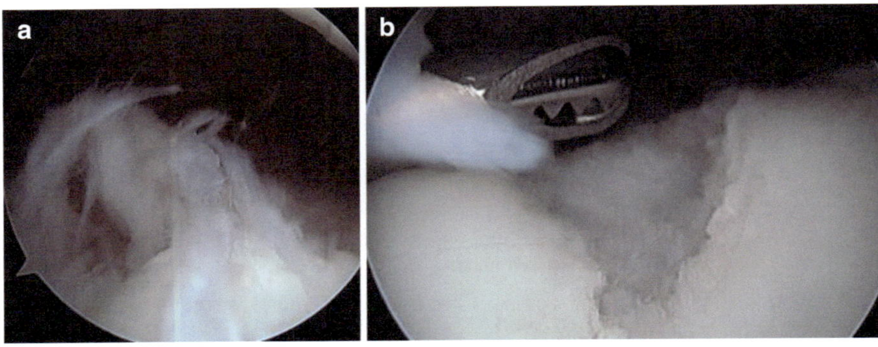

Fig. 9.11 (**a**, **b**) Associated loose fragment and chondromalacia 1-year status post-trochleoplasty with pre- and post-debridement images

instability. To date, midterm follow-up studies by Dejour and von Knoch showed 0% and 30% arthritic findings from trochleoplasty, respectively [33, 34]. However, it was reported that in the latter group, the articular changes were noted at the time of the index procedure and were thought to be attributable to the patellar dislocation history.

How to Avoid It

Patient selection is critical in avoiding complications. Pre-existing arthritis makes the likelihood of an intra-articular fracture and propagation higher and thus should be avoided. Depending upon the type of surgical technique used, always pay attention to burr use and the proximity to the subchondral plate and cartilage to help limit heat-induced necrosis during sulcus deepening. Should this occur and be appreciated, then local arthroscopic debridement can be performed as needed, and depending upon its size, location, and involvement, then possible additional cartilage restoration procedures can be entertained. When creating the trochlea's new morphology and trough/groove, as stated above settling can occur postoperatively at the medial and lateral margins. To help combat this, place small segments of bone autograft, which can be saved during osteotome use to open a window for the burr, to soften the transition from the burr cavity to intact bone along the outer edges. This will help prevent settling as the trochleoplasty heals and keep the crafted morphology intact.

Take-Home Points

1. Patient selection is key.
2. Pay attention to depth of burr; irrigate as needed to reduce effects of heat.
3. Bolster the medial and lateral corticocancellous trochlear edges to help prevent settling of the edges, which will maintain sulcus angle and congruency.

Generalized Complications (Trochleoplasty)

Beyond the above-listed more commonly encountered complications associated with trochleoplasty procedures, postoperative superficial wound complications have been reported [37]. Given the intra-articular nature of the procedure and potential fixation devices used for trochleoplasty flap reduction, hardware removal has been reported in the literature as well [31, 32]. Continued patellar instability and increased pain from baseline have also been reported from the potential over- or under-correction resulting in patellar incongruence [38, 39] at the time of surgery.

References

1. Ahmad CS, Stein BE, Matuz D, Henry JH. Immediate surgical repair of the medial patellar stabilizers for acute patellar dislocation. A review of eight cases. Am.J. Sports Med. 2000;28:804–10.
2. Arendt EA, Moeller A, Agel J. Clinical outcomes of medial patellofemoral ligament repair in recurrent (chronic) lateral patella dislocations. Knee Surg Sports Traumatol Arthrosc. 2011;19:1909–14.
3. Christiansen SE, Jakobsen BW, Lund B, Lind M. Isolated repair of the medial patellofemoral ligament in primary dislocation of the patella: a prospective randomized study. Arthroscopy. 2008;24:881–7.
4. Schiphouwer L, Rood A, Tigchelaar S, Koeter S. Complications of medial patellofemoral ligament reconstruction using two transverse patellar tunnels. Knee Surg Sports Traumatol Arthrosc. 2016;25(1):245–50.
5. Shah JN, Howard JS, Flanigan DC, Brophy RH, Carey JL, Lattermann C. A systematic review of complications and failures associated with medial patellofemoral ligament reconstruction for recurrent patellar dislocation. Am J Sports Med. 2012;40:1916–23.
6. Mulliez A, Lambrecht D, Verbruggen D, Van Der Straeten C, Verdonk P, Victor J. Clinical outcome in MPFL reconstruction with and without tuberositas transposition. Knee Surg Sports Traumatol Arthrosc. 2017;25(9):2708–14. https://doi.org/10.1007/s00167-015-3654-0.
7. Panni AS, Alam M, Cerciello S, Vasso M, Maffulli N. Medial patellofemoral ligament reconstruction with a divergent patellar transverse 2-tunnel technique. Am J Sports Med. 2011;39:2647–55.
8. Parikh SN, Nathan ST, Wall EJ, Eismann EA. Complications of medial patellofemoral ligament reconstruction in young patients. Am J Sports Med. 2013;41:1030–8.
9. Mountney J, Senavongse W, Amis AA, Thomas NP. Tensile strength of the medial patellofemoral ligament before and after repair or reconstruction. J Bone Joint Surg Br. 2005;87:36–40.
10. Russo F, Doan J, Chase DC, Farnsworth CL, Pennock AT. Medial patellofemoral ligament reconstruction: fixation technique biomechanics. J Knee Surg. 2016;29:303–9.
11. Russ SD, Tompkins M, Nuckley D, Macalena J. Biomechanical comparison of patellar fixation techniques in medial patellofemoral ligament reconstruction. Am J Sports Med. 2015;43:195–9.
12. Steensen RN, Dopirak RM, Maurus PB. A simple technique for reconstruction of the medial patellofemoral ligament using a quadriceps tendon graft. Arthroscopy. 2005;21:365–70.
13. Vavalle G, Capozzi M. Isolated reconstruction of the medial patellofemoral ligament with autologous quadriceps tendon. J Orthop Traumatol. 2016;17:155–62.
14. Schottle PB, Romero J, Schmeling A, Weiler A. Technical note: anatomical reconstruction of the medial patellofemoral ligament using a free gracilis autograft. Arch Orthop Trauma Surg. 2008;128:479–84.

15. Burrus MT, Werner BC, Conte EJ, Diduch DR. Troubleshooting the femoral attachment during medial patellofemoral ligament reconstruction: location, location, location. Orthop J Sports Med. 2015;**3**:2325967115569198.
16. Stephen JM, Kaider D, Lumpaopong P, Deehan DJ, Amis AA. The effect of femoral tunnel position and graft tension on patellar contact mechanics and kinematics after medial patellofemoral ligament reconstruction. Am J Sports Med. 2014;42:364–72.
17. Elias JJ, Cosgarea AJ. Technical errors during medial patellofemoral ligament reconstruction could overload medial patellofemoral cartilage: a computational analysis. Am J Sports Med. 2006;34:1478–85.
18. Ronga M, Oliva F, Longo UG, Testa V, Capasso G, Maffulli N. Isolated medial patellofemoral ligament reconstruction for recurrent patellar dislocation. Am J Sports Med. 2009;37:1735–42.
19. Burrus MT, Werner BC, Cancienne JM, Gwathmey FW, Diduch DR. MPFL graft fixation in low degrees of knee flexion minimizes errors made in the femoral location. Knee Surg Sports Traumatol Arthrosc. 2016;25(10):3092–8.
20. Hughston JC, Deese M. Medial subluxation of the patella as a complication of lateral retinacular release. Am J Sports Med. 1988;16:383–8.
21. Shellock FG, Mink JH, Deutsch AL, Fox JM. Patellar tracking abnormalities: clinical experience with kinematic MR imaging in 130 patients. Radiology. 1989;172:799–804.
22. Sanchis-Alfonso V, Montesinos-Berry E, Monllau JC, Merchant AC. Results of isolated lateral retinacular reconstruction for iatrogenic medial patellar instability. Arthroscopy. 2015;31:422–7.
23. Teitge RA, Torga SR. Lateral patellofemoral ligament reconstruction. Arthroscopy. 2004;20:998–1002.
24. Payne J, Rimmke N, Schmitt LC, Flanigan DC, Magnussen RA. The incidence of complications of tibial tubercle osteotomy: a systematic review. Arthroscopy. 2015;31:1819–25.
25. Pidoriano AJ, Weinstein RN, Buuck DA, Fulkerson JP. Correlation of patellar articular lesions with results from anteromedial tibial tubercle transfer. Am J Sports Med. 1997;25:533–7.
26. Bellemans J, Cauwenberghs F, Witvrouw E, Brys P, Victor J. Anteromedial tibial tubercle transfer in patients with chronic anterior knee pain and a subluxation-type patellar malalignment. Am J Sports Med. 1997;25:375–81.
27. Zura R, Xiong Z, Einhorn T, Watson JT, Ostrum RF, Prayson MJ, et al. Epidemiology of fracture nonunion in 18 human bones. JAMA Surg. 2016;151(11):e162775.
28. Magnussen RA, De Simone V, Lustig S, Neyret P, Flanigan DC. Treatment of patella Alta in patients with episodic patellar dislocation: a systematic review. Knee Surg Sports Traumatol Arthrosc. 2014;22:2545–50.
29. Fisher TF, Waterman BR, Orr JD, Holland CA, Bader J, Belmont PJ Jr. Tibial tubercle osteotomy for patellar chondral pathology in an active United States military population. Arthroscopy. 2016;32(11):2342–9.
30. McNamara I, Bua N, Smith TO, Ali K, Donell ST. Deepening trochleoplasty with a thick osteochondral flap for patellar instability: clinical and functional outcomes at a mean 6-year follow-up. Am J Sports Med. 2015;43:2706–13.
31. Verdonk R, Jansegers E, Stuyts B. Trochleoplasty in dysplastic knee trochlea. Knee Surg Sports Traumatol Arthrosc. 2005;13:529–33.
32. Donell ST, Joseph G, Hing CB, Marshall TJ. Modified Dejour trochleoplasty for severe dysplasia: operative technique and early clinical results. Knee. 2006;13:266–73.
33. von Knoch F, Bohm T, Burgi ML, von Knoch M, Bereiter H. Trochleoplasty for recurrent patellar dislocation in association with trochlear dysplasia. A 4- to 14-year follow-up study. J Bone Joint Surg Br. 2006;88:1331–5.
34. Ntagiopoulos PG, Byn P, Dejour D. Midterm results of comprehensive surgical reconstruction including sulcus-deepening trochleoplasty in recurrent patellar dislocations with high-grade trochlear dysplasia. Am J Sports Med. 2013;41:998–1004.
35. Burrus M, Tompkins M, Hinckel B, Diduch DR, Arendt EA. Repair and reconstruction of the medial patellofemoral ligament for treatment of lateral patellar dislocations: Surgical tech-

niques and clinical results. In: Scott WN, editor. Insall and scott: surgery of the knee. 6th ed. Philadelphia: Elsevier; 2017. p. 939–53.
36. Burrus M, Carstensen S, Diduch DR. Trochleoplasty. In: Browne J, Owens B, editors. Operative techniques: knee surgery. Philadelphia: Elsevier. In Press.
37. Utting MR, Mulford JS, Eldridge JD. A prospective evaluation of trochleoplasty for the treatment of patellofemoral dislocation and instability. J Bone Joint Surg Br. 2008;90:180–5.
38. Dejour D, Saggin P. The sulcus deepening trochleoplasty-the Lyon's procedure. Int Orthop. 2010;34:311–6.
39. Fucentese SF, Zingg PO, Schmitt J, Pfirrmann CW, Meyer DC, Koch PP. Classification of trochlear dysplasia as predictor of clinical outcome after trochleoplasty. Knee Surg Sports Traumatol Arthrosc. 2011;19:1655–61.

Chapter 10
Imaging in Patellofemoral Instability

Vivek Kalia and Douglas N. Mintz

Introduction

Recurrent patellar instabilities, both subluxations and dislocations, often occur in the setting of trochlear and patellar dysplasia. Between 17% and 69% of patients who have a primary patellar dislocation go on to have a recurrent dislocation; after a second dislocation event, the chance of additional dislocations increases significantly [10, 17]. Recurrent dislocations increase the risk of cartilage injury [19].

Patellofemoral alignment and *patellofemoral tracking* are often confused. Patellofemoral alignment refers to the static relationship between the patella and trochlea, at a given flexion angle. Patellofemoral tracking describes a dynamic relationship of these structures and their associated soft tissue stabilizers during knee motion. *Patellofemoral maltracking*, then, results from a complex interplay of osseous and soft tissue anatomy with biomechanical stresses placed on the knee. Abnormalities of dynamic muscle strength, soft tissue stabilizers, patellar height and tilt, and trochlear morphology all play an important role in patellofemoral kinematics and the ability of the patella to glide congruently through the trochlear groove through the entire range of knee flexion and extension [22]. Abnormalities involving any of these components may lead to pain and clinical dysfunction. Trauma or specific movements/positions such as a pivoting mechanism can trigger a maltracking episode (i.e., an acute patellar subluxation or dislocation), and patients with predisposing anatomic or mechanical factors, the most common of which are trochlear dysplasia, patella alta, and lateralization of the tibial tuberosity, may experience recurrent episodes [7].

V. Kalia (✉) · D. N. Mintz
Hospital for Special Surgery, New York, NY, USA
e-mail: MintzD@hss.edu

B. E. Shubin Stein, S. M. Strickland (eds.), *Patellofemoral Pain and Instability*,
https://doi.org/10.1007/978-3-319-97640-2_10

Imaging of Instability

Radiography

Radiographic evaluation of the knee for instability traditionally involved a measurement of the quadriceps angle (or *Q angle*), first described by Brattstörm [3]. Two lines are drawn, one from the ipsilateral anterior superior iliac spine (ASIS) to the center of the patella and the second from the center of the patella to the tibial tubercle (Fig. 10.1). Knees with Q angles greater than 20° are at higher risk for patellar instability and have also been associated with anterior knee pain [23]. Q angles are

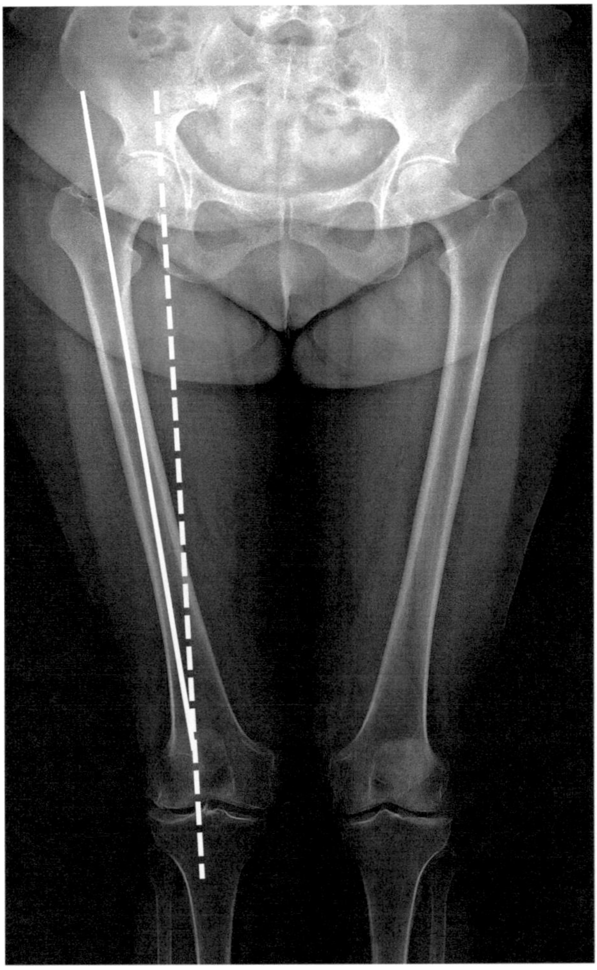

Fig. 10.1 Frontal radiograph of the lower pelvis through the proximal tibias demonstrates measurement of the Q angle. One line (*solid white line*) is drawn from the anterior superior iliac spine to the central patella, and the second line (*dashed white line*) is drawn from the central patella to the tibial tuberosity and then extended superiorly. The angle between the two lines is the Q angle

increased in various clinical scenarios, such as genu valgum, increased femoral anteversion, laterally positioned tibial tuberosity, and external tibial torsion. The reliability and validity of the Q angle remain controversial. Radiographs can evaluate static alignment of the patellofemoral joint, with patellar position and height seen on frontal and lateral radiographs respectively. Axial radiographs are obtained with the patients' knees in some degree of flexion, which engages the patella in the trochlea. Axial views vary tremendously in terms of the information they provide, based on the degree of knee flexion they are taken at. At higher degrees of flexion, less information can be obtained regarding patella position relative to the trochlea (tilt and subluxation). True lateral radiographs are the most appropriate views to assess trochlear morphology.

After patellar dislocation, radiographs may reveal effusion and soft tissue swelling which dissipate, as well as lateral patellar tilt and subluxation. The typical medial patellar fleck of the bone is present on radiographs in about one third of acute dislocators [21].

Cross-Sectional Imaging (CT and MRI)

A more reliable and validated measurement which can be done on cross-sectional imaging is the *tibial tuberosity-trochlear groove* (TT-TG) *distance* [25]. Since patellar position and alignment vary on static CT and MR imaging exams, the TT-TG has become a commonly used surrogate marker of patellar alignment which is relatively stable between imaging modalities and in various pathologies and is thus used most often now to help determine treatment options [4, 5]. On MRI, it is measured from the deepest point of the trochlear sulcus to the midpoint of the patellar tendon at its insertion on the tibial tuberosity on a direct axial image [25, 26] (Fig. 10.2). An increased TT-TG distance has been shown to be associated with the presence of lateral patellar facet chondrosis [25] and patellar instability [2, 18]. The *trochlear angle*, the angle between the medial and lateral trochlear facets on axial image, can also be used to indicate propensity for dislocation, such as in a shallow trochlea with a higher trochlear angle (Fig. 10.3).

In the setting of *transient lateral patellar dislocation*, reduction often occurs prior to imaging, and the clinical presentation of acute pain and knee swelling can be nonspecific. For this reason, the presence of hallmark features on imaging is necessary to make or confirm the diagnosis of a patella dislocation. MRI of the knee is frequently performed to evaluate underlying anatomy, characteristic bone marrow contusions indicative of dislocation, location of disruption of the medial retinaculum and medial patellofemoral ligament (MPFL), and extent of any fractures, as well as to identify osteochondral injury and fragments [14] (Fig. 10.4).

When the patella dislocates laterally or on its way back in, the inferomedial aspect of the patella impacts against the anterior lateral aspect of the extra-articular lateral femoral condyle [8], causing *bone marrow contusions* which present as focal

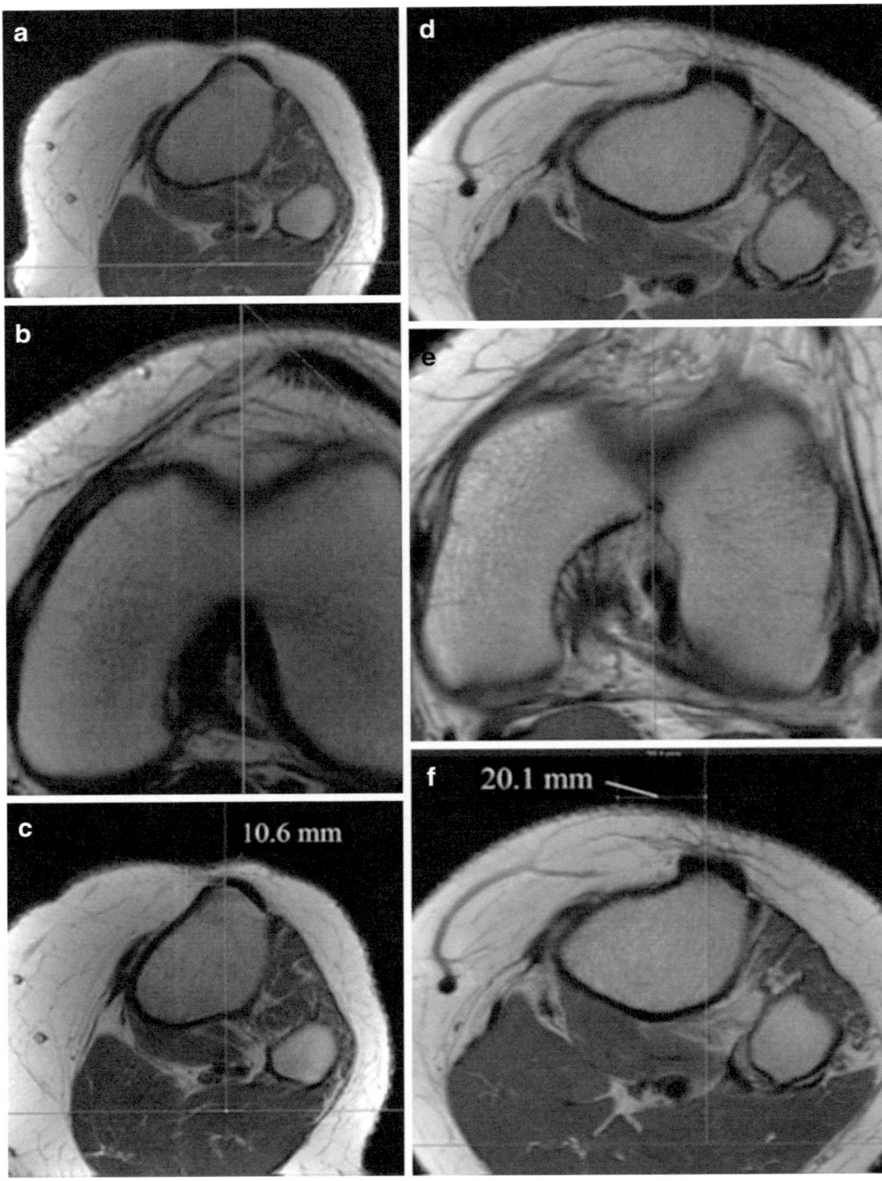

Fig. 10.2 Axial proton density-weighted images of the knee demonstrate measurement of the TT-TG distance. A vertical line is drawn through the tibial tubercle (**panel a**), a second vertical line is drawn through the center of the trochlear sulcus (**panel b**), and the distance between those two lines is measured (**panel c**), which is normal in this case (10.6 mm). In **panels d–f**, using the same method as in panels a–c, an abnormal TT-TG distance of 20.1 mm is seen

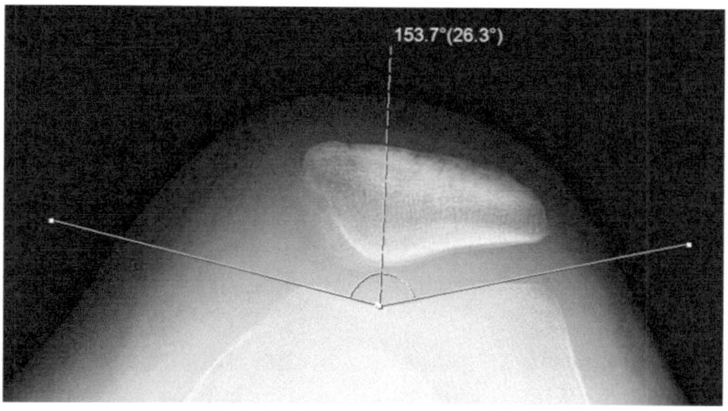

Fig. 10.3 Axial radiograph of the knee demonstrates a shallow trochlear angle of 153.7° (normal <145°)

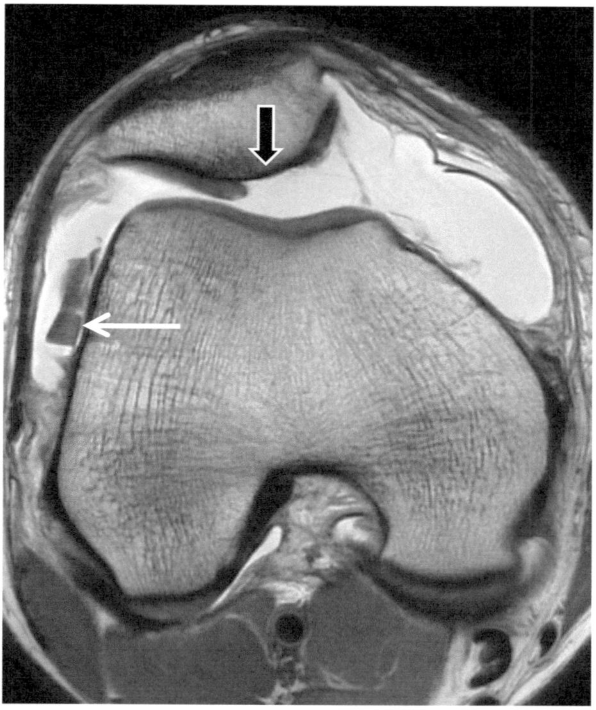

Fig. 10.4 Axial proton density-weighted image demonstrates a grade IV chondral injury at the patellar median ridge (*black block arrow*), with a displaced chondral fragment (*white arrow*) and large knee effusion visible in the same slice. Chondral injury dictates early surgery

areas of bone edema (Fig. 10.5). The contusion on the lateral femoral condyle is more anterior, superior, and lateral than those seen in the pivot shift of anterior cruciate ligament tears [15, 27]. Inferomedial patellar *osteochondral injuries* are present in about 70% of patellar dislocation patients [9]. More rarely, a shear-type fracture may occur along the lateral femoral condyle [24]. With dislocations that occur at higher degrees of flexion, there is higher risk of injury to the lateral femoral condyle rather than the lateral trochlea.

In the acute setting, the location (femoral vs. patellar) of *MPFL/medial retinacular complex* tear can be difficult to discern as almost every patient will have some injury pattern on the patellar side. Femoral injury is indicated by proximal edema at the anterior aspect of the proximal medial collateral ligament. The MPFL itself is often difficult to discern [7].

Intra-articular bodies, which are seen in as many as 33% of patients after patellar dislocation [7, 9, 15], usually present as separated fragments of chondral tissue or osteochondral fragments from the medial patella or lateral femoral condyle.

The majority of patients who have dislocated and spontaneously relocated their patellae will have persistent patellar subluxation or tilt due to concomitant MPFL/ medial retinacular complex injury and joint effusion [7].

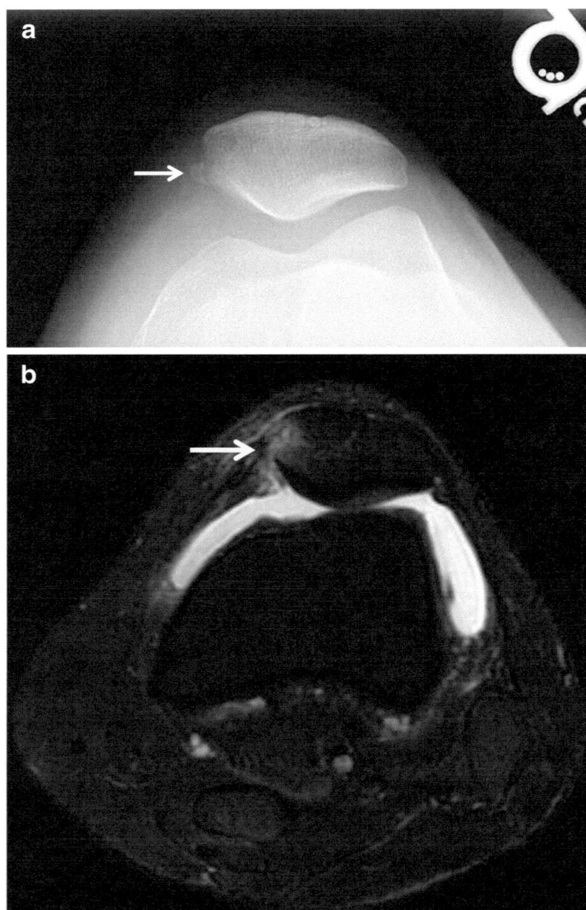

Fig. 10.5 Axial radiograph and fat-suppressed MRI sequences demonstrate classic findings of acute transient lateral patellar dislocation. **Panel a** shows a small fracture fragment (*white arrow*) at the medial patellar facet corresponding to an area of bone marrow contusion (*white arrow*) on MRI (**panel b**). In a different patient, another classic bone marrow contusion pattern is seen along the medial patellar facet (*white arrow*, **panel c**) and lateral femoral condyle (*white arrow*, **panel d**)

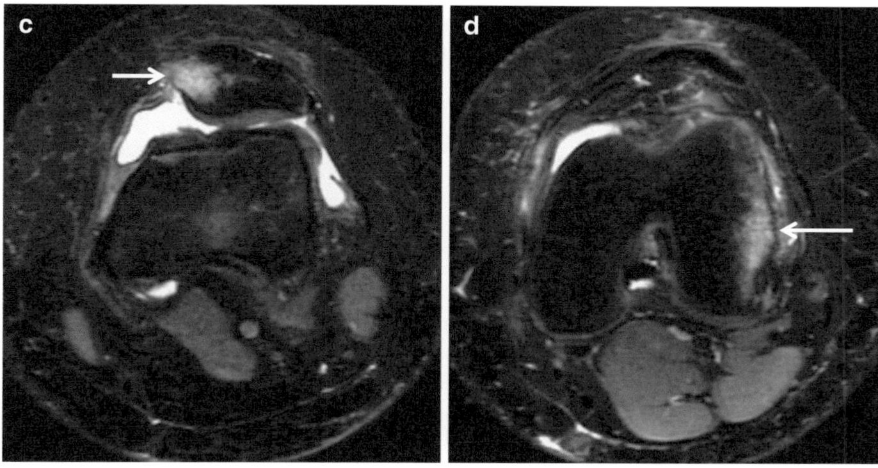

Fig. 5 (continued)

Normal Postoperative Imaging Appearance After Patellofemoral Procedures

Proximal Realignment Procedures

Proximal soft tissue realignment procedures can be lateral sided or medial sided. The medial sided include medial plication, repair, and reconstruction. The lateral side can undergo a soft tissue release or lengthening.

Trochleoplasty is a proximal bony procedure.

Medial Capsular Plication

Medial capsular or retinacular plication procedures are typically based off of the patella and attempt to reduce the redundancy and thus increase stability of the medial structures [1, 12]. These procedures have been shown to have a higher post-procedure re-dislocation rate than MPFL reconstruction [28]. Plication may be difficult to identify on MRI but is characterized by scar along the medial joint involving the MPFL/retinaculum/capsule (Fig. 10.6).

MPFL Repair and Reconstruction

The normal MPFL attaches between the adductor tubercle and medial epicondyle (Fig. 10.7). There are abundance of options for MPFL reconstruction surgical techniques. The normal postoperative MPFL should be (1) anatomically located, (2) continuous, and (3) low signal intensity on MR imaging (Fig. 10.8).

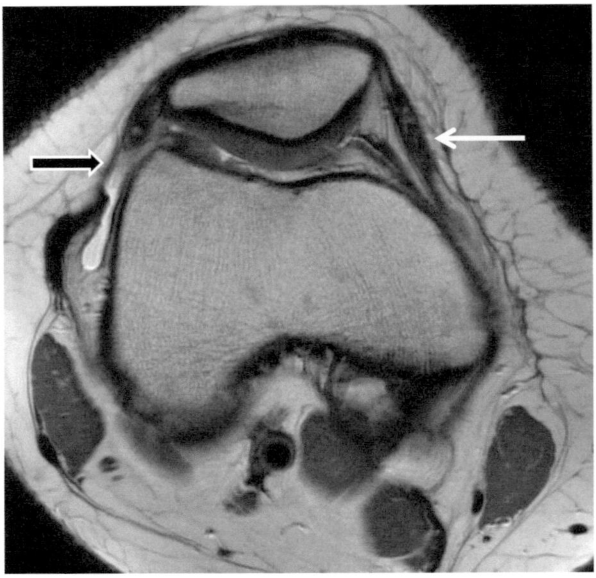

Fig. 10.6 Axial proton density-weighted image demonstrates postoperative scarring of the medial soft tissue stabilizers (*white arrow*) after a medial capsular plication procedure, as well as a gap in the lateral capsule after capsular release (*black block arrow*)

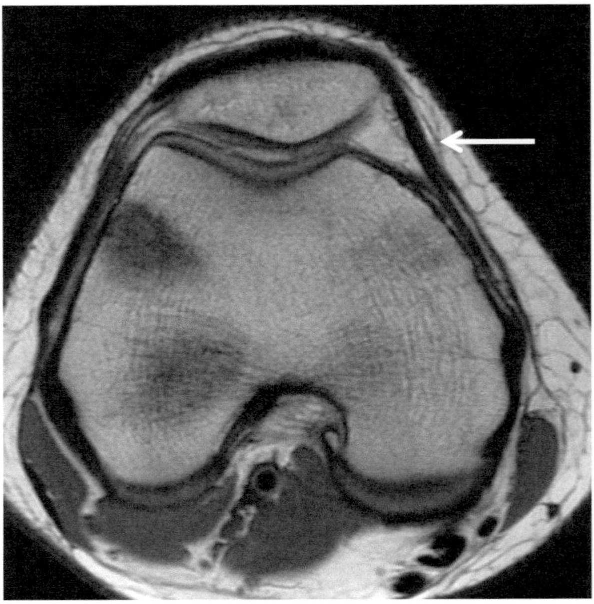

Fig. 10.7 Axial proton density-weighted image of the knee demonstrates a normal appearance of the medial patellofemoral ligament (MPFL) (*white arrow*)

Complications which may occur post-MPFL reconstruction include patellar fracture, graft malposition on either the femoral or patella side, graft failure from reinjury, and fixation failure (Fig. 10.9). The graft should be placed to be nearly isometric in its range of motion. The femoral side of the graft should be placed at Schottle's point (Fig. 10.10). A starting point that is too proximal will become too

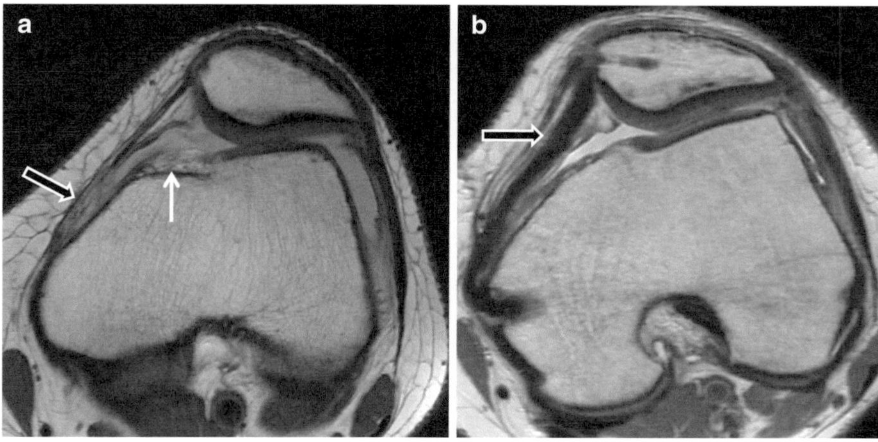

Fig. 10.8 Axial proton density-weighted MR images pre- and post-MPFL reconstruction in a 33-year-old woman with history of recurrent patellar subluxation. **Panel a** demonstrates chronic lateral subluxation of the patella with features of trochlear dysplasia including medial trochlea facet hypoplasia (*white arrow*). The MPFL is diminutive (*black block arrow*). **Panel b** demonstrates a contiguous, low-signal-intensity MPFL graft (*black block arrow*) with improved patellar alignment

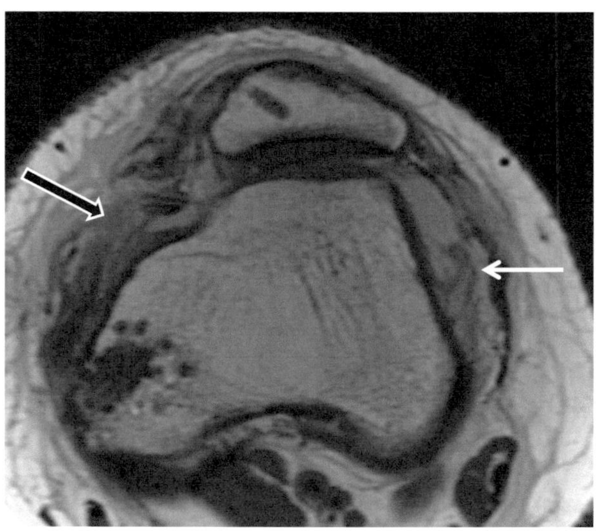

Fig. 10.9 Axial MR image in an 18-year-old female post-MPFL reconstruction demonstrates mid-substance disruption of the MPFL graft (*black block arrow*) and synovitis (*white arrow*)

tight in flexion and significantly increase pressures on the patellofemoral joint. A graft placed too distal will loosen too early in flexion and predispose to recurrent instability. *Patellar-side graft malpositioning* may result in fixation devices violating and injuring the patellar cartilage as well as fracture if the tunnels or anchors are positioned too anterior or too proximal.

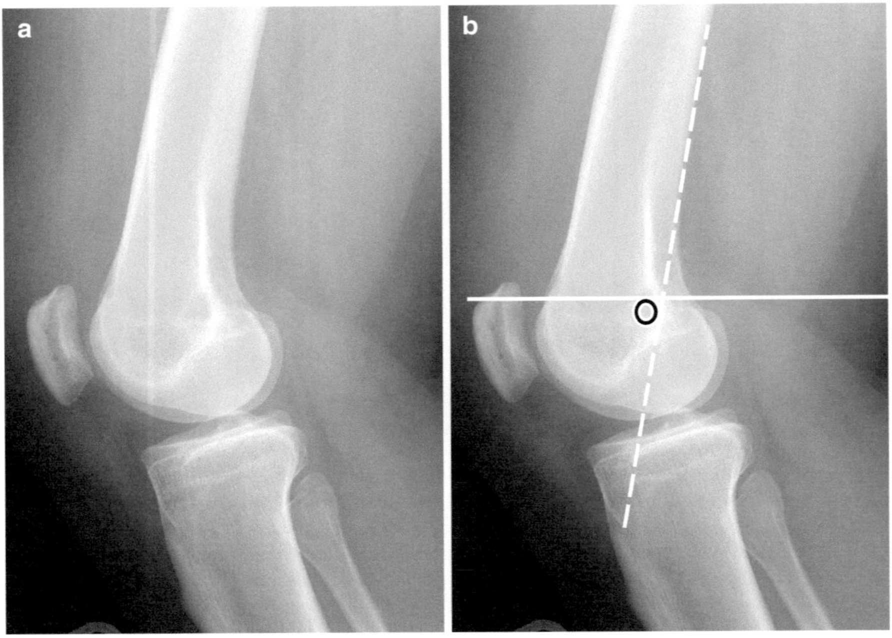

Fig. 10.10 Lateral radiographs of the knee without (**panel a**) and with (**panel b**) annotations demonstrating Schottle's insertion point for tunnel placement in MPFL reconstruction procedures. One line (*dashed white line*) is drawn along the posterior femoral cortex, and another line (*solid white line*) is drawn horizontally at the superior margin of the femoral condyles. Schottle's insertion point (*black circle*) then sits in the anteroinferior quadrant at the intersection of the two lines

Lateral Release

On the lateral side, release of the potential constraint by retinaculum and capsule is used to better center the patella and decrease the possibility for dislocation. This can be done by lateral release or lateral lengthening.

On imaging, there is a focal defect in the lateral capsule (Fig. 10.11) if a release has been performed. It may be difficult to distinguish from a lateral arthrotomy. With time, the defects can fill with fibrous tissue.

Trochleoplasty

Trochleoplasties indications, techniques and complications are described in other chapters. Trochleoplasty may be performed in skeletally mature patients with severe trochlear dysplasia. In skeletally immature patients, MPFL reconstruction procedures may be performed safely by avoiding the growth plate with the femoral fixation [6]. As trochleoplasty may significantly increase post-procedure baseline pain levels in patients with severe patellofemoral osteoarthritis, it is contraindicated in such settings [16].

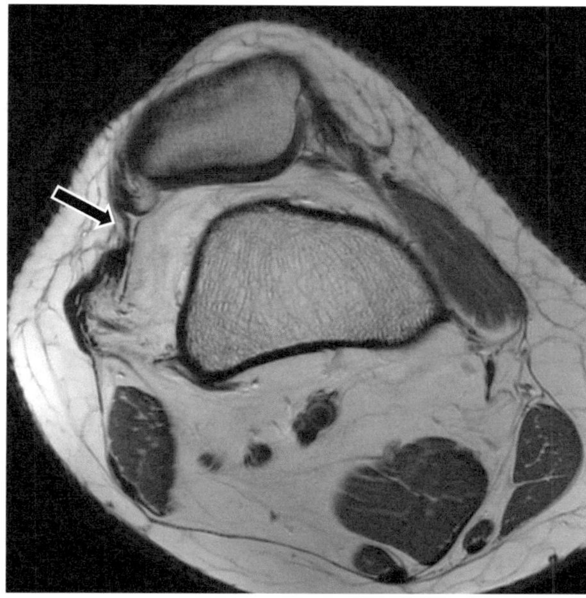

Fig. 10.11 Axial proton density-weighted image demonstrated a focal defect in the lateral capsule at the site of lateral release (*black block arrow*)

Trochleoplasties remain uncommon and are best identified by comparing a pre- and postoperative image for change in shape of the trochlea (Fig. 10.12). Preoperative radiographs and to a better degree cross-sectional images often demonstrate a supratrochlear spur (Fig. 10.13), and the goal of the trochleoplasty is to eliminate the spur and, to the extent possible, deepen the trochlear sulcus. On MRI, artifact and other evidence of surgery will be present.

Distal Realignment Procedures

Tibial Tubercle Osteotomy

Tibial tubercle osteotomy (TTO) procedures are considered for patients who experience pain and/or lateral patellar dislocations and have either (1) an increased TT-TG distance or (2) patella alta [13]. In patients with patellar instability, a TTO can be used to correct for elevated TT-TG by medializing the tubercle, and in addition, the TTO can also be used to distalize the patella tendon attachment in cases of severe patella alta. In patients with severe patella alta, the tubercle may be moved distally, which results in some degree of tubercle medialization [20]. Although there is no consensus based on the literature of when the TTO should be used in patients with recurrent patellar instability, medialization of the tibial tubercle should be considered in patients with TT-TG distance >20 mm to help correct coronal plane malalignment and decrease the lateral force on the patella [16]. The 20 mm number is

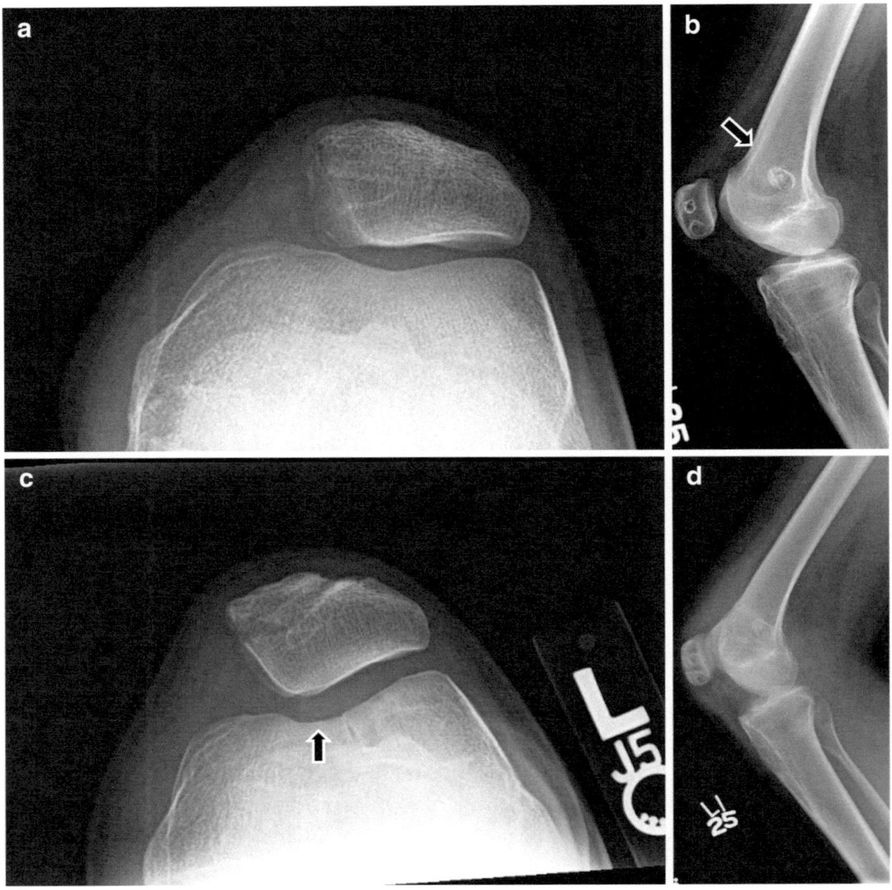

Fig. 10.12 Merchant and cross-table lateral radiographs in a 17-year-old patient taken pre- (**panels a, b**) and postoperatively (**panels c, d**) after trochleoplasty procedure. Postoperative images show elimination of the supratrochlear spur best seen in preoperative lateral image (*black block arrow*, panel **b**) and accompanying axial CT (not shown) as well as deepening of the trochlear sulcus (*black block arrow*, panel **c**)

currently under investigation, and more studies are needed to determine exactly when a patient should undergo a TTO vs. when an isolated MPFL may be sufficient.

The degree of anterior or medialization can be varied by the angle of the osteotomy or the size of the interposed bone. Fixation screws will cause artifact on MRI more than CT and may make it difficult to look for healing. Lateral radiograph is most commonly used to assess healing, looking for cortical continuity. Complications of tibial tubercle osteotomies include delayed or non-union (Fig. 10.14), fracture, and infection. Pain from screws may necessitate their removal.

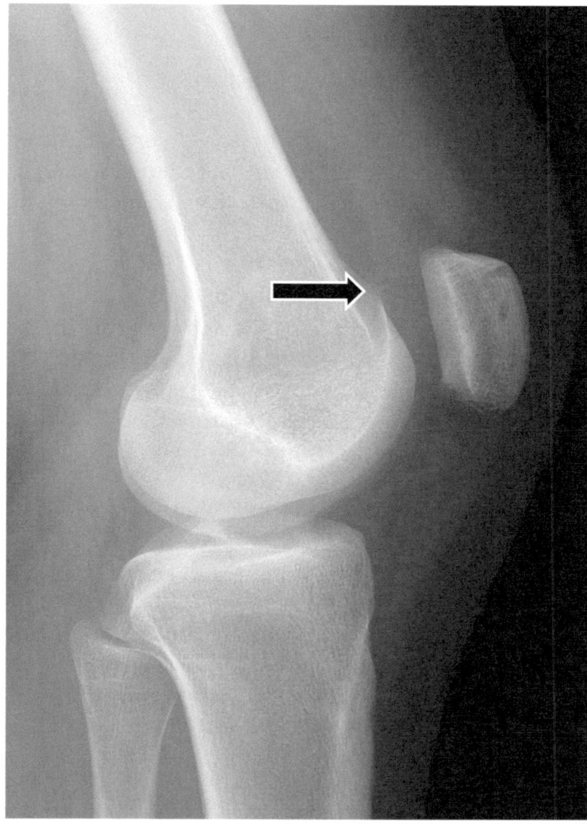

Fig. 10.13 Lateral radiograph of the knee demonstrates a subtle small supratrochlear spur (*black block arrow*)

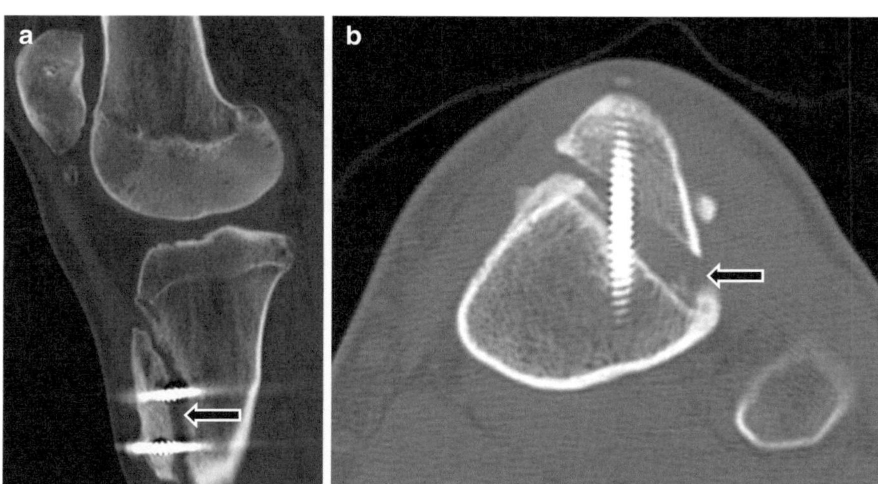

Fig. 10.14 Sagittal (panel A) and axial (panel B) CT images in two different patients who underwent tibial tubercle osteotomy for distalization of the tibial tubercle. Both images show a gap (*black block arrows*) between the osteotomy fragment and tibia with sclerotic margins of the fragments, consistent with non-union

Cartilage Procedures

Pinning for Osteochondral Fractures

For defects or injuries in which at least a layer of subchondral bone is attached to a chondral fragment, the fragment can be replaced into its native position and pinned. Bone-to-bone healing is the goal, working better in younger patients.

Chondral Regenerative Techniques

For small defects, picking or drilling, the so-called microfracture technique, can be used to stimulate bleeding from which pluripotential cells can differentiate into cartilage to fill the defect. These techniques yield fibrocartilage fill, not hyaline cartilage, and have shown poor results in the patellofemoral joint due to high shear forces.

Various scaffolds can be infused with chondrocytes implanted (MACI), or autologous cartilage implantation (ACI) can be used to fill defects. A more recent repair technique that is available is the placement of particulated juvenille allograft cartilage into the defect with fibrin glue (DeNOVO) (Fig. 10.15). This technique produces a cartilage refill that seems to mature over time to cartilage with similar MRI signal characteristics to adjacent normal cartilage at 2 years [11].

Plug

Osteochondral plugs can be used as autografts [*OATS* (*osteochondral autograft transfer system*)] or allografts [OCA – osteochondral allograft] (Fig. 10.16). Because of the unique topography and thicker cartilage in the patella than in the rest of the knee, OATs autograft will result in the bony part of the plug being proud in order that the chondral surfaces are flush.

Osteochondral allografts (OCAs) are typically used for the larger defects. In the recent few years, there is increased availability and thus a growing use of OCAs. With large patellar chondral lesions, OCAs are better taken from other donor patellae to match the unique topography and thickness of the patella cartilage. The specific risk with both autograft and allograft osteochondral plugs is potential failure of the bone plug to heal or incorporate and resulting cartilage delamination.

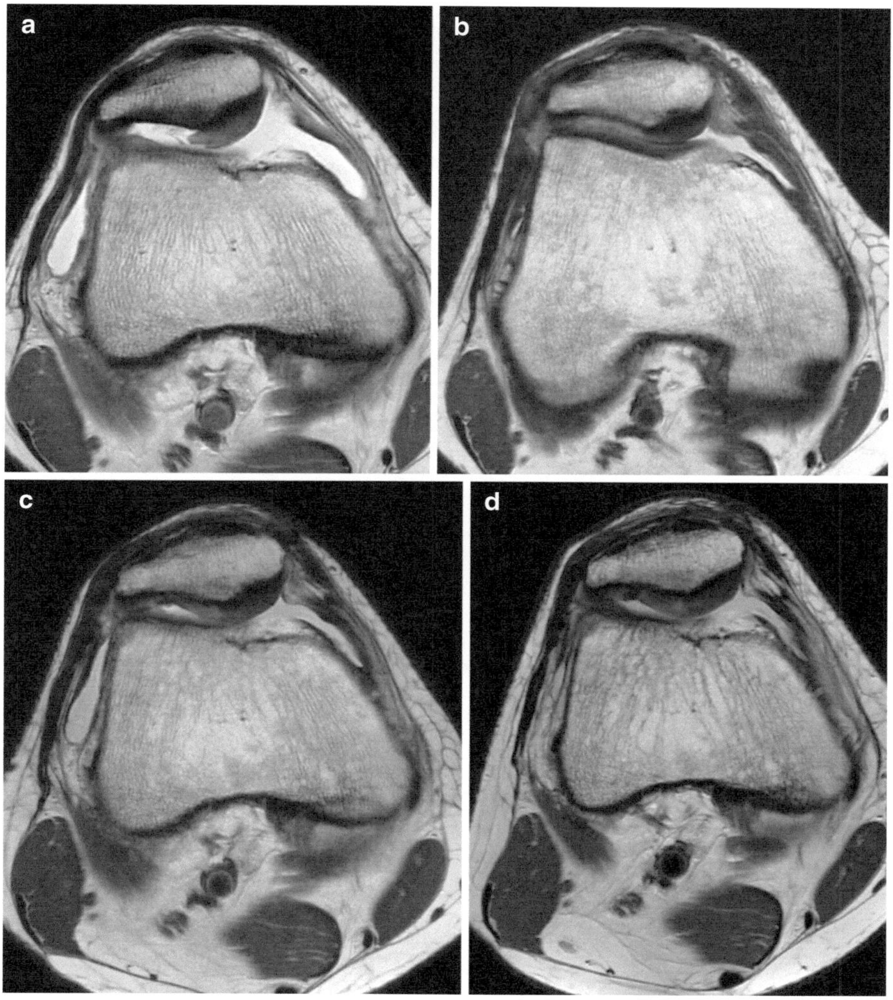

Fig. 10.15 Four serial axial proton density-weighted MR images from four different exams in the same patient. **Panel a** shows the patient has sustained a grade IV cartilage defect along the lateral patellar facet, after which he underwent a cartilage repair technique where the defect was filled with particulated juvenille allograft cartilage in a fibrin glue. Panels b through d show successive stages of healing at the graft site, with the graft initially appearing hyperintense (**panel b**) and successively losing hyperintense signal (**panel c**) and later more closely resembling the adjacent native cartilage in thickness and signal intensity (**panel d**), though never quite back to baseline appearance

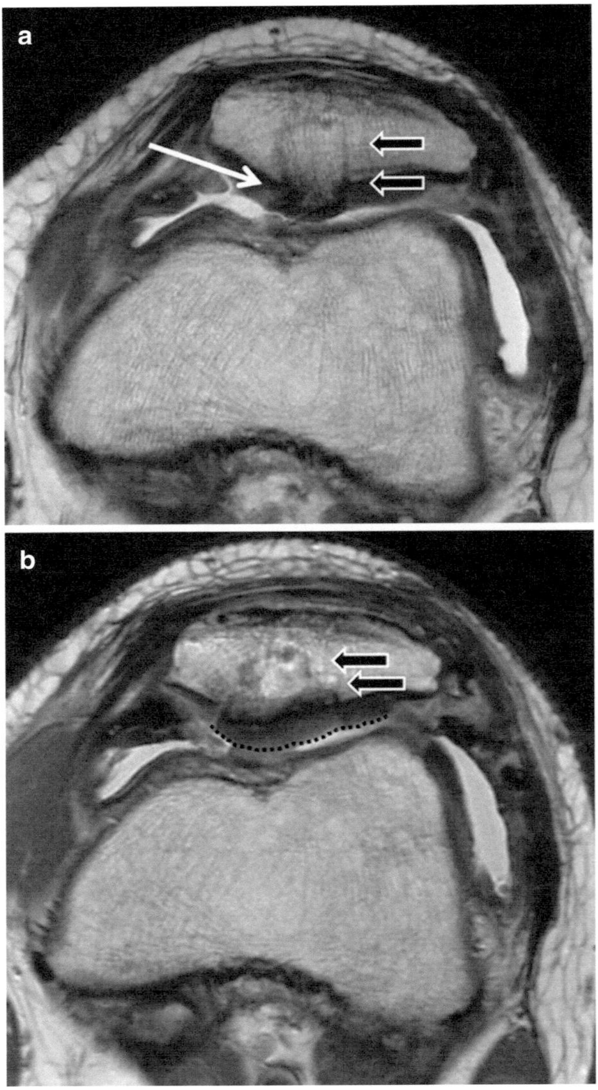

Fig. 10.16 Axial proton density-weighted MR images in a patient who underwent an osteochondral autograft transfer system (OATS) procedure (**panel a**) and subsequently returned and underwent an osteochondral cadaveric allograft (OCA) procedure (**panel b**). Panel a shows the autograft (*black block arrows*) with a small offset at the bone-cartilage interface (*white arrow*). Panel b shows replacement of the autograft with an OCA (*black block arrows*), showing an excellent reapproximation of normal cartilage surface/ architecture (*dashed black line*) with minimal residual offset at the bone-cartilage interface

Conclusion

Imaging is critical in evaluating individual patient anatomy which can help to determine the patient's risk for recurrence as well as to help guide surgical treatment. It will often determine whether or not surgery is indicated in patients with acute first-time dislocations, in whom a loose body or osteochondral fracture is identified. As we develop improved ways of addressing the high number of cartilage injuries seen in the setting of patella instability, imaging plays a key role in determining the success of our surgeries to repair or regenerate cartilage. In addition, imaging in the setting of failed surgery will help to determine how to better and more successfully perform the revision required.

References

1. Ahmad CS, Lee FY. An all-arthroscopic soft-tissue balancing technique for lateral patellar instability. Arthroscopy. 2001;17(5):555–7.
2. Askenberger M, Janarv PM, Finnbogason T, Arendt EA. Morphology and anatomic patellar instability risk factors on first-time traumatic lateral patellar dislocations: A prospective magnetic resonance imaging study in skeletally immature children. Am J Sports Med. 2017;45(1):50–8.
3. Brattstörm H. Patella alta in non-dislocating knee joints. Acta Orthop Scand. 1970;41:578–88.
4. Chhabra A, Subhawong TK, Carrino JA. A systematised MRI approach to evaluating the patellofemoral joint. Skelet Radiol. 2011;40(4):375–87.
5. Cooney AD, Kazi Z, Caplan N, et al. The relationship between quadriceps angle and tibial tuberosity–trochlear groove distance in patients with patellar instability. Knee Surg Sports Traumatol Arthrosc. 2012;20:2399–404.
6. Dean CS, Chahla J, Serra Cruz R. Patellofemoral joint reconstruction for patellar instability: medial patellofemoral ligament reconstruction, trochleoplasty, and tibial tubercle osteotomy. Arthrosc Tech. 2016;5(1):e169–75.
7. Diederichs G, Issever AS, Scheffler S. MR imaging of patellar instability: injury patterns and assessment of risk factors. Radiographics. 2010;30(4):961–81.
8. Earhart C, Patel DB, White EA, et al. Transient lateral patellar dislocation: review of imaging findings, patellofemoral anatomy, and treatment options. Emerg Radiol. 2013;20(1):11–23.
9. Elias DA, White LM, Fithian DC. Acute lateral patellar dislocation at MR imaging: injury patterns of medial patellar soft-tissue restraints and osteochondral injuries of the inferomedial patella. Radiology. 2002;225(3):736–43.
10. Fithian DC, Paxton EW, Stone ML, et al. Epidemiology and natural history of acute patellar dislocation. Am J Sports Med. 2004;32(5):1114–21.
11. Grawe B, Burge A, Nguyen J, Strickland S, Warren R, Rodeo S, ShubinStein B. Cartilage regeneration in full-thickness patellar chondral defects treated with particulated juvenile articular allograft cartilage: an MRI analysis. Cartilage. 2017;8:374–83.
12. Henry JE, Pflum FA Jr. Arthroscopic proximal patella realignment and stabilization. Arthroscopy. 1995;11(4):424–5.
13. Ho CP, James EW, Surowiec RK, et al. Systematic technique-dependent differences in CT versus MRI measurement of the tibial tubercle-trochlear groove distance. Am J Sports Med. 2015;43:675–82.
14. Hong E, Kraft MC. Evaluating anterior knee pain. Med Clin N Am. 2014;98:697–717.
15. Kirsch MD, Fitzgerald SW, Friedman H, et al. Transient lateral patellar dislocation: diagnosis with MR imaging. AJR Am J Roentgenol. 1993;161(1):109–13.
16. LaPrade RF, Cram TR, James EW, et al. Trochlear dysplasia and the role of trochleoplasty. Clin Sports Med. 2014;33(3):531–45.
17. Lewallen L, McIntosh A, Dahm D. First-time patellofemoral dislocation: risk factors for recurrent instability. J Knee Surg. 2015;28(4):303–9.
18. Munch JL, Sullivan JP, Nguyen JT, Mintz D, Green DW, Shubin Stein BE, Strickland S. Patellar articular overlap on MRI is a simple alternative to conventional measurements of patellar height. Orthop J Sports Med. 2016;4(7):2325967116656328.

19. Nomura E, Inoue M, Kuimura M. Chondral and osteochondral injuries associated with acute patellar dislocation. Arthroscopy. 2003;19(7):717–21.
20. Robin J, Neyret P. Tuberosity surgery: what is the role of distalization? Oper Tech Sports Med. 2015;23:107–13.
21. Seeley MA, Knesek M, Vanderhave KL. Osteochondral injury after patellar dislocation in children and adolescents. J Pediatr Orthop. 2013;33(5):511–8.
22. Sherman SL, Plackis AC, Nuelle CW. Patellofemoral anatomy and biomechanics. Clin Sports Med. 2014;33(3):389–401.
23. Smith TO, Hunt NJ, Donell ST. The reliability and validity of the Q-angle: a systematic review. Knee Surg Sports Traumatol Arthrosc. 2008;16:1068–79.
24. Swischuk LE, Hernandez JA, Hendrick EP, et al. Lateral femoral condylar shearing fractures. Emerg Radiol. 2003;10(1):19–22.
25. Thakkar RS, Del Grande F, Wadhwa V, et al. Patellar instability: CT and MRI measurements and their correlation with internal derangement findings. Knee Surg Sports Traumatol Arthrosc. 2016;24(9):3021–8.
26. Wittstein JR, Bartlett EC, Easterbrook J, et al. Magnetic resonance imaging evaluation of patellofemoral malalignment. Arthroscopy. 2006;22:643–9.
27. Zaidi A, Babyn P, Astori I, et al. MRI of traumatic patellar dislocation in children. Pediatr Radiol. 2006;36(11):1163–70.
28. Zhao J, Huangfu X, He Y, et al. The role of medial retinaculum plication versus medial patellofemoral ligament reconstruction in combined procedures for recurrent patellar instability in adults. Am J Sports Med. 2012;40:1355–64.

Index

B. E. Shubin Stein, S. M. Strickland (eds.), *Patellofemoral Pain and Instability*,
https://doi.org/10.1007/978-3-319-97640-2

FSC
www.fsc.org
MIX
Papier aus verantwortungsvollen Quellen
Paper from responsible sources
FSC® C105338

If you have any concerns about our products,
you can contact us on
ProductSafety@springernature.com

In case Publisher is established outside the EU,
the EU authorized representative is:
Springer Nature Customer Service Center GmbH
Europaplatz 3, 69115 Heidelberg, Germany

Printed by Libri Plureos GmbH
in Hamburg, Germany